TREATMENT PLANNING
in Psychiatry

Edited
by
Jerry M. Lewis, M.D.
Gene Usdin, M.D.

Published by

AMERICAN PSYCHIATRIC ASSOCIATION

1700 18TH STREET, N.W.
WASHINGTON, D.C. 20009

Library of Congress Cataloging in Publication Data
Main entry under title:

Treatment planning in psychiatry.

Bibliography: p.
1. Psychotherapy. I. Lewis, Jerry M., 1924-
II. Usdin, Gene L. [DNLM: 1. Mental disorders—Therapy.
2. Psychotherapy—Methods. 3. Patient care planning.
WM 400 L674t]
RC480.T68 616.89'14 82-3985
ISBN 0-89042-045-9 AACR2

Cover and text designed by Jessica Morgan
Printed and bound in the U.S.A.

ISBN 0-89042-045-9

ACKNOWLEDGMENTS

It is often difficult in retrospect to identify precisely both the moment in which an idea is born and the circumstances giving it form and substance. As early, however, as the fall of 1978, the American Psychiatric Association Task Force on Nomenclature and Statistics, led by its chairman, Robert L. Spitzer, M.D., was actively encouraging and giving initial form to the idea of a volume on treatment planning. Publication of DSM-III was imminent; it was apparent that DSM-III diagnoses, including Axes IV and V, were not, in and of themselves, sufficient for treatment planning.

The form of the volume was to have chapters prepared by committees, each committee chosen by national organizations representing five major treatment perspectives: the psychodynamic, the somatic, the behavioral, the group, and the family and marital therapies. The American Psychoanalytic Association and the American Academy of Psychoanalysis were invited to develop jointly a chapter on psychodynamic therapies. The Association for the Advancement of Behavior Therapy, the Society for Biological Psychiatry, and the American Group Psychotherapy Association were invited to appoint committees representing those treatment perspectives. The family and marital therapies were included by involving the American Family Therapy Association and the American Association for Marriage and Family Therapists.

These organizations agreed to submit chapter drafts. In the two instances wherein national organizations reflected similar treatment perspectives, committees were formed including either members from both organizations or individuals with membership in both groups.

It became apparent that information regarding treatment planning for special age groups would be needed. As a consequence, the American Academy of Child Psychiatry and the American Association for Geriatric Psychiatry were contacted and asked to appoint individuals to each of the five committees to add sections to each chapter reflecting those special considerations necessary for effective treatment planning for children, adolescents, and the elderly.

In the summer of 1980, the Board of Trustees of the American Psychiatric Association decided that the volume required editors, and we (Jerry M. Lewis and Gene Usdin) were selected.

Several decisions were made by the editors that altered the form of the volume. An introductory chapter was developed. The material regarding special perspectives on treatment planning for children, adolescents, and the aged were removed from the text of each chapter; it was decided to add three additional chapters to give sufficient depth to the perspectives needed for each of these age groups. In addition, an organizing format common to each of the initial five chapters was proposed along with a different format for the three age group chapters.

All of this is by way of sharing with the reader something of what must have been the confusing experience of the various contributors. To their credit, each of the eight committees responded with productivity and patience through the inevitable negotiations that comprise the relationship between writers and editors. Each committee chairperson, however, made the decision as to just how a particular committee was to function. As a consequence, some of the chapters reflect a committee process in which all members participated; others were written by one or two members of the committee with other members playing only reactive or supportive roles.

Throughout the process, the editors were helped by a number of persons. Many members of our Association offered support and counsel. Henry H. Work, M.D. supplied excellent staff support, and the guiding hand of Melvin Sabshin, M.D. was always available. A committee composed of two Assembly officers and three members of the Board of Trustees, chaired by H. Keith H. Brodie, M.D., monitored the work throughout. As the editorial work reached its final stage, Ronald McMillen of the American Psychiatric Press was particularly helpful. We again wish to emphasize the crucial role of Robert L. Spitzer, M.D. in giving life to this project. Finally, our secretaries, Mrs. Nannette Bruchey and Mrs. Cathy Culmone, made our own efforts possible, and we are indeed most grateful to them.

Careful treatment planning is, we believe, a distinguishing characteristic of the highest level of the clinical care of patients. We feel that the efforts of those colleagues who did the actual writing of the chapters have resulted in a volume from which all can learn and, as editors, we are in their debt.

Jerry M. Lewis, M.D. and Gene Usdin, M.D.

TABLE OF CONTENTS

INTRODUCTION

Jerry M. Lewis, M.D.
Gene Usdin, M.D.

Introduction

Publication of a new classification system in psychiatry has led to an expressed need for a volume on treatment planning. In the early process of planning this book, a decision was made to invite experts in five major treatment modalities to contribute chapters.

The five treatment modalities were: psychodynamic psychotherapy, group therapy, behavior therapy, biological treatment, and marital and family therapy. Later, the decision was made to develop chapters relating to children, adolescents, and the elderly.

Questions posed to the experts included:

1. What are the basic theoretical premises underlying each treatment modality?
2. What are the specific treatment techniques that are a part of each treatment modality?
3. What information, in addition to a diagnosis, is necessary to plan treatment?
4. What are the processes or techniques for obtaining that information?

The goal of this volume is to provide psychiatrists with a broad and general guide regarding clinical procedures that may be useful in deciding if a particular treatment modality might be applicable in the treatment of a given patient.

The *Diagnostic and Statistical Manual, Volume III* (DSM-III) is a descriptive typology which classifies syndromes on the basis of signs and symptoms. Although psychiatrists of various theoretical orientations may disagree about which clinical phenomena should be the basis for classification, the use of signs and symptoms is in accord with the diagnostic process in medicine for diseases in which etiology is incompletely understood.

A DSM-III diagnosis is, however, not sufficient for treatment planning in most clinical situations. Psychiatrists need more data with which to plan clinical interventions. These data are obtained through a variety of clinical procedures, which collectively are called a psychiatric evaluation.

Psychiatric Evaluation

As part of the process of making a diagnosis, psychiatrists obtain a comprehensive history from the patient and, often, another informant. A mental status examination is accomplished, and physical and neurological examinations either are done or arrangements are made for another physician to do these. Special studies may be required also in order to arrive at a diagnosis.

Although diagnosis focuses on shared symptoms and signs, the aim of the psychiatric evaluation is to discover individual differences in patients with the same syndrome and to assess the etiology of a particular patient's syndrome. It encompasses a broader group of clinical activities than does the process of diagnosis. As it is most frequently undertaken, the psychiatric evaluation speaks to the role of multiple etiologic factors in the production of psychiatric syndromes. Those biological, psychological, and social factors which, in concert, play predisposing, precipitating, and sustaining roles in the patient's psychopathology are assessed.

First, the individual patient is understood as a biological organism. As such he or she has a current general level of physical health, specific physical disabilities, and a family pedigree that may include a genetic diathesis either to certain physical diseases or to specific psychiatric syndromes. There may be evidence of central nervous system dysfunction, an unusual pattern of development, or the suggestion of residual deficits from earlier developmental difficulties. Past episodes of psychiatric syndromes and, in particular, response to biologic treatments are important data.

A patient's psychological status is a critical aspect of the psychiatric evaluation. Many psychiatrists think of it as a psychodynamic appraisal. From this perspective the clinician is interested in the patient's conflicts, defense mechanisms, coping styles, character type, level of ego organization, quality of object relationships, nature of the self-system, specific personality strengths, and other aspects of the patient's conscious and unconscious life.

In understanding a patient from a developmental perspective, the continuity of his or her evolution as a person is emphasized: information about early development and current developmental challenges is sought.

A psychiatrist also strives to understand the individual patient's past and current social contexts. Characteristics of the patient's enduring interpersonal relationships are evaluated. The presence of a central dyadic relationship and its characteristics are important aspects of the patient's social context. Distinguishing features of the patient's current family and the family of origin are considered. Family characteristics that encourage intimacy, clear ego boundaries, and autonomy are evaluated. The role of the patient's symptoms in maintaining a precarious family equilibrium is explored. Forces within the family that either push for recovery or pull for continuing dysfunction are appraised.

A psychiatrist also evaluates the presence and nature of the patient's network of friends and occupational stresses and satisfactions. Recent life stress is explored and, in the larger social context, the effects of socioeconomic, ethnic, and cultural factors.

These and other biological, psychological, and social forces are explored in the psychiatric evaluation. In addition, clinicians need to attend important threads running through the tapestry of the patient's life that cannot easily be considered as exclusively biological, psychological, or social: intelligence, motivation, and basic value orientation are examples.

A psychiatric evaluation results in the psychiatrist's constructing a model of the patient, often called a "clinical formulation." A large number of factors are usually involved, and these interact, frequently in ways that are unknowable. Despite the attempt to construct a holistic model, a formulation is invariably only a partial representation of the patient, never complete. Rather, psychiatrists must be open to constant revision of the model as new data are uncovered in the course of treatment. Although a clinical formulation resulting from a psychiatric evaluation is an orienting structure necessary for treatment, it must be considered tentative and approximate.

The clinical processes used in the psychiatric evaluation are multiple and diverse. Many clinicians consider a few exploratory interviews a crucial part of the evaluation process. Often these are interviews designed to evaluate the patient's suitability for some form of individual psychotherapy or psychoanalysis. Such interviews may be particularly concerned with the patient's affective availability, capacity for self-reflection, or ability to free associate. Other interviews have a specific goal such as obtaining a detailed past history, constructing a family genetic pedigree, or testing a provisional hypothesis about the patient's psychopathology by noting his or her response to specific therapeutic interventions.

Some psychiatrists consider a psychiatric evaluation incomplete unless the patient is interviewed in his or her major interpersonal context. Interviews of the patient with spouse or family are, therefore, considered by some to be a routine part of the psychiatric evaluation. The persons comprising the interpersonal context are not, in this regard, considered informants but possible participants in the patient's psychopathology.

As data from the psychiatric evaluation emerge, other evaluative procedures may be indicated. These may range from specific procedures such as psychological testing, electroencephalography, brain scans, or neuroendocrine studies to broader inquiries such as an internal medicine or neurology consultation.

The psychiatrist is interested also in making observations about the potential for an effective treatment alliance. Regardless of the form of treatment, opportunity for success is augmented by the development of a strong alliance between the psychiatrist and the patient. As a consequence, psychiatrists are sensitive to data both from the patient and from himself or herself regarding the likelihood that they will be able to trust each other and work together.

Clinicians differ in regard to procedures that are considered essential for a psychiatric evaluation. Although there are many reasons for this diversity, a major factor is the lack of a single, unifying theory of psychiatric disorders. There is considerable agreement that most often multiple etiologic factors are involved in the production of psychiatric syndromes, but there are significant differences of opinion among psychiatrists regarding the importance of different factors.

Regardless, however, of an individual clinician's theoretical orientation, a growing body of data implicating biological, psychological, and social variables in the etiology of most psychiatric syndromes mandates an evaluation process of sufficient breadth to detect critical variables in each of the three areas. To be heavily committed to a single theoretical orientation may do disservice to patients if variables emphasized by other orientations and overlooked during the evaluation process are relevant.

FACTORS INFLUENCING THE PSYCHIATRIC EVALUATION

Other factors may impinge upon the process of the psychiatric evaluation. One is the psychiatrist's management of the inevitable uncertainty involved in evaluating a patient. More often than not, the clinical data are insufficient for certainty, and decisions of profound importance must be made at a time when there is some doubt in the physician's mind. The urgency of the patient's situation as, for example, with the suicidal patient, adds to the clinician's dilemma. Such forces may push the psychiatrist in the direction of a strong sense of certainty, a conviction of the correctness of the clinical observations, and a commitment to a particular plan of action. The resulting danger is premature closure and subsequent inattention to emerging data that would alter the original formulation.

Although these forces may push clinicians toward a level of certainty that interferes with an appropriate degree of clinical flexibility, there are also problems in the other direction. With too little certainty, the clinician may be immobilized and have difficulty in getting any treatment started.

There is evidence that clinicians tend to develop characteristic styles of evaluation which appear to reflect two basic dimensions.[1] One involves the degree of structure brought to the evaluation process. This can be seen as a continuum ranging from an orderly, systematic approach in which each patient is studied the same way, to a much less structured evaluation in which each patient is seen as a unique clinical adventure. The second dimension is the type of thought processes used by the clinician, and these range from an almost complete reliance on logical, inductive thinking to a major reliance on intuitive thinking. Some of the resulting styles of evaluation can be seen to deal with the inevitable uncertainty by premature closure, others by interminable rumination, and still others by a more comfortable acceptance of a reasonable level of tentativeness.

Another factor that influences the nature of a psychiatric evaluation is the psychiatrist's awareness of the ways in which he or she influences the data that emerge during the evaluation process. A clinician needs to understand how he or she may either subtly encourage or discourage particular behaviors of patients. To assume that one is always the same may influence the results of the evaluation process.

Each psychiatrist's value system is a particular aspect of his or her person that can influence the psychiatric evaluation. The practice of medicine and psychiatry cannot be value-free; concepts of health, illness, and disease are shaped and molded by the social, cultural, and historical context in which they are embedded and to which they contribute. Ideas of what "ought to be" are invariably part of what the clinician brings to the psychiatric evaluation. Many clinicians have developed mainstream, cultural values. These include a higher regard for "doing" than for "being," emphasizing the future more than present or past, and assigning higher priority to the individual than to the couple, family, or community.[2] These values are such an integral part of the world views of many clinicians that professional contact with individuals who do not share them may not go well. For example, the patient from a different cultural, ethnic, or socioeconomic background who values "being" and the present may be seen as sick or disturbed rather than as having a different set of values. In situations in which the clinician's values conflict with the patient's, there is an increased possibility that the evaluation process may be influenced adversely. It is important, therefore, that psychiatrists maintain a clear awareness of their value orientations.

Constraints generated by reality often influence the process of psychiatric evaluation. Regardless of a psychiatrist's theoretical orientation, management of uncertainty, awareness of his or her own impact upon the process of evaluation, and sensitivity to value conflicts, he or she may work in a professional context in which time is too limited, patients too many, and funding too little. These circumstances may preclude a complete psychiatric evaluation. In such settings there may be strong pressure on psychiatrists to function only as diagnosticians and to base treatment solely on patients' diagnoses. Treatment based on a descriptive diagnosis alone is inadequate for many patients. There is, for example, increasing evidence that combinations of psychotropic drugs and certain forms of individual, group, or family therapy produce better outcomes for some patients than either drugs or therapy alone. Prescribing such combinations of treatment requires more clinical data than a descriptive diagnosis.

Such reality constraints may be most obvious in the public sector, but are not rare in the private sector. In the former, psychiatrists may be pressured to function in a narrowly defined way, while in the latter, economic considerations or availability of services often dictate the choice of a less than optimal treatment plan. In either situation, the message is clear: psychiatry, like other branches of medicine, is practiced in a social context that influences decisively what is possible. For a psychiatrist, this may pose a serious conflict among values involving responsibility to patients, to professional standards, and to self.

Treatment Planning

The clinical formulation arising from a psychiatric evaluation is basic to treatment planning. The psychiatrist asks himself or herself whether or not there are biological, psychological, and social treatment modalities which alone, or in combination, can be of help to the patient. This requires that the psychiatrist be knowledgeable about a broad array of treatment modalities and, if a specialist in only one, be willing to work collaboratively with colleagues of differing expertise. Most psychiatrists, however, are expert in several treatment approaches and are able to provide a broad range of therapeutic interventions.

The process of considering multiple approaches and combinations of treatments distinguishes the competent professional. The ability to plan a treatment program that is related to the clinical data about a particular patient, his or her specific problems and strengths, is essential. This sets the psychiatrist apart from those who offer all patients the same treatment regardless of clear biological, psychological, and social differences in the etiology of their illnesses.

The opportunity to consider multiple therapeutic approaches will be illustrated by the use of the following clinical vignette.

A 42-year-old businessman presented with complaints of loss of interest in his business, hobbies, and family over a period of six weeks. He acknowledged periods of profound sadness, reduced appetite with significant weight loss, insomnia, fatigue, and recurrent thoughts of death without, however, suicidal ideation.

He described himself as unusually serious, conservative, and relatively unable to express affection. He also acknowledged trying to be perfect, needing to be in control of every social situation, and having an excessive commitment to work.

The patient indicated that his marriage had been worsening for several years and described his wife as flighty, overemotional, and helpless under stress. For the past several years she had been angry, distant, and had declined to be involved sexually with him. Since the onset of his symptomatology, however, she had been solicitous and obviously concerned.

He described his family of origin as very poor. His father deserted his mother when the patient was twelve years of age and, as the oldest child, he had to take considerable responsibility for younger siblings, as well as to work part-time while attending school. He knew that his maternal grandfather had committed suicide and that two maternal uncles were alcoholic. A paternal uncle had died in prison after a long period of antisocial behavior.

Physical, laboratory, and neurological studies were negative.

After two evaluation interviews, the attending psychiatrist arrived at the following DSM-III diagnoses:

AXIS I —296.22—major depressive episode
AXIS II —301.40—personality disorder, compulsive
AXIS III—no relevant current physical disorder
AXIS IV—4—moderate psychosocial stress, marital
AXIS V —4—fair level of prior adaptive functioning

In the first five chapters, the reader will have the opportunity to follow experts from five major treatment modalities as they review basic theoretical premises and treatment techniques and then apply them to this patient. The clinical vignette is deliberately brief in order that these experts may develop the data that are useful in deciding whether a particular form of treatment may be helpful.

Publication of DSM-III was a landmark in the mental health field. It has received considerable attention, not only from clinicians, but also from legislative, insurance, and legal authorities. It has spawned a variety of books—case studies, training manuals, and others. With its emphasis on reliable diagnostic criteria, it promises to promote the increased scientific study of various treatment approaches to psychiatric syndromes. In this book, emphasis is on the process of treatment planning crucial to the psychiatrist's decision regarding the choice of treatment.

References

1. Garvon, E. F., and J. K. Dickson: Diagnostic Decision Making in Psychiatry: II. Diagnostic Styles, *Archives of General Psychiatry*, 14:233-237, March, 1966.
2. Spiegel, J.: *Transactions: The Interplay Between Individual, Family, and Society*, New York: Science House, 1971.

Chapter One

Treatment Planning and Psychodynamic Psychiatry

William Offenkrantz, M.D., Chairperson
Sol Altschul, M.D.
Arnold Cooper, M.D.
Allen Frances, M.D.
Robert Michels, M.D.
Allan Rosenblatt, M.D.
John Schimel, M.D.
Arnold Tobin, M.D.
Miltiades Zaphiropoulos, M.D.

All are members of the American Psychoanalytic Association, except Drs. Schimel and Zaphiropoulos, who represent the American Academy of Psychoanalysis.

Introduction and Theoretical Premises

The psychodynamic understanding of behavior had its origins in the discoveries of Sigmund Freud and his collaborators. Throughout this century the methods of psychodynamic inference about normal and abnormal human behavior have provided a powerful instrument for research and treatment and have led to an evolving general theory of human development and behavior. The psychoanalytic point of view concerning human behavior has become an integral part of the world view of Western culture, with wide applications in general psychiatry and medicine, as well as in all fields of humanistic study. Although training in psychoanalysis as a treatment technique is conducted in postgraduate institutes, the teaching of psychodynamics is included in virtually all residency training programs and represents the major theoretical orientation in American psychiatry today.

This chapter attempts to supplement the descriptive approach of DSM-III with the psychodynamic diagnostic point of view and to indicate how the two perspectives may enrich each other. A knowledge of psychodynamics can provide an organizing principle for phenomenological data and assist in evaluation and treatment planning, even if the choice should be other than psychodynamic therapy.

The word psychodynamic is used here in its broadest sense, referring to all the propositions that derive from the application of the psychoanalytic point of view. There is a narrower sense of the word in which the term psychodynamic refers only to a specific psychoanalytic hypothesis—the assumption of intrapsychic conflict.

The psychodynamic point of view has contributed to the understanding of an enormous range of human behaviors—normal and abnormal, waking and sleeping, intended and unintended, significant and trivial, frequent and unique, fantasied and experienced. This explanatory power has derived from the application of a few relatively simple principles; in fact, the basic propositions of psychodynamics codify and organize methods of understanding human behavior that traditionally have been used unsystematically by creative writers as well as the public in general.

Psychodynamic psychiatry has developed a conceptual framework of hypotheses and constructs—some very close to clinical data, others quite distant, some generally agreed upon by psychodynamic psychiatrists, and others the source of much controversy. However, the basic propositions are few, have been affirmed by a great deal of clinical experience, are data-close, and are so much a part of most psychiatrists' thinking that many people often fail to realize that they are thinking along psychodynamic lines. The value of psychodynamic hypotheses lies in the fact that they can be used both to organize large amounts of clinical data that might otherwise seem unrelated and to direct attention to significant behaviors that might be overlooked.

The basic propositions of the psychodynamic point of view are:

1) All psychological behavior can be understood in terms of psychological causes—the concept of *psychic determinism.*
2) All behavior is designed to fulfill human needs that originate at various levels of development and range from basic biologically determined needs (e.g., attachment to the parent) to those that represent complex goals and values (e.g., the willingness to die for a cause). Thus, behavior can be understood as *motivated* and generally tending toward the avoidance of pain and the maintenance of pleasure and security—*the pleasure-unpleasure principle.*
3) These needs and wishes often conflict with each other or with inner values and prohibitions. Because this state of *intrapsychic conflict*, although inevitable and ubiquitous, can be painful and frightening, a variety of defense mechanisms develop for removing these conflicts from the realm of conscious awareness. These mechanisms involve an active process, *repression*, and result in important aspects of thinking, feeling and decision-making becoming *psychodynamically unconscious*; i.e., not available to awareness by an act of will.
4) Early life experiences, the vicissitudes of maturation and de-

velopment, have a lasting effect on behavior; the adaptations made during each developmental stage affect the succeeding stages. This *genetic point of view* dictates that an understanding of the antecedents of any behavior is necessary for a full understanding of current behaviors. Significant failures to develop the appropriate phase-specific capacities at each stage of development can result in life-long arrest of these capacities.

5) The individual is always engaged in making the best adaptation possible out of the mix of inner needs, values, and fears, and the requirements of outer reality. These adaptive efforts often require unconscious compromises among opposing needs, and these compromises may present as *symptoms*.

6) The individual's repertoire of available behaviors is limited and repetitive. Therefore, a detailed examination of these behaviors in a relatively neutral setting, e.g., the psychodynamic treatment situation, can yield evidence concerning the person's behavior in other settings. The term *transference* refers to the perceptions, needs, and quality of interactions that the individual tends to create in relationship with the therapist and other significant persons. These reflect past experiences and ongoing needs imposed upon current relationships and are often markedly discrepant with the realities of the relationship.

7) It is useful to view many functions of mental life as coalescing into a group of *structures*—i.e., stable ways in which groups of experiences are organized. In psychoanalytic theory, such comprehensive structural systems of mental life are organized around the major functions of wishing (id), restraining (superego), mediation of conflict and recognition of reality (ego), and maintenance of a cohesive inner organization (self). Psychopathology may occur either as a result of failure of adequate structure formation due to developmental vicissitudes or as a result of conflict between or within structures.

These basic psychodynamic principles are shared by psychoanalysts of varied schools, despite differences they may have on other issues. They lead the psychodynamic psychiatrist to view all behavior, normal and psychopathological, as the result of interactions between endowment and environment, past and present, wishes and fears, fantasy and reality, and conflict and defenses. From this point of view, behavior is psychopathological when 1) it causes conscious distress, i.e., symptoms occur; 2) is maladaptive and inflexible, inhibiting the capacity for pleasure, self-fulfillment and optimal social functioning; or 3) brings the individual into conflict within the self or with the environment.

Range and Description of Specific Treatment Procedures

Treatment selection is not a matter of absolute indications and contraindications, but rather involves the weighing of complex variables that render psychodynamic psychotherapy more or less likely to be successful. The following outlines the criteria for suitability, first in a general way and then more specifically for the five psychodynamic psychotherapies: symptom-relief, supportive, focal, long-term exploratory, and psychoanalysis.

When considering psychodynamic psychotherapy, the psychiatrist must also evaluate the possible usefulness of medication, behavioral modification, group psychotherapy, environmental manipulation, and other therapies. For optimal psychiatric treatment, however, there must be an understanding of the relevant psychodynamic factors. These determine the primary themes of treatment and illuminate the doctor-patient relationship regardless of whether psychodynamic or other forms of treatment are to be the primary modalities. The changes resulting from psychodynamic psychotherapy have been attributed to a number of factors: the patient's insight into and resolution of psychological conflict, growth in the process of treatment, identification with the therapist, corrective emotional experiences, and positive conditioning, or some combination of these. The psychiatrist must evaluate the weight of these factors in a wide variety of treatment modalities, e.g., the role of identification and positive conditioning, as well as pharmacologic effects when medication is utilized.

There are a number of patient attributes that increase the likelihood of benefit from psychodynamic psychotherapy. Although they may seem to suggest a healthy or even ideal person, it should be emphasized that no one ever meets all the optimal requirements for suitability for psychodynamic psychotherapy. However, when either many unsuitable features or just a few extreme ones are present, psychodynamic psychotherapy is more difficult, and at times risky, unwise, or impossible.

Although some psychodynamic treatment techniques are often useful in crisis situations, the long-term techniques are ideally begun in a context of a relatively stable current and prospective life situation. Psychodynamic techniques may be useful, however, for many of the problems that emerge throughout the life cycle, and adaptations of techniques are often appropriate. Some patients may benefit from psychotherapy by one psychotherapist but not by another, or benefit from one form of psychodynamic psychotherapy and not others.

Five models of psychodynamic psychotherapy—symptom relief, supportive, focal, long-term, exploratory, and psychoanalysis—can be delineated. The indications for the different types of psychodynamic psychotherapy are not mutually exclusive, but form a continuum and overlap with one another. The following emphasizes their differences, however, and is organized around the dimensions of clinical setting, goals, selection criteria, and techniques.

These five modalities of therapy, themselves, may overlap and interpenetrate to a considerable degree in actual practice. The reason for this becomes clear if one considers each modality as representing not a monolithic approach, but a *cluster* of interrelated techniques. The more each cluster is employed exclusively and consistently, the more the resulting therapy will approach the model for that modality. In any actual therapeutic endeavor, however, there will be some, though perhaps slight, admixture of clusters of techniques and some variation in consistency of employment within each cluster, resulting in a blurring of the ideal types. Therapeutic efficacy may, at times, be enhanced when techniques serving *complementary* goals are mixed. However, when differing techniques serve *antithetical* goals, their admixture can impede or even negate therapeutic progress. It is, therefore, important that the psychotherapist keep clearly in mind the theoretical rationale and the related tactical and strategic goals of each modality or cluster of techniques.

SYMPTOM RELIEF PSYCHOTHERAPY

In this form of treatment, the psychotherapist attempts primarily to relieve quickly and directly the symptom or other form of distress for which the patient seeks help. Relief often results when the patient is able to experience and express previously unacceptable feelings in the presence of a psychotherapist who is experienced as a benign authority figure. It may only be necessary, however, for the feelings to be experienced, with little verbalization occurring. The resulting rise in self-esteem is reinforced if the patient learns that the expression of such feelings outside the treatment situation is acceptable. The effectiveness of this modality does not necessarily involve the acquisition of insight into the patient's past, unconscious mental life, or relationship to the therapist, but probably occurs through corrective emotional experiences, positive conditioning, and magical fantasies of the psychotherapist's power and caring. The corrective emotional experiences may include an unconscious identification with the loved or admired therapist's more benign conscience.[1] Similar modalities have been called Reparative Psychotherapy, and "focused, brief, psychodynamic psychotherapy."[2,3]

The psychotherapy sessions are generally held once a week for one to six months. Attempts are made to define the relief for which the patient has sought help.

Symptom relief psychotherapy is used in other forms of psychotherapy, especially the supportive variety, and occurs as well in the course of psychodynamic diagnostic interviewing. When the distress is eliminated or alleviated, the psychotherapist makes it as easy as possible for the patient to terminate, while clearly indicating that a return is possible without humiliation. If the patient wishes to continue, the psychotherapist makes an explicit agreement to work toward one or more goals in stated areas such as intimacy, work, or general interpersonal relations.

The first group of criteria for selection include: acute symptom formation in Affective, Anxiety, Somatoform, and Dissociative Disorders (categories grouped together as the Neuroses in DSM-II); adolescent crises (delinquency or acute inhibition of schoolwork); and acute grief reactions. A second group involves more chronic and characterological forms of psychopathology in which social, economic, geographic, and other factors make longer-term psychotherapies impossible. The third group involves those severe illnesses in which a major treatment approach is pharmacologic, and symptom relief psychotherapy is seen as an integral component of the pharmacologic approach. Finally, symptom relief psychotherapy may occur during the diagnostic or exploratory interviews. If the acute distress subsides during this procedure, the psychiatrist may consider the usefulness of a longer-term psychodynamic psychotherapy.

SUPPORTIVE PSYCHOTHERAPY

There are many forms of supportive psychotherapy, but this chapter addresses only that supportive psychotherapy in which the use of psychodynamic principles is primary. It is important to emphasize both that supportive techniques are utilized and are essential, at times, in all the psychodynamic psychotherapies. Also, no psychotherapies are totally supportive, in that elements of support and uncovering are intermixed inextricably in any form of psychodynamic psychotherapy. In this chapter, however, supportive psychotherapy is discussed as if it exists in a pure state, although this does not reflect the complexity of the psychotherapeutic process.

The goal of supportive psychotherapy is to help maintain or restore the individual to the highest previous level of functioning while attempting to alleviate symptoms and improve self-esteem. The goal does not include character change, increased self-awareness, or the confrontation of defenses.

Supportive techniques are designed to strengthen defenses. Psychodynamic psychotherapists use their understanding to plan appropriate interventions, and their verbal activity is often greater than in other forms of psychodynamic psychotherapy. It may be useful for the psychotherapist to communicate feelings and personal information in order to provide the patient with a model and to avoid the development of transference distortions. The psychotherapist may suggest alternative courses of action, help in problem solving, and use instruction and advice.

Supportive psychotherapies may be the shortest or the longest of all psychotherapies. Brief supportive treatment may be necessary for those caught in life crises in order to help restore functioning and to inhibit regression. At the other extreme, life-long, supportive psychotherapy may be necessary for those for whom the maintenance of functioning requires an ongoing relationship with a psychotherapist. The frequency of psychotherapeutic sessions may vary from several times a week in crisis situations to once every several weeks (or even months) for many years. Family members and other significant persons, including community networks, may be involved in the psychotherapy.

Some patients eventually may develop a readiness to shift to a more uncovering type of psychotherapy.

FOCAL PSYCHOTHERAPY

Focal or brief psychotherapy is an increasingly well described and researched application of psychodynamic principles and techniques to a planned short-term treatment. Although differing in details, the major proponents of this method generally agree about its appropriate duration, goals, techniques, and selection criteria.

The goal of focal psychotherapy is limited to the exploration and resolution of a specific area of intrapsychic conflict, selected both as central to the patient's suffering and amenable to insight. The goal is for the patient to derive increased understanding of his or her contribution to what had previously been experienced as mostly external problems. The patient is helped to recognize both the vulnerability and repetitive responses to particular stresses and to learn new and more adaptive coping and problem-solving skills.

Some authorities believe that focal psychotherapy may facilitate an extensive character change in some patients, similar to that produced by the more intensive psychodynamic psychotherapies. They suggest that focal psychotherapy can lead to a beneficial circle of mastery, increased problem-solving skills, and augmented self-esteem that generalize to foster structural change as well as an amelioration of conflicts other than the one chosen for exploration and resolution.

Focal psychotherapy is conducted most often at a frequency of once or twice weekly for 12 to 40 sessions. Most authorities agree on the importance of a predetermined and agreed-upon time limit. Some suggest that the termination occur on a fixed calendar date agreed upon at the outset of treatment, while others limit the total number of sessions allowing for flexible spacing over time. Others suggest that treatment extensions and/or follow-up visits may be useful and that, in some instances, focal psychotherapy may lead to long-term psychodynamic psychotherapy. Some, however, insist that it is essential for the termination date to be irrevocable in order to highlight the experience of the separation.

This treatment modality requires a high level of planning, activity, and data selection by the psychotherapist. Patient and psychotherapist collaboratively choose a specific problem area, and the psychotherapist attempts to establish a psychodynamic focus that connects the patient's chief complaint, recurrent interactional patterns, early experiences, and the evolving transference and resistance manifestations.

Some authorities suggest that effective focal psychotherapy is characterized by the active interpretation of the transference, while others emphasize the need to focus upon early resistances and to relate them to the factors involved in the patient's chief complaint. Mann recommends that focal therapy concentrate on the issue of separation.[4] Sifneos prefers to find an Oedipal focus.[5,6]

Ideally, the patient should possess a considerable degree of psychological mindedness, an attribute that can be developed in the early phase of the longer therapies. Also, the patient should begin with a strong motivation in wanting increased self-understanding and changes in attitudes and behaviors. There should be a clearly delineated problem that can be understood as the manifestation of an intrapsychic conflict. The patient must be able both to tolerate considerable anxiety and to experience quickly transference distortions while studying their roots. As the patient's roots are explored, there must be an ability to separate from the psychotherapist while simultaneously understanding his or her reactions to separation.

Focal psychotherapy should not commence during a life crisis that may require immediate action or support. During the evaluation process, the psychotherapist may offer tentative interpretations in order to determine the patient's capacity to respond with increased understanding.

LONG-TERM EXPLORATORY PSYCHOTHERAPY

Long-term exploratory psychotherapy is the most varied and difficult psychotherapy to define. The designation has been used to describe treatment processes with a wide range of frequency, duration, intensity, goals, techniques, and selection criteria. At one extreme, long-term exploratory psychotherapy may approach psychoanalysis; at the other, it may merge into brief psychodynamic or focal psychotherapy. Synonyms in common use include "intensive psychoanalytic psychotherapy" and "long-term uncovering psychotherapy."

It can be helpful to use the dimensions of depth, duration, and frequency to describe various types of psychotherapy. Depth refers both to the extent to which the therapist tries to explore the patient's attitudes and feelings that have been excluded from conscious awareness, and the extent to which a regressive transference is mobilized and explored. This type of treatment usually lasts more than 50 sessions or longer than 12 months.[7] The frequency may vary from one to as many as three or more sessions weekly.

Although the resolution of intrapsychic conflict and the resumption of arrested development usually are aspects of the treatment, the goals are more often symptom relief and improved self-esteem with subsequently improved interpersonal relationships. A major mechanism of positive change may be the patient's positive identification with the psychotherapist. In psychoanalysis, this development is considered to constitute a possible limitation of the patient's ultimate autonomy and hence subject to interpretation and working through before termination.

Techniques tend to be more flexible than those used in either psychoanalysis or focal psychotherapy, e.g., the couch is not used, ambiguity is not enhanced, and detailed exploration of unconscious fantasies is not promoted. The major feature, however, that distinguishes long-term exploratory psychotherapy from psychoanalysis is the avoidance of systematic regressive transference experiences. Transference distortions generally are interpreted as they become manifest and comprehensible. This procedure clarifies and intercepts the patient's regressed and distorted feelings about the psychotherapist as they emerge.[8] In the early stages of psychoanalysis the therapist uses transference interpretations to help the patient understand how the past is alive in the present and to deal with the anxieties involved in such regressions. This conveys the implicit message that these are worthwhile experiences and are to be encouraged. Long-term exploratory psychotherapy tends to rely less than does psychoanalysis on the use of transference interpretation as a major technical tool and is likely to employ more nontransference-related interpretations.

In long-term exploratory psychotherapy there is leeway for such activities as the giving of information, reassurance, and advice. There is an opportunity for the analysis of the resistance to the emergence of unconscious material and the working through of its emotional impact. The uncovering techniques confront rather than strengthen defenses (as in the supportive psychotherapies), promote rather than suppress the emergence of anxiety provoking fantasies and feelings, and clearly provide less reassurance.

Patients who experience their transference feelings as real and not subject to the need for understanding may fare better in long-term exploratory psychotherapy than in psychoanalysis. In contrast to focal psychotherapy, the patient in long-term psychotherapy need not be so immediately and strongly motivated, because this issue can be dealt with during the early phase. The patient need not have so clear a focal conflict since many conflicts can be dealt with and at a less rapid pace. In contrast to the supportive psychotherapies, the patient must have or develop during psychotherapy a greater tolerance for anxiety, a greater ability for introspection, greater internal resources, and a stable life situation that does not require immediate or repeated emergency interventions.

PSYCHOANALYSIS

Psychoanalysis is the most intensive and the most ambitious of the psychotherapies. Its goals include the relief of chronic symptoms, characterologic distortions, and other maladaptive behaviors by promoting fundamental intrapsychic changes. These changes ameliorate the severity of the patient's conflicts, soften the rigidity and restrictiveness of defenses and character traits, and promote the maturation of psychic structures. Patients selected for psychoanalysis may present with acute symptoms imposed upon or reflecting an exacerbation of chronic psychopathology. The patient who has successfully completed psychoanalysis will have acquired significant autonomy from the psychopathological patterns that have ruled his or her past life, from many unconscious and irrational wishes and fears, from the distortions that have formed an inevitable part of interpersonal relationships (including the relationship with the psychoanalyst), as well as freedom from the identifications with the psychoanalyst that have been helpful in achieving symptom relief.

The distinguishing feature of the psychoanalytic process is that it can provide an opportunity for the full development and systematic interpretation of regressive transference patterns which, in the paradigmatic case, develop into the transference neurosis. This occurs when the patient's transference reactions become organized around the psychoanalyst, recreating the psychopathogenic experiences most salient to the neurotic conflict and replacing the neurotic symptoms. Some psychoanalysts, while questioning the central importance of this concept, nevertheless agree that the systematic exploration and not just the interception of transference reactions is crucial. This structured, controlled, and adaptive psychotherapeutic regression requires a highly specialized treatment environment that must be intense, prolonged (usually three or more years), and intentionally ambiguous. The ambiguity is fostered by the psychoanalyst's systematic avoidance of social conversation, reassurance, or advice about the patient's problems. Some psychoanalysts believe three sessions a week are sufficient; others believe four or more sessions are necessary.

Psychoanalysts generally conduct the treatment with the patient lying on a couch so that the psychoanalyst cannot be seen, thus increasing the degree to which the patient's associations are a response to internal fantasy rather than to external reality. The intensity and duration of the treatment are required for two reasons. Time is required to achieve a significant degree of reconstruction and re-experiencing of earliest developmental stages as a precondition to the development of stable new adaptations. In addition, time is required for the powerful unconscious resistances to this process of change to be overcome.

The goal in the first phase of psychoanalysis is to foster a situation in which the patient can experience, within the treatment, intense feelings in order to discover how the past is still alive in current perceptions and behavior. The experience of regression provides the patient with an opportunity to regain access to warded off conflicts, distortions, and psychopathological solutions as they become manifest in the immediacy of the psychoanalytic relationship and may culminate in the transference neurosis. With the emergence of the transference regression, an increasingly strong alliance develops between the psychoanalyst and the relatively conflict-free, rational aspects of the patient. This indispensable alliance is characterized by the patient's ability to experience the regressive transference reactions with full intensity and yet be able also to observe and understand them. The psychoanalyst's stable, predictable, and friendly neutrality with regard to the patient's conflicts permits the patient to arrive at new and more satisfactory resolutions of intrapsychic conflicts and to resume the arrested process of psychic development. Transference interpretation, the making conscious and subjecting to scrutiny the patient's transference wishes, fears, and distortions, is a major technical device toward the achievement of these goals. A fully developed interpretation involves the clarification of current, distorted perceptions of the psychoanalytic situation and/or the psychoanalyst, which are then related both to antecedents in the patient's early life experiences and to behavior in recent experiences outside of treatment, as well as to hopes for the future. Complete interpretations and their ensuing insights are rarely accomplished by single interventions, but require frequent repetition and elaboration in what is called the "working through" process. As the patient comes to understand previously unconscious motivations, fears, and distortions, he or she is less influenced by conflict and better able to replace the automatic repetition of past behaviors with new and more adaptive ones.

The primary indicators for psychoanalysis are, first, chronic symptoms that reflect intrapsychic conflict and, second, arrested or deviant development.[9] In addition, there are three qualifying indicators, only one of which need be present for prescribing psychoanalysis. First, the chronic symptoms will not respond to other treatment methods because they are either embedded in a rigid character structure or occur in the presence of fragile or brittle defenses. Second, these symptoms can be relieved by other treatment methods only at excessive personal or social cost, e.g., the risk of chronic dependency upon antianxiety medication. Third, although temporary relief may be obtained with other treatment methods, it is believed that the presenting chronic symptom or inhibition, or an equivalent disability such as psychosomatic illness, is likely to recur. Finally, the patient should also fulfill a group of criteria for analyzability that predict both the ability to form a suitable therapeutic alliance by alternately experiencing and observing the regressive responses to the anticipated treatment and the ability eventually to give up the therapeutic relationship entirely.

These criteria also require the construction of a psychodynamic formulation that makes use of all the data drawn from the presenting chronic symptom(s) and other psychopathology. This includes the recent and early history; the mental status encompassing the patient's total behavior in the interview, especially reactions to various historical items; and the quality of interaction between the patient and the psychiatrist. When the indications for psychoanalysis and criteria for analyzability are applied to a large group of patients, the appropriateness of psychoanalysis varies from optimal to contraindicated. The various combinations of primary and qualifying indicators, criteria for analyzability, and diagnostic categories that enable the psychoanalyst to determine where psychoanalysis fits on the spectrum of suitable treatment modalities have been published.[9] Applying these selection criteria suggests that the majority of psychiatric patients are not considered suitable for psychoanalysis. Indeed, in considering only those patients treated by psychoanalysts, and setting aside financial factors, a recent survey indicated that only 47 percent of those studied were considered appropriate for psychoanalysis, with the remainder being treated by other forms of psychotherapy.[10]

Table 1 summarizes the modalities for convenient comparison.

Nature of Clinical Data Necessary for Treatment Planning

The psychodynamic psychiatrist conducting diagnostic interviews or psychotherapy will attempt to understand the patient from the viewpoint of the levels of structural personality organization and their defects, the types of motivation that are operating in areas of major conflict, the nature of the defenses, and the quality of the patient's object relations, particularly as they are manifested in the transference. The psychodynamic formulation will attempt to integrate this understanding of the patient's psychopathology with its genetic antecedents, the level of integration and structure formation that has been achieved, and the nature of the unconscious conflicts and the efforts to resolve them.

TABLE 1

Modality	Clinical Setting	Goals	Selection Criteria	Technique	Major Therapeutic Factors
Symptom relief	1/week for 4-25 sessions usually outpatient	relief of symptoms	1) acute symptoms 2) chronic character pathology when long-term therapies inappropriate 3) severe illness as part of pharmacologic therapy	encourage patient to express hitherto unacceptable feelings	1) expression of feelings to accepting therapist—"catharsis" → rise in self-esteem 2) identification with therapist's benign conscience 3) magical fantasies of therapist's power and caring 4) genetic or transference insight unnecessary
Supportive	wide variation—outpatient and inpatient	maintain at or restore to highest previous level of function	1) life crises 2) severe chronic illness when other modalities unacceptable	1) advice, instruction, reassurance, etc. 2) designed to *strengthen* defenses 3) *avoid* transference distortions 4) provide real relationship and model	1) identification with therapist 2) magical fantasies regarding therapist's power and caring 3) provision of structure 4) provision of realistic information

TABLE 1 (CONTINUED)

Modality	*Clinical Setting*	*Goals*	*Selection Criteria*	*Technique*	*Major Therapeutic Factors*
Focal	1-2/week for 12-40 sessions —usually present time limit— outpatient	resolution of specific area of intrapsychic conflict	1) chronic symptoms 2) clearly delineated intrapsychic conflict 3) considerable psychological mindedness 4) high motivation to understand and change 5) ability to tolerate considerable anxiety	1) choose specific problem area 2) interpretation is major tool 3) *confront* defenses 4) *active* interpretation of transference	1) insight 2) identification with therapist
Long-term exploratory	1-4/week— more than 50 sessions —no time limit —usually outpatient	resolution of intrapsychic conflict— improved self-esteem and interpersonal relationships —symptom relief	1) chronic symptoms 2) need *less* initial motivation than for psychoanalysis 3) need *less* focused conflict than for focal therapy	1) interpretation is major tool, though advice, reassurance, etc. is used 2) confront defenses. More flexible than focal therapy or psychoanalysis	1) insight 2) identification with therapist

			4) need *more* anxiety tolerance, introspective ability, internal resources, and stable life situation than for supportive therapy	3) regressive transference discouraged by interceptive interpretations 4) *not* confined to focal conflict	
Psychoanalysis	3-5/week for 3 years or longer — outpatient (see pg. 17)	fundamental intrapsychic change → resolution of conflict and maturation of psychic structure → relief of chronic symptoms and characterologic problems	1) chronic symptoms reflecting intrapsychic conflict *and* arrested or deviant development, which 2) will not respond to other therapies, or will only with excessive personal cost, or will recur and 3) fulfill criteria for analyzability (see Psychoanalytic Peer Review section in APA Manual)	1) interpretation is major tool 2) encourage controlled therapeutic regression → transference neurosis	1) insight

Some of the clinical data that emerge when these basic psychodynamic propositions are used as guidelines are elaborated in the following discussion.

MATURATION AND DEVELOPMENT

One achievement of the infant is the gradual unfolding of the capacity to distinguish within its mind between representations of self and other object representations. The establishment of self-boundaries is manifested in a clinical interview by the individual's ability to discriminate between fantasy and reality, or between thoughts, feelings, and actions initiated by self as contrasted with those originated by others. Absent or severely defective self-boundaries in the adult are associated with vulnerability to psychosis. A further step in development requires the integration of primitive self and object experiences and images so that the child comes to experience the self and inner objects as stable and cohesive over time; good and bad self and object representations are experienced as unified rather than separate entities. Crucial for healthy development is the ability to develop and maintain a stable internal representation of the loved object (e.g., mother) even when absent or frustrating, and later to be able to realize the needs of another in a reciprocal relationship. These are also capacities visible in the clinical interview. Arrested or deviant development leading to fixation or regression in forming an integrated self or object representation are manifest in adult Borderline Personality Disorders.

If there is a failure to relinquish the grandiose and/or omnipotent fantasies that accompany the earlier phases of the child's tie to the mother, this is often followed by a failure in acquiring the ability to acknowledge the autonomy of significant others. Once again this failure is visible in the clinical interview. When these deficiencies result in a failure of psychological structure formation and persist into adult life, the condition may be termed a "developmental arrest" and designated a Narcissistic Personality Disorder. Those personality structures of a person with a Borderline Personality Disorder or a Narcissistic Personality Disorder that do develop tend to be unstable under conditions of psychological stress.

With reasonably adequate mothering and an involved father, the child will extend his or her ties beyond the original mother-child dyad to the triadic mother-child-father relationship. In the setting of love, competition, desire, and fear involved in the Oedipus complex, further psychic structures develop. External prohibitions and values begin to be internalized as the superego, which includes both the development of conscience and the unfolding of the ego ideal. Language acquisition, pleasure in mastery, self-representation, and reality-testing coalesce as the ego. The set of powerful desires conceived as the id, at work since earliest infancy, take on a new coherence during the Oedipal period.

The clinical data concerning the degree of structure formation are important in determining the diagnosis, in treatment planning, and in conveying vital information concerning the patient's ability to cooperate in and to tolerate the frustrations of a psychotherapeutic relationship, whether or not the primary treatment modality is medication, psychotherapy, or some combination of treatment modalities. The required data for making this assessment can usually be obtained in the initial interview(s) as the history, the mental status (including the patient's reaction to the items of the history), the behavior of the patient, and the quality of interaction in the interview situation are examined.

The more severe disturbances of development that may result from grossly inadequate parenting, severe early traumata, or constitutional defects can lead to a serious failure of structure development. The early loss of a loving parent, for example, may lead to a failure to develop a capacity for loving ties to others and/or to a grossly deficient conscience.

Under less dire circumstances, deficiencies of psychic structures may interfere with important regulatory functions needed for successful adaptation. These functions may include the regulation of self-esteem, shame, and guilt; the regulation of the relations between fantasy and action and the capacity for delay and thought; and the ability to tolerate strong affects such as hate, fear, or love.

MOTIVATION

Psychodynamic psychiatry has traditionally studied the quality, intensity, and balance of three motivational systems: sexual (sensual, pleasure-seeking), aggressive, and dependency-attachment. In more recent years, motivations deriving from needs of the self have been emphasized. These include self-esteem, ideals, mastery, safety, pleasure in functioning, and others. They can be viewed as derivatives of the first three systems. In most clinical situations, the unconscious fantasies of danger, the ensuing anxiety, and defensive operations, can be understood as a result of conflicts related to the unconscious and unacceptable wishes that derive from one of the major motivational systems. The patterning of an individual's motivational systems is fairly enduring over time and may find expression in ways that, though symptomatic, are compatible with current circumstances. A patient with agoraphobia, for example, may have one or more conflicts underlying the symptom. For the patient whose control of sexual impulses is fragile, becoming housebound protects against temptation. For the patient struggling with angry feelings, it is a way to remain securely attached to an ambivalently regarded partner. For the patient with strong dependency needs and a fear of autonomy, agoraphobia allows continual attachment to the person and place seen as safe and nurturing. For the patient with a defective or deviant self, remaining at home may serve to prevent fragmentation. In general, unconscious needs and anxieties do find indirect expression. The manner of detecting their derivatives in a psychodynamic diagnostic interview will be illustrated in a later section.

ANXIETY

Psychoanalytic theory postulates that the experience of needs and desires occurs very early in the infant's psychic experience and is related to a frightening expectation of danger. These expectations evolve in a manner parallel to the motivational systems. Freud described the typical fantasies of danger that lead to conflict and anxiety. These include fears of: 1) loss or separation from a person on whom the child depends for love and care (object loss); 2) anger or disapproval on the part of such a person (loss of love); 3) physical punishment or mutilation for transgressions, real or imagined (castration anxiety); and 4) punitive conscience (guilt, superego anxiety, disapproval of oneself on the basis of internalized parental standards). Subsequent workers have delineated other anxiety-provoking fantasies: 1) fear of fusion with the object; 2) fear of disintegration of the self; and 3) shame, feelings of humiliation, or feelings of inferiority based on disapproval by significant others or oneself for not living up to ideal standards.

A knowledge of the maturational level from which the anxiety originates is an aid in planning treatment. For example, patients suffering conscious or unconscious feelings of guilt will often be eager to confess their sins in the interview situation and may, in words or behavior, attempt to elicit from the therapist the sympathy and/or condemnation they feel they deserve. Self-condemnation correlates well with both the anticipation of the condemnation by others and with the conscious and/or unconscious tendency to condemn others. A patient with a conscious or unconscious sense of shame, on the other hand, may experience the interview as a source of real or threatened humiliation and attempt to withhold embarrassing thoughts, fantasies, and behavior from the therapist.

A description of the defense mechanisms is not included in this chapter because it is assumed that the reader is familiar with them.

TRANSFERENCE

The nature of the relationship between patient and doctor, and its moment-to-moment changes, are a special focus of the psychodynamic psychotherapist in both diagnostic and psychotherapeutic activity. With a reasonable sense of the actualities of the interview situation, including, importantly, his or her reactions to the patient, the therapist can note the distortions introduced by the patient and make deductions concerning their meaning, importance, and motivation. The patient's ability to form meaningful ties to others, the developmental level of the relationship, and the nature of the failure in the capacity for relationships can be assessed. The psychotherapist evaluates whether the initial transference distortions are a result of conflict or of structural deficit.

The patient who complains about the doctor because the appointment was set for a week after the initial phone call is likely to reveal a series of narcissistic difficulties in accepting the fact that others have needs. Similarly, a patient who describes never having experienced a feeling of being in love often will come to feel that treatment is disappointing and without interest or meaning and will not appear to develop a tie to the psychotherapist. Whether or not this precludes psychodynamic psychotherapy will depend upon the evaluation of additional aspects of the patient's personality.

The Psychodynamic Interview: The Major Clinical Procedure Used in Obtaining Data for Treatment Planning

In order to clarify the decision-making process that inclines a clinician to recommend a particular psychodynamic treatment or to choose a nonpsychodynamic one, the following description of the method of obtaining a psychodynamic data base is offered.

The traditional psychiatric interview is one in which the interaction is structured and the goal is the collection of various categories of data. Although interested in these data, the psychodynamically oriented interviewer regards the interviewing procedure as a psychodynamic process and as a source of interactional data in itself. This perspective is fostered by a relatively nondirective approach that permits the sequence and kinds of data revealed and the manner in which they are offered to be determined primarily by the patient rather than by the interviewer.

The inevitable difficulty the patient may have in spontaneously revealing himself or herself allows the interviewer to identify, explore, and, perhaps in some instances, to point out defensive operations as they occur in the interview situation. The ambiguity of a nondirective approach fosters the emergence of such behavior. By observing this behavior the clinician is in a position to make inferences about the patient's early and subsequent modes of relating, the nature of his or her fantasy life, and an estimate of the patient's ability to utilize a psychodynamic treatment modality.

In measuring the patient's ability to participate in a therapeutic alliance, the clinician observes how well the patient is able both to communicate emotions and fantasies and to reflect upon them. The clinician attends to the trends in the patient's associations in order to understand the unconscious connections that link contiguous thoughts. The patient's nonverbal and paraverbal behaviors are observed for the additional light they may shed on the verbal content. This is important because the patient will unconsciously attempt to mold the relationship with the psychiatrist to fit the unconscious needs he or she has for certain qualities in all relationships. These unconscious efforts by the patient evoke feelings in the psychotherapist that are a stimulus for him or her to respond in particular ways. The psychodynamically oriented psychiatrist, by using empathy and introspection, learns to detect these efforts and to experience and understand the evoked feelings and tendencies to act. This regular use of empathy by all psychodynamically oriented psychiatrists has been of particular interest in recent years as disorders in the regulation of self-esteem (e.g., Narcissistic Personality Disorders and Borderline Personality Disorders) have received broader attention. The crucial necessity of verbalizing empathic understanding to the patient has recently been demonstrated in the psychotherapy of patients with these disorders. The psychiatrist considers his or her own evoked feelings and tendencies to act as diagnostically reflecting the "quality of interaction" that suggests different forms of the patient's psychopathology and associated underlying patterns of unconscious conflict and conflict resolution. There is, of course, no single or "proper" reaction a psychiatrist "should" have in response to a patient. Other diagnostic data may accrue from the patient's reaction to a trial confrontation or interpretation.

The psychiatrist traces the threads that connect nuclear conflicts and the quality of object relations. The patient's early memories, dreams, and fantasies are correlated with each other. The knowledge of the development of motivational systems and their typical derivatives permits the clinician to predict the patient's probable response to various treatment modalities. An example: a pretty female patient reported in a diagnostic interview with a male psychiatrist an early memory of dancing to her family's applause. The chief complaint was that she had become depressed after her boyfriend had left her for another woman. During the next interview she reported a dream of being shut outside a locked door and of having a bitter sense of missing the fun that others were having. The clinician might postulate even from these scant data that her sense of self-esteem had been closely related to being appreciated as sexually exciting (and that primal scene fantasies or experiences were an important part of her early development) and that this theme continues to operate. The accuracy of these postulates can be checked by making short-term predictions and determining how well they are borne out by the clinical material, i.e., the patient will form an erotic, exhibitionistic transference or manifest a reaction formation against sexual wishes. It might also be predicted that she will express curiosity about the male psychotherapist's wife. The erotic, exhibitionistic transference feelings can be predicted as a defense against aggressive and dependent wishes as well as an expression of her continuing effort to bolster shaky self-esteem.

There are other ways of collecting psychodynamic data. In projective psychological tests, for example, the data of the clinical interview are made more systematic by standardizing the stimuli offered to the patient. Psychodynamic data can also be gathered in a number of settings; examples are the hospitalized patient in group or occupational therapy, the child in a nursery or at school, and the patient's drawings, sculpture, or writings.

A more comprehensive description of the psychodynamic interview and the useful data it generates is illustrated in the following clinical vignette:

A 26-year-old, single male complained that he has experienced little or nothing when sexual or angry feelings would have been appropriate and that this had been so for as long as he could remember (an example of what is meant by a chronic symptom). He has been relatively unsuccessful in business and unable to sustain intimate relationships with women. It is noted from his history that for several years the patient has "fallen in love" rapidly and repeatedly. However, he quickly depreciates the woman (another chronic symptom). The patient stated that he has always seen his mother as the perfect woman and has consciously continued to search for her equal. Although the patient seems unaware that there might be a connection between his relationships with women and his feelings about his mother, the psychotherapist infers that these short-lived affairs reflect, in part, a maladaptive attempt to deal with an unresolved intrapsychic conflict (presumably overdetermined) between earlier positive feelings toward his mother and incompatible feelings. Examples of incompatible feelings are guilty fears over childhood wishes for sexual intimacy with her, or anger at her excessive control or neglect of him, or fear of abandonment by her, etc. During the interview, the patient expresses shame at the way he has "used" women and becomes visibly uncomfortable when describing the repetitive pattern. This tends to confirm the existence of unresolved intrapsychic conflict.

The patient had undergone psychotherapy six years earlier after he had flunked out of a second college. This period of treatment had involved 18 months of once- or twice-weekly sessions. He expressed the feeling that his previous therapy had been for his parents' sake, rather than his own, because he did not pay for it himself. As a result of psychotherapy, however, he had completed college and entered an occupation similar to that of his father. Thus, symptom relief had been achieved. The old problem, however, reappeared in a milder form; although able to work regularly and to enthusiastically plan many business ventures with his father, he withdrew from each before completion. When the interviewer suggested the possibility of a problem with competition, the patient related that he had experienced conscious feelings of conflict over succeeding on his own or joining his father in business. He commented sadly that he realized he had chosen his vocation solely to please his father.

During the course of the initial interview, the psychotherapist became aware that in the interaction with the patient, he was responding to the patient's expressed enthusiasm for psychotherapy with reciprocal feelings of optimism. The psychotherapist realized that this was a reaction to the seductive aspect of the patient's pattern of "falling in love" rapidly, now re-enacted with the interviewer. He also realized that the immediate idealization of the psychotherapist would probably be followed by depreciation and possible premature termination of treatment by the patient. It was crucial to recognize that this repetitive self-defeating pattern, both with women and in business ventures with his father, would threaten the successful completion of the treatment if not adequately dealt with by timely interpretation. Data from three sources (history, mental status, and quality of interaction) supported the presumption that the chronic symptoms reported by the patient reflected intrapsychic conflict and that, although his previous psychotherapy had helped, the chronic symptoms had recurred.

At the age of five, the patient had cut himself severely with a knife while attempting to help his mother in the kitchen. Although there was no permanent damage, the patient had always believed that this had occurred because his mother was too preoccupied at the time with decorating her new home to pay attention to him. He became fearful of any separation from her and exhibited clinging behavior and the inhibition of any expression of assertion, anger, or hostility. In circumstances where anger might have been appropriate, he had resorted to babyish clowning. This pattern has continued in modified form. He still responds to authorities, when rejection is possible, by idealizing the authority and playing the clown, without conscious awareness of anger. The interviewer concluded that the physical trauma had triggered a psychological reaction and that the normal developmental line of separation from the mother had become arrested. Confirmation is apparent from the patient's interview behavior in which he expresses the fear that closeness makes him vulnerable to the other person. In spite of his expressed eagerness to begin treatment, the patient's behavior implied that he was experiencing similar fears in regard to the psychotherapist.

The patient ruminated about whether he would be able to keep his appointment times. The psychotherapist believed that the patient's behavior reflected an internal struggle between the need to please and rebellion against an appointment schedule that is experienced as a demand on the part of the psychotherapist. The psychotherapist became aware of some surprise as the patient shifted from clinging idealization of him to an ostensible loss of interest in psychotherapy. This was manifested, for example, by requests for additional sessions during the evaluation interviews, followed immediately by an apparent sudden loss of interest and by monotonous speech. Noting that he was experiencing a spectrum of feelings, starting with compassion and friendly amusement, but including boredom and annoyance, the psychotherapist inferred that there was an angry element in the patient's sudden shifts of attitude. He was reminded of the typical behavior of a child struggling with the separation from a parent, in which the child alternately clings to and then ignores the parent. Unlike a child in a normal developmental phase, however, this patient is much more tyrannical and demanding, without the appealing quality that characterizes a normal child.

The psychotherapist realizes that beneath the patient's apparent cooperation lurks a pervasive oppositional tendency, the feeling that

> *any agreement with another's expectations is equivalent to a surrender of his autonomy. The patient appears to experience this, even if initiated by himself, as a capitulation that he must then resist. The psychotherapist infers that the patient is thereby able to avoid the frightening prospect of taking responsibility for assertive or competitive action on his own. Although his previous therapy had resulted in some improvement, it did not enable him to avoid returning to his regressive patterns.*

After a brief reconnaissance of the terrain of intrapsychic conflict, arrested development, and the quality of his interaction, the psychiatrist assessed the following items as diverse manifestations of the same problem: the patient's flunking out of two colleges, his difficulty living up to his potential in business, his inability to sustain intimate relations with women, and his potential for dropping out of treatment.

The psychotherapist determined that psychoanalysis may be required to effect a lasting resolution of these problems. To help make this decision, the criteria for analyzability were assessed. Favorable criteria include evidence of successful social functioning and the ability to use his intellect in school and on the job, despite his failures. He can communicate adequately, has an accessible fantasy life, and has some capacity for introspection. There is at least a modest tolerance for anxiety, frustration, and depression, as well as some ability to form reciprocal and nurturing relationships. Even in the face of conflictual competitive strivings, the patient has been able to sustain mutually gratifying relationships with male friends and is attracted to women. He has demonstrated a stable current and prospective life situation that provides a basis for the possibility of change.

The unfavorable aspects of the assessment include his fear of loss of control resulting in overcontrol, a rigid focus on external reality, and an impaired potential for sublimation, since his creative activities are limited to new business ventures. Similarly, his capacity to utilize therapeutic regression may be less than optimal. He is able to form reciprocal relationships with women, but only until they fall in love with him at which point he withdraws. Thus, his capacity for intimacy is limited and, to the extent that he does not realize his unconscious manipulation of women until later, his capacity for self-object differentiation is intermittent.

On balance, the psychotherapist views the criteria for analyzability as favorable. In addition, the patient demonstrates the primary indication for psychoanalysis (chronic symptoms reflecting intrapsychic conflict and arrested development) and one qualifying indicator, i.e., only temporary relief had been obtained with long-term exploratory psychotherapy. The interviewer's conclusion is that psychoanalysis may well be the optimal treatment for this patient. If an accurate diagnostic assessment for recommending psychoanalysis has been made, it is unlikely that major changes in technique will be necessary during the course of treatment.

There are, however, other variables. For example, if this patient had presented with only one of the several problems he actually described and was highly motivated toward change in that area, focal psychotherapy might have been considered. This is particularly so if it can be shown that he is able to form a transference quickly and to respond introspectively to interpretive comments. He and the psychotherapist may have been able then to arrive at a definition of a circumscribed or focal conflict and a reasonably clear, if tentative, formulation of the psychodynamics. Another factor in this clinical decision is the availability of a psychoanalyst or a low-cost psychoanalytic clinic. The rapid development of transference reactions may, however, also be a sign of relative weakness of internal personality structures (intrapsychic regulatory mechanisms), and, if so, the psychotherapist must be ready to shift to another form of psychotherapy if other conflicts begin to surface in the treatment.

The patient's previous 18 months of treatment had been in long-term exploratory psychotherapy. It was successful, as measured by his completion of college, and it is likely that an important mechanism of this change was the fact that his need to frustrate his parents became more ego-alien. This change separated him from them to some extent and enabled him to discontinue psychotherapy because they were paying for it. Long-term exploratory psychotherapy directed at his fear of his anger both at women and his father might again be appropriate under some circumstances. If, for example, assessment of criteria for analyzability indicated that the patient had not been able to finish college despite previous psychotherapy, had a limited ability to communicate through speech, presented himself as incurious about himself, and seemed to have a low tolerance for anxiety, the clinician might consider long-term exploratory psychotherapy.

Supportive psychotherapy directed at maintaining functioning, with improvement in self-esteem primarily through the mechanism of identification with an admired therapist, might have been indicated if, in addition to the findings in the preceding paragraph, his history and mental status revealed other features. Examples of such features might be paranoid thinking when angry, perhaps alternating with suicidal ruminations, and a history of no reciprocal relations with women and few, if any, male friends.

Either focal or supportive psychotherapy may lead to one of the longer-term psychotherapies. The patient in focal psychotherapy, unless it is expressly time-limited, may well become interested in a wider exploration of his symptomatology and personality as the psychotherapy progresses. The patient undergoing supportive psychotherapy may gain sufficient ego strength, curiosity, and motivation to seek deeper understanding.

Although the patient presented in this case report would seem to fit well into the category of Compulsive Personality Disorder, it should be apparent that more than the diagnosis is required in treatment choice and planning. For the psychodynamic psychotherapist, the clinical interview is the primary instrument for data collection and treatment planning. Although there is overlapping among the psychodynamic psychotherapies, and one may merge into another during the course of treatment, the resourceful psychotherapist will be well versed in the indications and contraindications of each, as well as attentive to the fluctuations and changes in the patient, in order to select appropriate measures during the course of treatment.

Clinical Vignette to Illustrate Treatment Planning

The clinical vignette presented in the Introduction of this volume might be approached from a psychodynamic point of view as follows:

The 40-year-old businessman or professional who presents himself as suffering symptoms of depression is a familiar figure in the psychiatrist's office. The story of a loss of interest in business, hobbies, and family is likewise familiar, often enough accompanied by what may appear to be signs of an endogenous illness: sadness, loss of appetite and weight, insomnia, and melancholic thoughts of death, without there necessarily being actual suicidal ideas. It is tempting simply to put him on an antidepressant, particularly since this can be conceived of as a life-saving measure, despite the absence of overt suicidal ideation. One may even be tempted to consider hospitalization or electroconvulsive therapy for such a patient who seems so clearly to have a major depressive episode. However, there is also the presence of a Compulsive Personality Disorder. It is noted that the patient is conservative, serious, and unable to express affection. He is concerned with perfection, with excessive control, and is preoccupied with his work. Psychiatrists have learned to expect a patient with a compulsive character disorder to respond with depression when there is diminished self-esteem occasioned by a perceived defeat or humiliation in the realm of work or love. During the evaluative interviews, the psychodynamic psychotherapist, like his or her colleague the internist, would be interested in discovering the precipitating stress(es) that may have thrown this patient into a depression. The clinical data presented are all long standing, and there is no indication in the vignette of altered circumstances that might account for the precipitation of depressive symptoms six weeks before the initial consultation. The ability to elicit the precipitating events and to explore them with the patient would be important criteria for: 1) defining the potential of this patient for psychodynamic psychotherapy, and 2) the possible rapid amelioration of the symptoms. The latter regularly occurs when patient and psychotherapist are able to define and agree upon the precipitating sources of stress.

One can only speculate on what might be found to account for the apparently sudden and rapid decompensation of an individual who had presumably functioned adequately under difficult personal (compulsive) and interpersonal (marital stress) problems. Particular attention would be paid to the mode of communication, the feelings, mood, and affect of both patient and interviewer, as they are evoked by the communication of the historical events regarding the immediate and distant past and the patient's reactions to them.

There could be failures in the vocational sphere—business reverses, struggles with a partner, or tax problems. Finally, a success that is threatening to the patient or a final realization that the long hoped for great success was not possible might be uncovered.

After some initial hesitation, with the patient expressing some distress and embarrassment at having to talk to a stranger about what he calls "minor problems," he begins tearfully to elaborate the following: his business has been successful, but he has recently had an offer from a larger firm to merge with them and accept the position of second in command of the new company. He is flattered that the offer has been made, but he is threatened by the fact that he hasn't "made it" completely on his own and will have to bow to the authority of an older man. The interviewer senses a feeling of wanting to reassure the patient that he has done well, while wondering what else the patient is complaining about. From this, the interviewer surmises that the patient's perfectionism and unresolved competitive feelings are interfering with his ability to enjoy his success and are operative in his depressive symptomatology.

There could be some new cachet in the marital situation, e.g., physical illness, newly manifest sexual impotence, infidelity desired or discovered, divorce threatened, or a perversion disclosed.

The patient quickly turns to his difficult marital relationship and wonders whether this may have brought on his depression. The early part of the marriage had been reasonably happy, with four children born in rapid succession, the oldest a son, about to become 12 years old. In the beginning, he enjoyed his wife's flighty attitude and thought it cute, but he became resentful of her as she became increasingly preoccupied and ineffectual under the pressure of family responsibilities. Their sex life had been all right, but never completely satisfactory to either. The patient tended toward premature ejaculation, but early in the marriage he had occasionally been able to maintain an erection until his wife achieved orgasm. Gradually, their sexual activity has deteriorated. In the last two years, his wife has often refused to participate, complaining angrily that she becomes aroused and then is left "high and dry." The patient complains bitterly that the premature ejaculation is his wife's fault because she is cold and unresponsive. The interviewer attempts a trial interpretation by asking whether the patient thinks his wife's complaints have any substance. The patient is taken aback, but upon reflection remembers that at times their sex life had been much better, certainly before they were married and before they had children. He begins to wonder whether all the women he has been attracted to have had this same flighty quality. This includes a young woman in his office with whom he has been carrying on a flirtation. He had been having intense fantasies that his wife would get so fed up with him that she would leave, allowing him to be free to marry the young woman. He remarks that his feelings cooled markedly toward her when she became engaged two months ago and he realized he still cared for his wife. He speculates on why his relationship with his wife has become so difficult when he obviously cares for her and realizes that she is concerned about his welfare. In so doing, he demonstrates a capacity for active fantasy life and an ability to reflect on his own thoughts. There could be some new stresses in relation to children, siblings, or parents. An earlier life situation may have been reactivated. The patient talks about the burden of four children and the decreased time available just for him and his wife. He shifts to his past and talks about the family problems when his father deserted, of his mother's helplessness, and his need to step in and be the man of the house. Life became a struggle, and his mother expected him to comfort her. The interviewer suggests that perhaps he had been feeling as though all the problems he had at 12 were going to be repeated again–an anniversary effect contributing to the depression. The patient elaborated on the hard times the family went through and how it had been his task to reassure his mother that they would make ends meet. He contributed financially to the family by working after school and during the summers. During this time, the patient did well in school and, by virtue of scholarship and loans, was able to work his way through college.

Perhaps more important for the psychodynamic psychotherapist than the discovery of the facts would be any evidence that a collaborative search for the facts would be possible. If the signs are positive for a collaborative relationship between the psychotherapist and the patient, further exploration along these lines is indicated. Generally speaking, psychopharmacology and/or hospitalization can be safely deferred, as can an evaluation of the value of marital or behavior therapy, while a psychotherapeutic test of treatability is conducted, if positive signs of a collaborative relationship with the psychotherapist are present. It is frequently found that many such acute depressive episodes are amenable to even brief psychodynamic psychotherapy. There are, of course, the usual caveats. Amenability to a purely psychodynamic psychotherapeutic intervention may vary with cultural background, language facility, social class, and psychological mindedness. When the criteria for a successful psychotherapeutic intervention are absent, the other modalities may indeed be indicated and even life-saving. In an earlier section it was noted that psychodynamic psychotherapy may be considered under the five rubrics of:

1) *symptom-relief psychotherapy*
2) *supportive psychotherapy*
3) *focal psychotherapy*
4) *long-term exploratory psychotherapy*
5) *psychoanalysis*

It was also noted that while there was considerable heuristic benefit in the delineations; in fact, there is considerable overlapping of the described modalities in actual practice. This will become more apparent as the encounter of our depressed compulsive patient with a psychodynamic psychotherapist is explored.

In regard to the specific forms of psychodynamic psychotherapy, it might well be found that the evaluation interviews in themselves result in considerable relief without any great insight being acquired on the part of either the psychotherapist or the patient. It may well be the case that a simple cathartic experience for the patient with a nonjudgmental psychotherapist may be sufficient for amelioration of the florid symptomatology, i.e., *symptom-relief psychotherapy*. Experience would indicate that this is a not uncommon result of a sympathetic exploration on the part of the psychodynamic psychotherapist. The result may be due to a corrective emotional experience, a positive conditioning, or magical fantasies of the psychotherapist's power and caring. It may be, in fact, that the patient experiences a form of absolution for perceived shortcomings or derelictions, particularly the suppressed rage that usually subtends depressive episodes.

> *During his college years, he had had a brief depression for which he sought psychotherapy from a school counselor. The counseling helped*

with reality issues, and the patient improved enough to be sufficiently relieved of his depression to complete his schooling. In retrospect, he feels he did not get to the root of his problems, although he became aware he was uncomfortable being the only member of his family to go to college. The patient also realized that he seemed to have trouble with girlfriends until he met his future wife with whom he immediately felt stronger and more in command. Ruefully, he comments that this time he wants to get better control of his problems so that he can function more comfortably and not be subject to the fits of depression he has been experiencing.

As suggested above, the evaluation interviews may serve as *supportive psychotherapy*. The psychodynamic psychotherapist can uncover stressful areas of conflict for the patient and counsel alternative courses of action, help in problem solving, and offer instruction and advice. He or she may offer useful insight into the psychology and motivations of others in the patient's environment with whom the patient is engaged in maladaptive struggles. In so doing, the patient's curiosity may be engaged, and he may come to feel more influential and potent in his dealings with spouse, children, or others. This effect, without necessarily involving any deep insight, can be supportive and far-reaching.

The interviewer feels that he can make a preliminary psychodynamic formulation. The patient is struggling with unconscious conflicts over competition and success. He has been able to perform successfully because of his intelligence and perfectionism, but as he approached a point in his life that reverberated with his own past history at age 12, old burdens and conflicts were reawakened that reflected intrapsychic conflicts and arrested development from the time of his father's desertion. These reawakened struggles coincided with the current conflict over merging his business. Although this meant a great financial gain for him, it also meant giving up being top man in his own business. The patient's previous psychotherapy was helpful, but since his symptoms had recurred, symptom-relief psychotherapy was not deemed to be the treatment of choice.

It may be that even in the evaluation interviews, psychotherapist and patient can define a focal area of conflict that has contributed to the patient's depressive symptoms. If the patient is sufficiently motivated, psychologically involved, and able to endure the transferential distortions, a great deal can be accomplished. It is sometimes possible, even within a time-limited psychotherapy program as in *focal psychotherapy*, to achieve remarkable results which, in some instances, may lead to structural changes. The growth process may well continue after formal psychotherapy is concluded.

Any of the aforementioned possible outcomes of the initial stages of patient-psychotherapist contact may lead to *long-term exploratory psychotherapy*. Even if the patient becomes stabilized and his acute conflict and the attendent defensive symptomatology relieved, the patient is left with a formidable obstacle to adaptive coexistence with himself and others: a compulsive personality. Often enough, when such patients recover from the frightening experience of a major depressive disorder, they are sufficiently motivated to continue in treatment in order to explore the basis of their difficulties in living. This wish may well be buttressed by the developing psychotherapeutic relationship with the psychodynamic psychotherapist who has helped lead the patient out of the worst of his or her acute, serious emotional difficulties. With such an induction into psychotherapy for the exploration of the rigid character structure found in the compulsive personality states, long-term exploratory psychotherapy, with its greater flexibility than psychoanalysis proper (as defined in this section) is often the most appropriate of the long-term psychotherapies aimed at character reorganization and the correction of deficient or deviant structures. Attention will be paid to the transference distortions occurring in the treatment situation because of their great importance in understanding the ongoing transactions with the psychotherapist and other significant individuals in the environment, as well as for the light that an understanding of the transference phenomena may throw on the genetic antecedents of the patient's difficulties. The psychodynamic psychotherapist will be aware of the facilitating effects of the positive transference, even if he or she chooses to interpret it during at least part of the course of long-term exploratory psychotherapy.

There is, also, the possibility of psychoanalysis. The psychoanalyst will wish, if it is at all possible, to psychoanalyze the transference finally and completely, understanding that this is the final pathway to an ending of the patient's dependence on the psychoanalyst and to the emergence of true autonomy not only in relation to the psychoanalyst, but also in relation to others in the patient's environment. Although this treatment outcome for a compulsive character disorder is often difficult to attain, it is held as a goal if psychoanalysis has been considered an appropriate form of treatment, according to the indications and criteria described earlier in this chapter.

Conclusion

Psychoanalysis and psychodynamic approaches in psychiatry contribute to the treatment planning process in three important ways. First, they provide the basis for a method of generating and collecting data—the psychodynamic interview. This is an interactive process between the patient and the psychiatrist that provides access not only to the facts that the psychiatrist is able to elicit, but also to the implicit, often unconscious, patterns that shape the patient's inner experience and outer behavior. The psychodynamic interview can be thought of as an experiment, with the interviewer actively intervening and testing hypotheses, creating possibilities, and observing how the patient (and the interviewer himself or herself) responds to them. This is in contrast to less psychodynamic approaches in psychiatric data gathering, in which the information is presumed to exist in the patient, with the interviewer's task being to collect and organize it, being careful not to overlook any area of possible importance, but not utilizing the interview situation itself as the setting in which new data can be created.

Second, psychodynamic approaches point to important areas of data—the patient's subjective world, inner representations of self and others, patterns of human relationships, characteristic modes of defense and coping, and early life experience and the persistence of that experience in the patient's contemporary adaptation. These data are all central to a psychodynamic assessment, although they have only varying relevance to a descriptive psychopathologic diagnosis. They are vital both in prescribing psychiatric treatments and in predicting treatment responses. This is particularly true for treatments that involve psychodynamically informed interventions, but also holds in broader terms for any treatment that requires even the patient's minimum participation in a relationship with the therapist.

Finally, psychoanalysis and psychodynamic understanding have led to the development of a wide array of therapeutic methods, including some of the most widely accepted treatments in contemporary psychiatry. These treatment approaches cannot be prescribed rationally without a psychodynamic assessment and evaluation process, in addition to a descriptive psychopathologic diagnosis. The two types of data and the two types of assessment are fully compatible; in fact, they tend to strengthen and enrich each other. Together they provide the basis of a scientific psychiatric treatment approach.

References

1. Offenkrantz, W., and Tobin, A.: Psychoanalytic Psychotherapy, *Archives of General Psychiatry*, May, 1974, p. 593.
2. Goldman, G.: Reparative Psychotherapy, in S. Rado, and G. Daniels (eds.): *Changing Concepts of Psychoanalytic Medicine*, New York: Grune & Stratton, 1956, pp. 101-113.
3. Horwitz, M: *Stress Response Syndromes*, New York: Jason Aronson, 1976, p. 6.
4. Mann, J.: *Time Limited Psychotherapy*, Cambridge, Mass.: Harvard University Press, 1973.
5. Sifneos, P.: *Short-Term Psychotherapy and Emotional Crisis*, Cambridge, Mass.: Harvard University Press, 1972.
6. Sifneos, P.: *Dynamic Psychotherapy: Evaluation and Technique*, New York: Plenum, 1979.
7. *Psychotherapy and Its Financial Feasibility Within the National Health Care System* (GAP Committee on Therapy), New York: GAP Publications, Report 100, Vol. X., February, 1978, p. 18.
8. Rado, S.: Adaptational Development of Psychoanalytic Therapy, in S. Rado, and G. Daniels (eds.), *Changing Concepts of Psychoanalytic Medicine*, New York: Grune & Stratton, 1956.
9. Psychoanalytic Peer Review, in *Manual of Psychiatric Peer Review*, Second Edition, Washington, D.C.: American Psychiatric Association, 1980.
10. Pulver, S. (Reporter) Panel on, "Survey of Psychoanalytic Practice in 1976. Some Trends and Implications," *Journal of the American Psychoanalytic Association*, Vol. 26(3), p. 621.

Bibliography

Alexander, F.: Principles and Techniques of Briefer Psychotherapeutic Procedures, *Proceedings of the Association for the Research of Nervous & Mental Diseases*, 31:16, 1951.

Balint, M., et al: *Focal Psychotherapy: An Example of Applied Psychoanalysis*, London: Tavistock Publications, 1972.

Bellak, L., and Small, L.: *Emergency Psychotherapy and Brief Psychotherapy*, 2nd Edition, New York: Grune & Stratton, 1978.

Bibring, E.: Psychoanalysis and the Dynamic Psychotherapies, *Journal of the American Psychoanalytic Association*, 2:745-770, 1954.

Brenner, C.: *Psychoanalytic Technique and Psychic Conflict*, New York: International Universities Press, 1976.

Davanloo, H.: *Basic Principles and Technique of Short-Term Dynamic Psychotherapy*, New York: Spectrum Publications, 1978.

Dewald, P.: *Psychotherapy: A Dynamic Approach*, Ed. 2, New York: Basic Books, 1970.

Dewald, P. A.: *The Psychoanalytic Process*, New York: Basic Books, 1972.

English, O. S.: The Essentials of Psychotherapy as Viewed by the Psychoanalyst, *Journal of the American Psychoanalytic Association*, 1:550-561, 1953.

Fenichel, O.: Brief Psychotherapy, in H. Fenichel, and D. Rappaport (eds.), *The Collected Papers of Otto Fenichel*, New York: Norton, 1954.

Freud, S.: Introductory Lectures on Psychoanalysis, Parts I and II (1915-1917), *The Complete Psychological Works*, Standard Edition, Vol. 15. Translated and edited by Strachey, J., London: Hogarth Press, 1963.

Freud, S.: An Outline of Psychoanalysis, *Standard Edition*, 23:139-205, 1938, London: Hogarth Press, 1964.

Fromm-Reichmann, F.: *Principles of Intensive Psychotherapy*, Chicago: University of Chicago Press, 1950.

Gaskill, H. S.: The Closing Phase of the Psychoanalytic Treatment of Adults and the Goals of Psychoanalysis "The Myth of Perfectibility," *International Journal of Psycho-Analysis*, 61:11-23, 1980.

Greenspan, S. I., and Cullander, C. C.: A Systematic Metapsychological Assessment of the Course of an Analysis, *Journal of the American Psychoanalytic Association*, 23:107-138, 1975.

Group for the Advancement of Psychiatry: *Psychotherapy and the Dual Research Tradition*, 1969, Vol. 7(73).

Horney, K.: *New Ways in Psychoanalysis*, New York: W. W. Norton, 1939.

Karasu, T. B.: Psychotherapies: An Overview, *American Journal of Psychiatry*, 134:8, 851-863, 1977.

Knight, R. P.: An Evaluation of Psychotherapeutic Techniques, *Bulletin of the Menninger Clinic*, 16:113-124, 1952.

Kohut, H.: *The Analysis of the Self*, New York: International Universities Press, 1971.

Kohut, H., and Seitz, P. F. D.: Concepts and Theories of Psychoanalysis, in J. M. Wepman, and R. W. Heine (eds.), *Concepts of Personality*, Chicago: Aldine Publishing Co., 1963.

Langs, R. J.: *The Technique of Psychoanalytic Psychotherapy, Vol. 1 & 2*, New York: Aronson, 1973, 1974.

Malan, D. H.: *A Study of Brief Psychotherapy*, New York: Plenum Press, 1975.

Malan, D. H.: *The Frontier of Brief Psychotherapy*, New York: Plenum Publishing Corp., 1976.

Mann, J.: *Time-Limited Psychotherapy*, Cambridge, Mass.: Harvard University Press, 1973.

Marmor, J.: New Directions in Psychoanalytic Theory and Therapy, in *Modern Psychoanalysis: New Directions and Perspectives*, New York: Basic Books, Inc., 1968.

Mendel, W.: *Supportive Care: Theory & Technique*, Santa Monica, CA.: Mara Books, Inc. 1975.

Menninger, K.: *Theory of Psychoanalytic Technique*, New York: Basic Books, Inc., 1958.

Munroe, R. L.: *Schools of Psychoanalytic Thought*, New York: Dryden, 1955.

Offenkrantz, W., and Tobin, A.: Psychoanalytic Psychotherapy, *Archives of General Psychiatry*, 30:593-606, 1974.

Paolino, Jr., T. J.: *Psychoanalytic Psychotherapy: Theory, Technique, Therapeutic Relationship and Treatability*, New York: Brunner/Mazel, 1981.

Rado, S.: *Psychoanalysis of Behavior, Selected Papers of Sandor Rado, Vol. II*, New York: Grune & Stratton, 1962.

Rangell, L.: Psychoanalysis—A Current Look, *Journal of the American Psychoanalytic Association*, 15:2, April, 1967.

Sifneos, P. E.: Short-term, Anxiety-provoking Psychotherapy: An Emotional Problem-solving Technique, *Seminars in Psychiatry*, 1:389-398, 1969.

Sifneos, P. E.: *Short-Term Psychotherapy and Emotional Crisis*, Cambridge, Mass: Harvard University Press, 1972.

Sifneos, P. E.: *Short-Term Dynamic Psychotherapy Evaluation and Technique*, New York: Plenum Publishing Corp., 1979.

Small, L.: *The Briefer Psychotherapies, Revised Edition*, New York: Brunner/Mazel, 1979.

Strupp, H.: Psychoanalytic Psychotherapy and Research, in L. Eron, and R. Callahan (eds.), *The Relation of Theory to Practice in Psychotherapy*, Chicago: Aldine Publishing Co., 1969, pp. 21-62.

Strupp, H.: Psychoanalysis, "Focal Psychotherapy" and the Nature of the Therapeutic Influence, *Archives of General Psychiatry*, 32:127-135, 1975.

Sullivan, H. S.: *Conceptions of Modern Psychiatry*, Washington, D.C.: William Alanson White Psychiatric Foundation, 1947.

Waelder, R.: *Basic Theory of Psychoanalysis*, New York: International Universities Press, 1960.

Wallerstein, R. S.: *Psychotherapy and Psychoanalysis: Theory, Practice, Research*, New York: International Universities Press, 1975.

Wallerstein, R. S.: Psychoanalysis and Psychotherapy (The Relationships of Psychoanalysis to Psychotherapy: Current Issues), *International Journal of Psychoanalysis*, 50:117-126, 1969.

Wolbert, L. R.: *Short-Term Psychotherapy*, New York: Grune & Stratton, 1965.

Chapter Two

The Group Therapies

Aaron Stein, M.D.
Howard D. Kibel, M.D.
Jay W. Fidler, M.D.
Henry I. Spitz, M.D.

The authors wish to thank the following for their assistance in the preparation of this chapter:

Priscilla F. Kauff, Ph.D., Jerome W. Kosseff, Ph.D., Max Rosenbaum, Ph.D., Clifford J. Sager, M.D., Shirley Schechter, M.S.W., Saul Scheidlinger, M.S.W., Ph.D., and Isaac Z. Youcha, M.S.W.

This chapter was prepared in cooperation with and under the auspices of the American Group Psychotherapy Association, Inc.

Theoretical Premises

The interpersonal and social field within which one lives is generally acknowledged as a factor conducive to producing psychopathology in some individuals. The professionally devised and organized social field represented by the therapeutic group may be used as an instrument to reduce symptomatology and to modify personality functioning. Groups have been used for centuries in medical, religious, and secular attempts to support the distressed, exorcise the possessed, and, more recently, to cure the mentally ill. While these group procedures had certain features in common, their differences were easily discerned. These differences arose from the variety of mechanisms believed to have been the cause of the "sickness" and the ways in which the group was used to deal with it. The work of social psychologists in defining the dynamics of human groups, and of the clinical theoreticians in explaining the effect of groups upon individual dynamics, has given specific form to these differences, with the result that several distinctive group approaches have emerged in the last 50 years. All of the mechanisms by which one individual communicates with another to bring about changes in internal psychological dynamics can be utilized in the group setting. Variations are frequently created by choosing different aspects of group dynamics and different levels of attention to the group as a whole or to the individuals in it; these variations are major tools for bringing about the desired change.

The development of a group by a professional therapist necessarily creates a special and unique social context. Clinicians who use groups become increasingly aware of the broader institutional, social, and cultural contexts as factors that establish expectations in both the patient and the therapist. An awareness that the therapist, as well as the patient, is immersed in a complex of social assumptions makes somewhat more comprehensible attitudes that exist toward the use of groups. In the days when physicians did most of their work in the homes of sick patients, it was unlikely that either patients or physicians would have been comfortable in a group setting. When the advantages of the hospital brought physicians into contact with several patients, and the physicians' offices brought patients to physicians, it became more likely that group phenomena would impinge on the awareness of both. Thus, early in this century, Dr. Joseph Pratt, who treated tubercular patients, discovered that those who got to know each other's concerns had the best clinical course.[1] He then began deliberatively to use groups to capitalize on this phenomenon.

Americans who value individuality and privacy presumably have expectations of the group that are different from those of the Soviets or, especially, the Chinese, who value the collective. Nevertheless, the awareness that man is a social creature encourages use of the social context for treatment. Some language historians, for instance, contend that words describing relationships between persons were invented before words describing individuals. Common sense tells us that the action of certain individuals upon the developing child produces many of the major personality features observed later. Indeed, one can see social facts as antecedents to psychic facts. Therefore, the group can be a tool of psychic change.

The therapist who looks to the group for assistance draws certain assumptions from these sociocultural perspectives, but the therapist is also influenced by his or her theoretical understanding of the nature of psychopathology. Psychodramatists consider that attention is most profitably applied to the social role rather than to the isolated individual. Recent developments in psychoanalytic theory emphasize object relations, i.e., the relationship patterns of internal objects compared to psychobiologic drives. Interpersonal theories emphasize therapist/patient interaction compared to the "objective" stance of a descriptive clinician. Regardless of theoretical orientation, the group psychotherapist is likely to define the goal of treatment as attainment of a hypothetical normal state, including both individuation and a syntonic immersion in society. The group is advantageous in working toward these interlocking goals.

SPECIFIC GROUP PHENOMENA

Many processes that are at the core of individual psychotherapy and psychoanalysis can be utilized in the group setting. In some instances, group therapy can be used equally as well as individual psychotherapy. The focus here, however, is on those features of the group that contribute additional mechanisms for impact and change.

Patients in a group almost uniformly become conscious of parallel events or themes in each other's lives. The realization that one's problems are not unique, that others have similar difficulties, a process called *universalization*, is emotionally liberating. Abreaction by one member is in effect shared by all and enriched by comparison as other members tell their versions of related material. Therefore, stimulation of group members by one another enhances ventilation compared to other forms of treatment.

The benefits of treatment do not derive simply from revealing one's problems. An individual who verbalizes only to a small extent gains much as a *spectator* by listening to and observing others, imitating them, and observing his or her own affective and behavioral responses. Helping others is beneficial; *altruistic acts* enhance self-esteem and may help vicariously. Merely belonging to a well-functioning group is therapeutic. The feelings of acceptance that derive from *group cohesion* help to establish a haven in which not only personal secrets can be revealed, but in which risks can be taken and where one can experiment with new modes of relatedness. A combination of active and passive involvement, and the interpersonal learning that allows for development of socializing techniques, are readily available in the group.

The social nature of the group permits *reality testing* in this relatively safe and unthreatening atmosphere. Through their mutual and usually successful efforts to help each other, group members *instill hope* in one another.

Projective identification as a mental mechanism allows patients to use the struggles of other members for their own benefit with reduced emotional distress and less interference from resistance. An individual uses peers in the group as psychological *mirrors* to examine his or her own personality. Through verbal feedback, members display their reflected appraisals of each other. An individual may have had reason to doubt the objectivity of parental judgments or employers' evaluations. Yet, when several peers, i.e., group members, who are also potentially as vulnerable as that individual express a judgment, it is often taken more seriously. The therapist uses these phenomena to break through the resistance of a given patient by highlighting these relevant issues in other group members.

Through feedback, individuals learn about themselves in a meaningful way; affective experience combines with intellectual understanding of the experience to produce insight and, hence, change. Groups are most useful for *interpersonal learning* through *group interactions*, including all of the emotional reactions of the members to any group event and all of the verbal and nonverbal interchanges among members. Thus, the *group process*, i.e., the sum total of all of these interactions, provides a fertile ground for treatment.

Knowledge of individual dynamics is clearly relevant to the transference phenomena that become manifest in the group. While observing the transference, the leader should watch for each person's unique responses to other individuals evoked by their physical characteristics or behavioral styles. Thus, a rich field of *multitransference* variations is available for observation and working through. Whereas some group members may represent parent figures for one member, to others they represent siblings. These interpersonal engagements recreate past interpersonal relationships to some degree, and each is part of a total *matrix of transpersonal processes* often characterized as *group transference.*[2] The group matrix creates a therapeutic field that allows for a *corrective recapitulation* of the experience of the family of origin.

An intricate network of communications creates a shared psychic life that takes on a character independent of each individual and more nearly approximates the impact of family, school class, adolescent "gang," or work group. This intimate connection of one member to all others affords a unique demonstration of patient behavior not readily available in other settings. One such feature is the ability to study in action the ways in which a given patient's mode of behavior manipulates others into behavior similar to that of the historical object. How a patient educes the behavior to which he or she then reacts adversely is seen as the pattern evolves. The beneficial effect of the discovery and understanding of the underlying psychodynamic factors is more likely to occur if such transference reactions are experienced in the presence of the group.

GROUP DYNAMICS

Many practitioners and theorists have observed that group events evolve from something more than the group process; they do not merely reflect the sum total of the interactions of group members. Additionally, the group leader must consider what has been labeled *group dynamics*, namely, the structure that emerges from individuals in constant interaction with one another, wherein these individuals are interdependent parts of a larger whole that is *different* from the sum of its parts.[3]

Discussion of group dynamics is beyond the scope of this chapter, yet suffice it to note that such dynamics help the practitioner of group therapy to go beyond the usual paradigms of dyadic treatment to explore personality in a unique way. Groups highlight conflicts around dependency, aggression, competition, and intimacy in ways no other treatment modality can. Members serve as spokesmen for one another, fill group roles, struggle for power, seek deviancy or conformity, scapegoat one another, identify with a subgroup, and so on, thereby revealing latent aspects of personality that would remain undiscovered through other treatment modalities. These dynamic aspects of groups can be used to advantage in treatment. For example, consider the strong impact of group forces that occurs in the reciprocal relationship between the group and the individual. As a set of expectations emerges in the group, it is useful to analyze the dynamic relationship of group functioning to induced individual behavior. The degree to which an individual responds to group norms as compared to stubborn resistance or open rebellion frequently correlates with the conflict situations underlying the symptoms. In groups, the positive side of conformity becomes of greatest importance when the individual has been unsuccessful at integration into family and other social alliances. The therapist will find the group a most revealing setting in which to demonstrate the dynamics of this process and to facilitate the experiential learning of corrective measures. On the negative side, conformity can obscure an individual's motivational patterns, thereby becoming a resistance to the psychotherapeutic process; this, too, must be analyzed.

As one individual responds to another, and finally each responds to all others, there is also amplification of an emotion or content in which a resonance occurs. When this serves as a reinforcement of resistance to individual self-disclosure, it takes on some aspects of mob psychology and requires redirection by the therapist. But more often, these resonating themes will bring out latent shared concerns as individual associations relate to those concerns and open the way for more associations of a similar kind in other group members. The group therapist should operate on the premise that the associative process is always at work, whether overt statements appear to be of a random or a unified nature. It is generally safe to assume that some aspect of a shared here-and-now situation will become apparent in the flow of conversation. Each member reacts in characteristic fashion to the collective theme of the moment. Some will participate actively and aggressively, some will be group spokesmen, some will be opponents to the underlying discussion, and some will attack and others will defend fellow members. Some will attack and others will defend the therapist. The value of this characteristic participation of each member in the here-and-now of the group discussion is that it brings out each member's underlying conflicts in object relationships without having to go into the individual history of each member.

DYNAMICS OF A THERAPY GROUP

The presence of the therapist is essential to the formation of the group because he or she is the focus of the interacting forces in the treatment.[4] The therapist is the focal figure for establishment of the group, for mutual identifications among the members, and for the multiple transference reactions that occur. This is true even in so-called leaderless groups and those that use alternate sessions, when the group meets without the therapist or no specific leader is designated; actually, whether or not present, there is always a central figure in the group.

Because of the presence of a number of persons in the group, the intensity of the transference to the therapist is lessened; it is deflected onto other group members. Nevertheless, leader transference continues to be a major factor in group interactions, as its deflection to other members of the group causes patients to interact therapeutically with one another.

Emotional ties in the group consist largely of a number of identifications. Most importantly, group members share the therapist. The patients see the leader as an idealized figure. Identification with the leader enables them to imitate him or her in their therapeutic efforts with one another. Additionally, the mutual identifications of the patients with each other permit the group to coalesce. Members share feelings, recognize similarities in each other, and reach out to one another for support and gratification. Coalescence of a group takes time, as members must divert their attention away from the leader as the sole source of help and learn how to work therapeutically together. In other words, over time, the group develops.

The way in which this happens is not random. Students of group dynamics and group process report consistently a specific series of phases of group development.[5] These key phases, which develop in accord with the issues found most useful for the individual therapist, vary from three to nine. The initial task of orientation of all members is considered by some to be one such phase, but others view this as a pregroup requirement. Once orientation is achieved, the group is confronted with the problem of learning to trust the leader.

During this early phase, each member tries to establish a special relationship with the group leader in order to satisfy dependency needs. Patients with severe psychopathology may even seek some type of symbiotic fusion with the leader. In these severely ill patients, group development does not go past this initial phase and, accordingly, affects the process of therapy. In groups of less severely ill patients, as the frustration of dependency needs increases, a rebellious anger toward the therapist emerges, the patients then turn away from the therapist and toward each other. In doing so, pathologic character traits, defenses, and attitudes become very quickly apparent.

The major therapeutic work occurs during this second phase of member interaction. Individuals enter into therapeutic relationships both with the therapist and with each other. They can now examine the pathologic aspect of these relationships and develop healthier ones. These interactions encompass this major phase of group development. Now transference manifestations, which are seen more clearly and rapidly in group therapy than in individual therapy, become available for therapeutic consideration. Resistances may be bypassed and certain defenses overcome because of the opportunity to observe certain characteristic attitudes, reactions, and interactions as they actually occur.

Whereas dependency dominated the earlier phase of group development, intimacy and closeness characterize this major phase. Finally, relative independence from the leader, and pursuit of independence and separation from the group, complete the phases. Along this developmental path, themes occur in sequence, focusing attention on specific intrapersonal conflicts residing in group members as they relate to those tasks of development.

GROUP PSYCHOTHERAPY

This more formalized and specialized type of group therapy uses to therapeutic advantage the phenomena and dynamics described above. Patients must be carefully evaluated and selected for this modality. Both patient and therapist should mutually agree to certain conditions (treatment contract) under which treatment will be conducted.

The group is designed for the treatment of psychopathology, and members acknowledge that they are ill and commit themselves to the group for treatment. The therapist undertakes to treat the patients, assuming responsibility for recommending or prescribing treatment and for seeing that it is carried out as effectively and safely as possible. This acknowledgment by both the members and the leader that the therapeutic group is set up for the sake of treatment is characteristic of a clinical model. In order for the group leader to be effective, he or she must undergo thorough training in group therapy beyond the usual requirements to be a mental health professional.[6]

Given these considerations, the term *group psychotherapy* should apply only to a treatment modality wherein a specially trained professional practitioner utilizes the interaction of a small, carefully planned group to effect amelioration of personality malfunctioning in individuals specifically selected for this purpose. A clinical orientation, which includes a diagnostic assessment of each group member's problems, is part of this picture. A continuing responsibility for care is assumed. Furthermore, each patient is cognizant of the treatment purpose and accepts the group as a means of obtaining help in modifying certain pathologic modes of functioning.

Classification of Groups

Prior to discussion of the application of group techniques, it is necessary to outline a few general principles concerning the parameters of group therapy. All effective groups share a minimum of three elements:

1) sound group composition and organization
2) careful attention to pre-group screening, diagnostic assessment, patient selection and preparation prior to group entry
3) active and responsible group leadership based on a firm grounding in group theory and dynamics

When these elements are managed effectively, the central ingredients for a positive group experience are enhanced and the risk of detrimental consequences is reduced.

As a way of thinking about the key dimensions of a group and to aid in appropriate member placement, it is helpful to have in mind a group classification scheme. Several such approaches have been advanced in the group therapy literature, two of which are summarized here.

MODEL A

This model classifies groups according to their properties, taking into account some of the elements noted above. Because of the heterogeneous nature of group properties, this model cannot neatly categorize the variety of treatment groups in use. Specific types of groups derive their character by drawing upon one or more properties to a greater or lesser extent. The clinician should be familiar with the properties used to characterize groups so that the group therapist's frame of reference can be understood and an informed referral made. In this model, four factors are taken into account:

1) The *theoretical orientation* of the group leader and style of group leadership significantly determine the nature of treatment. Examples include psychoanalytic, Gestalt, transactional, eclectic, group-as-a-whole, behavioral, existential, encounter, and sensitivity group models.
2) The process of treatment is very much affected by the *group*

composition, with particular regard to homogeneity and heterogeneity. Most groups have a heterogeneous population with respect to factors such as age, sex, socioeconomic status, race, religious background, and vocation. Many groups, however, are composed of members who share one trait from which the group derives its descriptive label, e.g., adolescent group, male homosexual group, heroin addiction group, alcoholic group, or married couples group. In general, heterogenous factors favor and facilitate group interaction, whereas homogeneous factors influence cohesion and dependency issues. The therapeutic implication of group composition will be discussed later in greater detail. Suffice it to note at this point, however, that groups which are not organized around one overriding trait both retain enough homogeneity to promote intermember trust, credibility, and identification, and possess sufficient dissimilarities in membership to create interpersonal tensions as the building blocks for group interaction.

3) The *time factor* suggests information relative to the goals of a given group. In this system, time has a dual meaning, referring both to total duration of the ongoing group experience and to length of each session. Many groups utilize a brief psychotherapy format employing realistically attainable goals within a fixed time span. Often these groups are task-oriented in nature, remaining in existence until the task is accomplished successfully. Ongoing or open-ended groups usually have more ambitious goals and begin to approximate those of psychoanalytically-oriented individual psychotherapy.

4) Group size, and whether or not *group membership* is fixed or open, are other areas of critical concern. Broadly speaking, fixed membership, shorter-term groups are geared to symptom removal and socialization goals, whereas open membership, longer-term groups aim for attainment of insight, increased self-awareness, and change in maladaptive behavioral patterns. Groups may vary in number from about five to fifteen members, and both types are suitable for management of patients taking psychotropic medications.

Selection of members and careful composition are essential ingredients in constructing groups that will realize their full therapeutic potential. In addition to the use of individual and interpersonal assessment for suitability of the group modality, one must evaluate the properties of a given group per se, to determine whether a prospective candidate will derive benefit from it and to help in matching members to specific groups.

MODEL B

An alternative method is to classify groups broadly according to their functions. Those that serve clinical needs but whose methods are not like those of traditional psychotherapy can be discussed as *group therapeutic methods.*[7] Those that both use psychotherapeutic techniques and aim to modify directly psychopathology can be discussed under *group psychotherapy proper.* In addition, there are groups that are found outside the province of treatment; these will be discussed as *non-clinical groups.*

GROUP THERAPEUTIC METHODS

Group therapeutic methods include activity groups and therapeutic participation groups. Activity groups are set up so that members can engage in a common activity, which itself is a therapeutic agent. While group discussion may be involved, the goal is to engage members in a common activity. Therapeutic participation groups are arranged to facilitate participation of the members in the work of the treatment setting (e.g., inpatient groups), or to provide a format for application of a specific method in a group. Participation is encouraged in order to activate the patient and facilitate socialization through interaction with others in the group. Many of these methods apply one particular theoretical orientation (e.g., transactional analysis, behavioral psychology) to a group format in order to treat the psychopathology of the members.

GROUP PSYCHOTHERAPY PROPER

Group psychotherapy uses small groups designed for the investigation and treatment of each member's psychopathology. Essential conditions of this group include the following:

1) the treatment relies solely on verbal communication

2) the individual member is the object of the treatment even though "group-as-a-whole" reactions may be discussed
3) the group interaction is the main therapeutic vehicle

As noted, the group is used to develop the relationships, through members' interactions, which are necessary to further spontaneous free-flowing discussions.

Varying degrees of intensity or uncovering are utilized in three different types of group psychotherapy, depending upon the extent to which resistance and transference are interpreted.[8] The most intensive type is psychoanalytically-oriented or exploratory group psychotherapy. In this type, conditions are set up so that the group interactions and the free-flowing group discussion help to uncover underlying unconscious conflicts and resistances; these are then interpreted. The interpretation, however, is not as thorough as in individual psychoanalysis. Some workers prefer to call this type of group psychotherapy "group psychoanalysis" or "psychoanalysis in groups" in the belief that infantile conflicts are focused on the therapist and can indeed be analyzed through transferences within the group. Most workers believe, though, that the transference that exists in group psychotherapy is different from and less intense than that which exists in psychoanalysis or intensive individual psychotherapy. Hence, they prefer to call this type of group treatment psychoanalytically-oriented or exploratory group psychotherapy.

The second type of group psychotherapy is termed modified or supportive. With this type, fewer efforts are made to uncover underlying unconscious psychopathology, and support is provided by leaving areas related to intragroup transferences uninterpreted.

Group counseling and group guidance represent the third type of group psychotherapy. Group counseling aims to help group members with solution of immediate, realistic problems. This is usually short-term; the group counselor, a trained mental health professional, is generally quite active. *Group guidance* is longer-term treatment in which the attitudes and feelings involved in the members' problems are exposed for consideration and evaluation, even though the underlying unconscious and preconscious motivations remain largely uninterpreted. Perhaps most group psychotherapy, as practiced today, is some form of group counseling or group guidance.

NONCLINICAL GROUPS

Nonclinical groups include the following:

1) problem-solving
2) experiential or encounter
3) sensitivity or laboratory groups

Although advocates of each type make widely different assumptions about human nature, they share the basic belief that experiences in groups are important aspects of learning and self-development.

To deal with reality problems, various problem-solving groups can be set up. Many of these may resemble group counseling or group guidance in helping the participants to become attuned to conscious emotional reactions. They are not, however, set up as treatment for uncovering and investigating each individual member's psychopathology. Two types of problem-solving groups are worth special mention: those that deal with alcoholism and those that deal with drug addictions. Although these may be established under medical auspices, their focus is nonclinical in the sense that their goals relate to the reality nature of problems rather than the modification of underlying psychopathology.

Experiential or encounter groups deal with the quality of encounters between individuals in the here-and-now. Hence, they focus on each participant's immediate experience in the group. They seek to enhance the capacity to live, to feel, to experience, and to grow or mature. The basic assumption is that free expression, exposure, and interaction in the group enhances growth and expansion, i.e., human potential, in and of itself. Techniques in these groups may vary. Many leaders rely on confrontation and mobilization of group pressure to elicit specific responses from members. Some use a time-extended format, i.e., sessions which run continuously for 12 to 24 or more hours. Yet, they have certain features in common. All are short-term and all utilize techniques to manipulate and to exert pressure on group members to participate in the group interaction as intensely as possible.

In the past, in most of these groups there was no selection of members. Also, in many of them the leaders had little or no formal training and the leadership role was relatively undifferentiated from that of the members. The active emotional participation of the leader, combined with the above-mentioned techniques led to rapid, forced reduction of defenses and stirring up of intense emotional reactions. When these reactions are severe, they can be dangerous; however, in the skilled hands of a sensitive, trained, clinical professional, such groups have been used successfully as an adjunct to traditional therapy.[9] Recently, however, there has been increasing recognition of the dangers in these methods, so that nowadays most groups do require training of their leaders, as well as some screening and selection of the participants, and recognize that the leader should be responsible for seeking consultation and for supervision and follow-up of members for possible detrimental effects.

In contrast, sensitivity or laboratory training groups use trained leaders. They are usually short-term, intense experiences and do not use a time-extended format. The leaders use techniques sometimes borrowed from encounter groups, but generally they rely on traditional methods. The goal is to teach participants about group dynamics through examination of collective themes, relationships to authority in groups, and each member's role in shared responses. Some leaders believe that these groups, like encounter groups, can enhance human potential.

TYPES OF GROUP PSYCHOTHERAPY GROUPS

Psychoanalysis in groups is the group therapy counterpart of individual psychoanalysis. The goals are ambitious and involve efforts to achieve major personality reconstruction. The method utilizes free association and analysis of transference, resistance, and dreams. The analyst interprets unconscious conflicts extensively as these become apparent in the group process.

Exploratory group therapy or psychoanalytically-oriented group psychotherapy is an insight-oriented form of treatment that employs modified traditional psychoanalytic techniques in conjunction with analysis of the intragroup dynamics. Examination of each member's present life situation, as well as past history, is also encouraged. These groups aim at moderate personality reconstruction and generally meet less frequently than psychoanalytic in groups.

Existential group therapy focuses primarily on the here-and-now and endeavors to help members deal with shared issues of human existence, such as birth, death, ambiguity, despair, and other aspects of the human condition. This point of view values confrontation and the development of affective experiences in the group. Leaders and members participate in somewhat similar ways in an attempt to realize certain general goals, e.g., enhancement of communication, authenticity, and individual growth.

Group-centered analytic groups focus on interpersonal processes and actively interpret intragroup tensions. Taken in large measure from the work of Bion, this form of group therapy relies on the understanding of whole group processes as a vehicle for self-awareness.[10] Leaders try to decentralize their position, functioning both as participant observers and interpreters of collective group interaction.

Concurrent individual and group therapy is a psychotherapeutic model in which a patient is seen in both modalities of treatment at the same time. The two forms of therapy may be conducted by the same therapist (combined therapy), or by two different therapists (conjoint therapy).

TYPES OF THERAPEUTIC GROUP METHODS

Structured group experiences include a range of group formats that are primarily supportive, educational, and nonstressful in nature. Examples include medication, supportive network, theme-centered, discussion/education, therapeutic community, and activity groups; the last may involve either quiet activities (e.g., music, poetry therapy), or physical activity groups (e.g., dance therapy).

Crisis groups are generally short-term experiences that utilize peer support, reality testing, and strengthening of existing individual defenses as vehicles for resolving a current life crisis. After the crisis is resolved, members may be transferred to another group in which selection is based on the primary personality diagnosis, rather than on the crisis situation that brought them to treatment in the first place (e.g., a marital crisis group).

Psychodrama is a technique developed by Moreno in which interpersonal relationships, individual personality conflicts, and group dynamics are examined using theatrical methods.[11] Specific ingredients of the psychodramatic technique include a stage, a subject (patient), a director (therapist), therapeutic aides (auxiliary ego), and an audience. These elements are employed in conjunction with a psychodynamic viewpoint that tries to promote insight, self-awareness, and individual growth.

Transactional analysis (T.A.) groups apply theoretical constructs from transactional analysis to a group matrix.[12] The focus is exclusively on the here-and-now. Certain intragroup transactions are highlighted in order to elucidate four major areas:

1) intrapsychic phenomena
2) parent, child, and adult ego states
3) interpersonal game analysis
4) script analysis or the attempt to understand the motivational basis for a member's emotional problems

Gestalt therapy, developed by Perls, aims to treat the person holistically in a biologic, perceptual, and interpersonal framework.[13] In order to accomplish this, the group concerns itself with the sensory awareness of members in the here-and-now rather than in past experience. Gestalt groups commonly employ exercises, role-playing, and other techniques to promote individual growth and development of potential personal resources.

Behavior therapy groups have their theoretical basis in learning theory and attempt to treat psychopathology by the application of its principles in a group setting. In contrast to other methods, behavioral groups are largely symptom-focused and have as their aim the removal of specific maladaptive behavior, symptom reduction, or other more circumscribed goals. These are often short-term, homogeneous groups with active, directive leadership of an educational nature.

Special patient population groups derive their descriptive level from the specific nature of the group composition. All members carry the same diagnosis or present the same symptoms for which they seek therapy. These groups rely on intermember support and identification, role modeling, and universality of experience to facilitate open discussion and sharing of mutual problems. An example is a group for members with egodystonic homosexuality.[14]

TYPES OF NONCLINICAL GROUPS

Repressive/inspirational groups are designed mainly to elevate members' morale and to create a positive group climate. This takes place because strong identification is encouraged. The group format includes discussions, testimonials, or relaxation experiences aimed at providing support and encouragement. An example of this type of group is Alcoholics Anonymous.

Self-help groups, which are often leaderless, are composed of members who share common problems. The goal of the group is to help members to understand and to cope with their areas of overlapping concern. These groups are educational and supportive in nature. One example is a group of recently discharged psychiatric patients dealing with the impact of hospitalization and of re-entry into the community. Recovery, Inc. and Schizophrenics Anonymous are examples.

Confrontation groups use group pressure, real or potential, to change specific maladaptive behaviors that are egosyntonic to the members. Frequently these techniques are reserved for situations in which an individual's attitude and behavioral patterns are rigid and long standing. High levels of affect are reached within these groups. Examples are Synanon and Daytop.

Time-extended groups use extended duration of sessions in an effort to break down psychological defenses and to accelerate group interaction. These groups place a high value on self-disclosure and psychological intimacy; they are centered mainly in the here-and-now. Such groups must be used with caution and require careful attention to pregroup screening, including diagnosis and adequate preparation of prospective participants. An example is marathon groups.

T-group is a general rubric for sensitivity training or laboratory training groups that are set up to teach group dynamics to students, mental health personnel, educators, executives, and so on. They are devoted essentially to the learning of group dynamics through discussion and evaluation of the here-and-now of the group interaction. Examples are the Bethel groups of the National Training Laboratory and the Tavistock study groups that began in England but are now being used in the United States.

COMPARISON OF DIFFERENT TYPES OF GROUPS

The following table compares several major types of groups along several central parameters. Listed are some frequently used types; the table is not meant to compare all those described in this section of the chapter. Note that the term "supportive groups" encompasses a broad range of treatments that have been described above.

Criteria For Treatment Planning

THE SCOPE OF TREATMENT PLANNING

A therapeutic group should be considered in planning treatment for most patients. Groups have a wide range of applications to a total treatment program. In addition to group psychotherapy proper, groups having therapeutic value include activity, socialization, counseling, and couples groups, as well as groups for those with the same symptoms or with similar problems. For some patients, group psychotherapy is at the hub of their treatment; for others, it is adjunctive to another modality; for still others, it is a part of a multifaceted approach. A group may be employed at any of several points during the course of treatment. For example, some practitioners have used group psychotherapy as a prelude to individual psychotherapy, others have used it to wean a patient from an intense transference relationship, and some routinely have their individual patients concurrently participating in a group.

No one practitioner can be familiar with all of the varieties of therapeutic groups, much less those available in a specific geographic area. Some familiarity with the clinical criteria of suitability for a group, however, facilitates intelligent referral. Discussion of criteria can be divided into three parts: those sufficient for an ancillary group that is part of a multimodal approach, those sufficient for a specialized or homogeneous group, and those sufficient for referral to a heterogeneous psychodynamic group (group psychotherapy proper).

Unlike the previous section of this chapter, which classified groups largely according to their methodology, this section categorizes groups by considering their relationship to the overall goals of treatment. Certain group treatments serve a specific but limited function as part of a comprehensive treatment program.

Such ancillary groups require a low order of specificity for selection criteria. Specialized or homogeneous groups serve broader and more specific treatment goals. These groups require an intermediate level of specificity of selection criteria, or what will be referred to as general criteria for inclusion. However, should group psychotherapy proper be considered as an optimal treatment modality, a high degree of specificity for selection is needed. In this case, specific inclusion criteria must be evaluated.

ANCILLARY GROUPS

The first category of criteria applies to groups that are part of a comprehensive treatment program, such as are found in inpatient settings, day treatment programs, and a variety of residential treatment centers. Some groups (e.g., activity, recreational, and dance therapy groups) often require only nonverbal participation; others (e.g., resocialization, supportive, and counseling groups) require more verbal participation. These groups have a defined task, be it an activity, formulation of discharge plans, or discussion of common problems and experiences. The criteria necessary for participation include only those facets of functioning necessary for the task. Thus, participation in a nonverbal group requires only the presence of certain motor functions and the absence of grossly disruptive behavior. In contrast, verbal groups require verbal coherency, rudimentary relatedness, intellectual comprehension compatible with that of other group members, and the absence of menacing, disruptive, or dangerous behavior. For these groups, selection criteria are minimal and are not dependent upon diagnostic categories. Thus, for example, a particular group may be suitable for both psychotic as well as nonpsychotic patients; diagnostic heterogeneity is appropriate, whereas functional homogeneity is required.

GROUP COMPOSITION

Before proceeding to specifics of patient selection, a few words are necessary about the degree of diversity in group membership, i.e., homogeneous versus heterogeneous groups.

Homogeneity of groups may be defined by diagnostic or

TABLE 1
COMPARISON OF DIFFERENT TYPES OF GROUPS

	Supportive Groups	*Analytically-oriented Groups*	*Psychoanalysis Groups*	*Transactional Groups*	*Behavioral Groups*
Frequency Duration	1-3x/wk. Limited or open-ended	1-3x/wk. Long term	1-5x/wk. Long term	1-3x/wk. Long term	1-3x/wk. Short term
Primary indications	Psychotic & neurotic disorders, transient situational reactions	Neurotic disorders, borderline states	Neurotic disorders	Neurotic disorders	Phobias, passivity, sexual problems
Individual screening interview	Usually	Always	Always	Usually	Usually
Communication content	Focus primarily on environmental factors	Present & past life situations, intragroup & extragroup relationships	Primarily past life experience, intragroup relationships	Primarily intragroup relationships, rarely past history, "here-and-now"	Specific symptoms examined without focus on causality
Transference	Positive transference encouraged to promote improved functioning	Positive and negative transference evoked and analyzed	Transference neurosis evoked and analyzed	Positive relationships fostered, negative feelings analyzed	Positive relationships fostered, no examination of transference

Dreams	Not analyzed	Analyzed frequently	Analyzed always, encouraged	Analyzed rarely	Not utilized
Dependency	Intragroup dependency encouraged, members rely on leader to great extent	Intragroup dependency encouraged, dependency on leader variable	Intragroup dependency not encouraged, dependency on leader variable	Intragroup dependency encouraged, dependency on leader not encouraged	Intragroup dependency not encouraged, reliance on leader is high
Therapist activity	Strengthen existing defenses, active, gives advice	Challenge defenses, active, gives advice or personal response in limited ways only	Challenge defenses, passive, no advice giving or personal response	Challenge defenses, active, gives personal response rather than advice	Create new defenses, active and directive
Interpretation	No interpretation of unconscious conflict	Interpretation of unconscious conflict	Interpretation of unconscious conflict extensive	Interpretation of current behavioral patterns in the here-and-now	Not utilized
Major group processes	Universalization, reality-testing	Cohesion, transference, reality-testing	Transference, ventilation, catharsis, reality-testing	Abreaction, reality-testing	Cohesion, reinforcement, conditioning
Socialization outside of group	Encouraged	Generally discouraged	Discouraged	Variable	Discouraged
Goals	Better adaptation to environment	Moderate reconstruction of personality dynamics	Extensive reconstruction of personality dynamics	Alteration of behavior via mechanism of conscious control	Relief of specific psychiatric symptoms

psychodynamic criteria: age, gender, cultural, or other characteristics of the members by the goals of the group, or, occasionally, by the setting in which the group occurs. When one of the foregoing criteria is central to the formation and life of the group, it is functionally homogeneous (i.e., it is specialized) even though the members are different from one another in many other respects. Thus, groups for those undergoing cancer chemotherapy will tend to focus around the circumstances of this illness and its treatment, even though the personalities of the members constitute a heterogeneous mix. Likewise, the thematic content of inpatient groups relates to the circumstances of hospitalization despite the varying individual diagnoses. Certain groups come into being within a homogeneous umbrella, but over time, they move toward heterogeneity as the initial purpose recedes in importance and the divergent personalities of the members become the prime focus of treatment. Examples include groups for postcardiac patients, for the aged, and certain mothers' groups.

In homogeneous groups, members readily identify with one another and soon with the group as a whole. Because group identification takes place fairly rapidly, cohesion is an important instrument for treatment. Members tend to reinforce mutual defenses, however, and the resulting collective resistances are relatively impermeable. When one member observes similar defenses in others, such behavior is then experienced as the norm; when everyone seems united in such a position, the therapist's lone protest seems like a voice in the wind. Consequently, specialized groups tend to be supportive but superficial; they reinforce defenses rather than promote change. As one moves along the spectrum of group diversity toward heterogeneous composition, opposite conditions prevail. In a group of heterogeneous composition, trends develop toward challenging symptoms and character structure, enhancement of reality testing, diversity of transference, and exposure of deeper levels of personality; therapy is more expressive and the opportunity for change is great.[15]

These considerations are crucial in treatment planning, because the nature of the group greatly influences both the nature and goals of therapy. Homogeneous groups are useful for many specific disorders when, for example:

1) the group is used as an adjunct to another form of psychiatric treatment
2) symptom relief takes precedence and other forms of treatment can be delayed
3) sharing problems with others who have similar conditions can relieve an unwarranted sense of uniqueness or embarrassment over one's condition, provided the group is used concurrently with or as preparation for another form of treatment
4) existing psychiatric disorders are not so severe as to require treatment in themselves and the major goal is symptom relief

Given these indications for a homogeneous group, general criteria are used for member selection, ascertaining only that an individual can function reasonably within the group. One need not determine that group therapy is the optimum modality, i.e., to be used as a primary treatment form.

GENERAL CRITERIA

Selecting members for a homogeneous group requires consideration only of broad criteria. Compatibility for a group method of treatment refers to those aspects of personality that must be present in order for an individual to function in a group.[16]

For purposes of consideration, it is helpful to categorize further these general criteria according to basic elements of group life. To make use of the group, members are required to relate to each other, to tolerate and work with the reactions of others, and to modulate their own behavior. Thus, for the sake of the discussion, criteria will be categorized as they relate to: the presence of other patients, group member interaction, and the quality of internal controls. As with any artificial compartmentalization of an integrated function (e.g., group compatibility), categories overlap and multiple criteria are needed to weigh the pros and cons of a group referral. It is hoped that categorization will help the clinician to evaluate referral potential systematically.

Presence of Other Patients

To be able to talk about one's problems with others, an individual must have had satisfying relationships with one or more persons, especially during childhood. Relatedness must have extended beyond parental relations to siblings or peers. Group treatment is not advised for those rare individuals whose relations with parents and siblings were nonexistent or extremely destructive.

The capacity for minimal object relatedness is predicated on the willingness and desire to reach out for interpersonal relationships. To be able to give as well as to receive, an individual must temporarily give up egocentricity and recognize commonalities with others. Even in a highly supportive group, one must possess some ability to identify regressively with others. Lack of these characteristics precludes group treatment.

Group Member Interaction

Once in a group, members need to do more than give and take; they need to learn to tolerate the idiosyncrasies of others and to tolerate the various intragroup tensions as these develop. Patients must have sufficiently strong egos to withstand the stress to which they will be subjected. They must possess enough flexibility to tolerate, or preferably to modulate, intragroup tensions. Individuals who need a skilled person to select topics for discussion, manage confrontations, and in general monitor tolerance for stress will find a group to be unendurable. Additionally, in the give and take of group life, an individual must eventually serve as a catalyst for others, either by virtue of direct action, or passively by the nature of his or her problems.

Quality of Internal Controls

In a group, an individual must be able to cooperate with fellow members to achieve a common goal. This implies the ability to share time, attention, and a willingness to delay work on one's own problems in deference to others. To be goal-oriented, an individual must have some motivation for improvement, as well as sufficient understanding of and commitment to the group method of treatment. In order to work with others, a patient must have full contact with reality and be reasonable. The latter requires minimal superego development; an individual must not be at the mercy of archaic impulses. Likewise, extreme tendencies to manipulate others ruthlessly, as occurs with several antisocial personalities, would contraindicate a group.

SPECIFIC CRITERIA

Psychodynamic therapy groups serve as primary treatment modalities, alone or in combination with individual psychotherapy. Referral to such a group requires comprehensive assessment of the patient and the presence of specific inclusion criteria. Candidates should possess a high degree of group compatibility. Therefore, the clinician needs to determine not only that the patient can function in a group, but that group psychotherapy is the best treatment. These groups, more than other types, capitalize on properties unique to the group process in order to treat the individual member's psychopathology. Again, for discussion's sake, these criteria will be categorized according to certain properties of group life: the emotional ties to the therapist, the effect of group interaction and relationships, and the relationship to the group. These categories are helpful for the purposes of evaluation, but are not functionally distinct.

Patients usually fulfill some, if not many, of these inclusion criteria. A high degree of group compatibility may be found both in a patient who scores moderately in most of the categories or highly in only one. Those suitable for a psychodynamic group satisfy several criteria or possess one central characteristic that makes group therapy the preferred treatment. Consideration of inclusion criteria requires the clinician to weigh the total assessment picture because certain aspects of the group provide support, others may serve as resistance to treatment, and still others facilitate the process of treatment.

Emotional Ties to the Therapist

Relationships in the group between the therapist and members, and between the members themselves, are important. Because the therapist must be shared by all group members, the nature and intensity of the relationships of the members to him or her are different than that formed in individual treatment. While collectively idealized, the therapist is less available for interaction with each member. Patients must depend upon each other for therapeutic interaction, confrontation, and insight.

The nature of these relationships in the group makes group psychotherapy specifically useful for the treatment of certain patients.[17] Patients with intense erotic conflicts, or those who have incapacitating anxiety in the one-to-one relationship with the therapist, do better in groups. Also, patients with submissive, passive, or oral dependent traits that often impede individual treatment are best treated in groups, as are those who rely on the defense of projections of blame because this mechanism is often mitigated when such patients are confronted by peers. An occasional patient who is destructively competitive or aggressive with authority is more approachable by fellow patients.

A 40-year-old engineer sought help for depression and vocational stagnation after his marriage had failed. He possessed excellent verbal ability, but upon interview demonstrated a narrow range of affect. A trial of individual treatment was unsuccessful because of marked intellectualization; he understood his problems thoroughly but meaninglessly. Only later did the therapist learn that the patient recited analytic constructs in the belief that he was a better therapist than the therapist himself. After transfer to a group, he was caught in the tide of interaction with the other patients. Competitiveness here was put to therapeutic use. As he pressed home with others his meaningless deductions, a new dimension of his personality unfolded–affect. This gave richness to his group experience and brought understanding to his marital and vocational problems.

Effect of Group Interaction and Relationships

Many patients for whom individual psychotherapy is nonproductive benefit from the mutual stimulation of a group. Members learn from each other, provide comfort and support, and help an individual to overcome feelings of loneliness. Some patients have strong beliefs that their conflicts are unique and shameful; realizing that others in the group have the same forbidden thoughts, feelings, and conflicts—a process called "universalization"—can be reassuring. Relatively unpsychologically-minded patients benefit from the sharing of feelings and reactions in the group.

Psychotherapy groups readily reveal character resistances as these are exposed within a social context. Many character problems are especially amenable to group psychotherapy, particularly when character traits are egosyntonic.[18] The social consequences of maladaptive patterns are readily apparent in a group and constructive feedback can ensue. Intellectualized defenses may give way under the affective impact of group interaction, making socially related symptoms more readily available for therapeutic work.

Problems manifested in sibling relationships are frequently resolved in group therapy. Patients with confused identity patterns use feedback within the group to clarify self-concepts and use group interactions to experiment with new social roles.

In a group, peer support permits banding together, thereby lessening unconscious fears of retribution for expression of guilt-laden conflicts. Thus, groups are especially suitable for many patients with severe consciences or a variety of related superego defects. The clinician should think of group therapy whenever significant obsessive-compulsive, masochistic, or depressive character traits are observed. Patients with rigid personalities and psychosomatic symptoms do well in group therapy because these traits are often a consequence of unconscious superego conflicts which additionally may produce relative psychological naivete.

Any patient who demonstrates character problems, psychosomatic symptoms, a rigid conscience, or lack of psychological mindedness should be considered for referral to a group.

Relationship to the Group

Individuals develop significant identifications with primary social groups, e.g., family, work, church, ethnic, neighborhood, and community groups. Examination of this phenomenon demonstrates that for certain individuals belonging to a group enhances self-identity and a sense of well-being. Psychotherapy groups utilize this effect to clinical advantage. Theoreticians speak of the group as a entity perceived in a benign, nurturing manner.[19] Patients usually refer to the group in a positive vein while re-enacting aggressive conflicts with the members and therapist. In this way, patients derive considerable support from the group while engaging in the rigors of treatment. Signs of emotional deprivation, isolation, and a need to belong often point to possible therapeutic benefits of a group experience.

In groups there is decreased pressure for active participation compared to other modalities. Patients often discuss their problems through others and regulate emotional distance. Thus, certain withdrawn patients and those afraid of self-expression can better tolerate therapy through a group experience.

In addition, the reality nature of the group interaction deters certain patients from unwarranted regression and retreat into fantasy. For those patients for whom regression would be antitherapeutic, e.g., those with relatively severe borderline disturbance, a group may provide a unique advantage.[20] In such instances, the clinician needs to evaluate the therapeutic advantage of fantasy elaboration versus reality orientation.

Contraindications

In contrast to inclusion criteria, the contraindications noted below usually mitigate against group therapy. Just one facet of personality may seriously impair group compatibility. This conclusion derives from examination of the nature of group treatment, wherein individualized attention is less possible compared to other modalities, and the individual must be able to tolerate group interaction. The group must also be able to tolerate the individual.

As noted, patients must tolerate the frustration of sharing attention; they must be able to show some ability to identify regressively with others and must have the desire (even if not the capacity) to reach out for interpersonal relationships. Consequently, patients unsuited for group psychotherapy include those who are extremely egocentric and demanding, those who are unable to tolerate a period of assimilation into the group culture, and those with highly unusual symptoms or life-styles that set them apart from others. Patients should have full contact with reality and be flexible enough to tolerate the give and take of group interactions without experiencing impairment of ego integrity. Additional contraindications include the presence of active psychosis, a history of recent uncontrolled acting-out behavior, and ego integrity so poor as to cause the patient to be extremely suggestible, excessively vulnerable to group pressure, or overly sensitive to criticism.

The period of assimilation into the group culture demands that patients possess the ability to delay problem-solving temporarily until new alternatives emerge through the group process. Obviously, then, group psychotherapy is unsuited for patients in acute distress or for those who are perpetually crisis-oriented.

Contraindications to group psychotherapy must also include

greater benefit from another treatment modality. Thus, for some patients, family therapy is the best treatment, whereas others are prime candidates for psychoanalytically-oriented individual psychotherapy or psychoanalysis.

Procedures for Obtaining Data and Planning Treatment

As yet there are no specialized procedures available to assess a patient's suitability for group treatment. The clinician must rely on traditional interviewing skills. A comprehensive history is invaluable, along with the usual examination of the patient's mental and psychological status. A comprehensive assessment includes a clear description of symptoms, the phenomenologic data obtained from several individual psychiatric interviews, and a psychodynamic understanding of both defenses and ego structures. Occasionally, psychological testing or an interview with a relative or close friend also proves useful.

Currently, there have been only rudimentary efforts to correlate descriptive diagnoses with the relative effectiveness of certain therapeutic groups. Perhaps DSM-III will encourage efforts along these lines. Group therapists, however, have characteristically stressed the more dynamic aspects of symptomatology and personology.

In terms of DSM-III axes, the clinician should include all five in assessment of a patient for group treatment. However, Axis II—Personality Disorders—will probably be relied on more heavily than the Axis I diagnosis. Axes IV and V may prove more useful in the future. Already one generalization can be made: a patient having a higher level of previous adaptive functioning (Axis V) is more likely to be appropriate for a psychodynamic group, whereas one having a lower level of adaptive functioning is usually more suited to an ancillary group.

THE EVALUATION

The depth of data needed varies depending upon whether one is considering a patient for an ancillary group, a homogeneous or specialized group, or a psychodynamic group. Inpatient, day treatment, and residential programs need only assign patients to their ancillary groups on the basis of most clinical data. Here a comprehensive psychological examination is not necessary and only certain parts of a mental status examination are useful. The latter includes motor and verbal functions, quality of the sensorium, and a global intellectual assessment. For proper placement, simple assessment of the patient's behavior and approximate level of functioning is needed. Sufficient data may be obtained from any of several mental health team members through observation alone; examination by a trained clinician is often not necessary.

In contrast, selection for either a homogeneous or psychodynamic group requires greater clinical skill. Examination should be performed only by a highly trained professional. In fact, as we move along the continuum from homogeneous to psychodynamic groups, greater clinical sophistication is required in order to make proper patient selection.

Group compatibility is measured by evaluating how the patient rates in the various subcategories under general and specific inclusion criteria. In certain instances, the history is revealing; in others, the interview is more fruitful; in still others, combining these two sources of data is necessary. The quality of object relationships can be assessed partially by reviewing the patient's past history of relationships. The patient's relatedness during the interview often proves telling. At times, however, the best indicator of how patients will relate to other group members comes from descriptions of the other persons in their lives and their relations with them.

In a specific way, assessment must focus on the patient's relatedness along an axis involving authority versus peer relationships. The history gives valuable clues in this area to the suitability for group therapy. Many patients give histories of incapacitating relationships with parents, teachers, superiors at work, and other authorities, but have demonstrated social facility with their siblings or peers. A history of the response to previous individual or group treatment is valuable, as is a history of response to various social situations. The relationship to the clinician during evaluation is often the initial predictor of a patient's response to authority.

Prediction of relatedness to peers in a group depends partly on the patient's potential to be catalytic to others and partly upon his or her tendency to respond constructively to intragroup tensions. The ability to serve as an active catalyst for others may be apparent during evaluation, but may remain an unknown quantity. The ability to serve as a passive catalyst should be evident during the interview as the clinician examines his or her own responses to the patient. The patient should be able to elicit empathy. Potential responses to group events, however, are difficult to foretell. Some clues may be gleaned from responses to social situations that can be derived from the history. The manner of reporting these past events is often instructive. During the examination, the patient's responses to questions, digressions, and confrontations are reasonable measures of tolerance for interpersonal stress.

Occasionally, the patient's initial presentation gives valuable clues to the usefulness of group treatment. The clinician should consider group psychotherapy when interpersonal difficulties are not evident in the dyadic interview, when symptoms are elicited only under social conditions, or when the patient comes for help primarily because of what others observe or how they react to him or her.

How a patient might function in a therapeutic group can often be gleaned by a history of past group relationships, particularly the first group experience—the family of origin. Obviously, the status a person had in his or her family of origin bears heavily on functioning in a group. Both the patient's fantasies about groups and his or her history of previous group relationships assist in the evaluation. The assessment should include the quality of relationships *to* a group as well as *within* a group. The patient's level of functioning in a primary social group can foreshadow his or her functioning in a psychotherapy group. Idealization of the group as an entity may motivate the patient to perform above his or her usual level. This helps to diminish resistance to the treatment process.

Clinical Example

The following case report illustrates how selection criteria are applied to the evaluation of a patient for whom a psychodynamic group was recommended. Only those aspects of the clinical material relevant to this discussion are presented. These data will be examined to determine the patient's suitability for group treatment.

> *A 32-year-old married homemaker sought treatment upon the urging of her husband and friends. They decried her reluctance to*

assume full responsibility for management of the household and care of the children, as she depended excessively upon her husband for guidance. Her friends had long been surprised by her childishness with her husband in contrast to her behavior with them; she had many friends, was socially engaging, and with them seemed mature. She complained that they overrated her; she felt empty inside and adapted too readily to others so that she presented a different facade to each group of friends. Friends flocked to her, but she did not know why.

The history revealed her to be an adopted, only child. As a youngster she always felt special and adored, not only by her parents but by several maiden aunts, and enjoyed this attention. Because she was pretty and had a flair for the theater, she was well known and popular in school. She was intelligent and academically successful. During adolescence, she grew especially close to her mother, whom she then considered to be her best friend.

She attended a local college and did well in all areas of endeavor. Afterward she lived at home and worked for a small theater company. She reported that this was the happiest time of her life; she was productive, carefree, and worked with very "exciting people."

She left home to marry and after the birth of the first of her three children became depressed and sought treatment. She reported that two years of individual, twice-weekly, psychoanalytic therapy helped her to resolve conflicts of dependency upon her mother. She terminated treatment abruptly by sending the therapist a note. Termination was not planned, and she had not mentioned it in sessions, but apparently had toyed privately with the idea for a few weeks. When the time seemed ripe, she acted.

During the intervening four years, the former feelings of sadness gradually returned. She felt acutely dissatisfied with herself and wanted to change, but was unable to say in what way.

Upon examination, this patient proved to be intellectually bright, articulate, and possessed both good motivation and insight for treatment. She displayed a good range of affect, but seemed somewhat sad at times. On other occasions, she seemed unusually happy, particularly when the psychiatrist appeared especially interested in what she said. In general, she was pleasing, affable, and cooperative. While she did appear to enjoy attention and had a flare for the dramatic, the basic character pathology was not striking and the interview did not explain her story. One unusual finding emerged: she felt very uncomfortable when the psychiatrist was silent, could not freely associate, and anxiously asked the examiner to resume questioning.

Pharmacotherapy was not considered. Although affective components were present, the findings did not fulfill the criteria for a dysthymic disorder. Marital therapy was considered in passing, but neither she nor her husband identified the marriage as problematic and her difficulties extended into other areas. Expressive psychoanalytic therapy had to be considered. She was well motivated, intelligent, psychologically minded, and demonstrated rich affect during the interviews. Basic identity and character problems such as hers are frequently amenable to individual treatment. A dyadic transference would create a mother-daughter paradigm that is generally associated with core problems. But would she find this useful or inhibitory?

Special features of this patient suggested the usefulness of a group:

1) her submissive dependency upon her husband
2) the presence of egosyntonic character pathology
3) her proclivity to be socially reactive and interactive
4) her hunger for peer relatedness and the history of a sense of well-being in groups (school and, especially, the theater company)

Two features made group referral equivocal. First, with her family of origin she felt special. Would she benefit from the universalization process or would her need to feel unique alienate her from her peers? Second, she was raised as an only child. Would she use the group to learn how to share with others, or would she demand too much of the group's time for herself?

Two other features weighed heavily. One of these related to transference and the other to the nature of her character pathology. Her dramatically precipitous termination from her previous individual therapy suggested that certain aspects of that transference were experienced as intolerable. Her response to the examiner's silence added evidence to the idea that such a regressive transference would be antitherapeutic. Not only was her character pathology egosyntonic, but she was generally unaware of her varied social faces. In addition, character pathology was less evident in the psychiatric interview and was felt to need a social stimulus.

With this patient the treatment recommendation was for

psychodynamic group psychotherapy, with supplementary individual sessions to be used on an as-needed basis when narcissistic defenses were unduly taxed. Subsequent treatment proved highly successful.

PREPARATION FOR A REFERRAL

More often than not, one clinician recommends group treatment as an appropriate modality and a second clinician carries out the actual therapy. The second clinician needs to re-evaluate the patient to determine compatibility for the particular group and to acquaint the patient with the formal arrangements (i.e., treatment contract) and the structure and operation of treatment. Transfer from one clinician to another is difficult; many patients resist referral or even drop out of treatment at this point unless the transfer process is handled judiciously.

The primary clinician has the tasks of imparting a recommendation to the patient and moderating initial resistance to treatment. These tasks should be handled with care and clinical understanding. In both instances, unconscious wishes (e.g., for exclusiveness) are frustrated and fears may be aroused. Healthy aspects of the ego must be allied with the goal of referral.

Patients usually seek treatment with unrealistic expectations. They present symptoms while the clinician evaluates the underlying processes. Even the most sophisticated patients both wish to change and, at the same time, seek unconsciously to gratify internal conflicts through the transference. A model for succor originates in early memory traces of dyadic experiences and is reinforced culturally (e.g., one goes for help to a physician, a clergyman, or a mentor, but rarely to a group). Thus, the recommendation for referral to a group is experienced, on some level, with disappointment; group psychotherapy carried with it an image of second-class treatment.

The recommendation should be made within the working alliance. After hearing the description of the present illness and taking a history, the clinician should convey his or her assessment of the patient's condition in understandable terms. From such a practical diagnostic formulation flows the recommendation. For example:

A 35-year-old attorney with chronic depressive features of ennui, fatigue, and impaired ability to experience pleasure sought treatment for a moderate failure of vocational productivity and unsatisfying interpersonal relationships. During the evaluation, he admitted that he had an unusually quiet adolescence and was passively dependent upon his parents for much of his life prior to marriage. The psychiatrist speculated that the patient's youthful patterns represented characterologic underdevelopment of normal assertiveness that now inhibited him vocationally and interpersonally. A group was suggested as a means through which the patient could explore and experiment with his feelings in the presence of others. Noting that every treatment format reactivates early patterns of relatedness, the patient was told that individual treatment would reactivate his earlier pattern with his parents. Both the patient and the psychiatrist saw this as undesirable because both appreciated the difficulty this man had in becoming independent. On the other hand, a superficial social facility and a keen interest in developing closer friendships suggested that the group format could tap latent assertiveness during interactions with peers. The clinician did not mention dependency wishes that were at the root of his problems and would eventually be revealed in a group.

It is important to make a recommendation in a positive manner with careful observation of the patient's reactions. Herein may lie important data that can enrich the evaluation. For example, previously unrevealed fears of social criticism may now emerge that might contraindicate a group referral. In contrast, reactions of curiosity or even mild wariness are positive signs. Some anxiety should be evident because, as previously noted, the recommendation is invariably received unconsciously with disappointment. Mild reluctance is usually expressed through queries about group, e.g., "Will I be able to talk?" "Will I be exposed?" "Will confidentiality be preserved?" "Will it be too superficial?" "Am I too sophisticated?" These questions should be answered factually and reassuringly. Education is a valuable tool to foster the working alliance and appeal to healthy aspects of the ego, and it can later sustain the patient during the anticipated stress of the acculturation period in the group. It is helpful to recognize and verbalize the anxiety that is ubiquitous in anticipation of entering a group. Recognition of the specific fears of an individual (e.g., a fear of neglect) is invaluable. Verbalization of fears provides reassurance, and education facilitates ego mastery.

The therapist who accepts a patient into a group needs to consider group balance, in addition to the patient's suitability for group treatment. Unfortunately, there is little research into or clinical understanding of this area. It is known that each group seems to have a character of its own; however, the components of that character are unknown. Every clinician recognizes that a well-functioning group has a balance of personality types within its membership. Thus, groups function well when they have an admixture of passive and active members, leaders and followers, outgoing and reserved types, and so on. Homogeneity of styles can be devastating, e.g., a group of extroverts is overly competitive, whereas a group of passive, schizoid members can devastate the therapist with silence. In addition, there must be limited compatibility with the particular group's culture, as marked deviancy usually results in early termination. Hence, even if a patient is deemed suitable for group and for a certain *kind* of group, the therapist still needs to determine compatibility with a particular group.

Should the patient not be accepted by the therapist for a particular group, he or she will be referred back to the primary psychiatrist. The patient may feel defeated or relieved by this unexpected turn of events. The psychiatrist must anticipate and be prepared to deal with such reactions. Should the patient be accepted for group therapy, it is important for the referring psychiatrist to make sure that the transition is smooth. The patient should never feel "dropped." Overlapping the sessions of the two clinicians is better than leaving a hiatus. The referring clinician should remain available if the referral proves unworkable.

Discussion of Clinical Vignette

The 42-year-old businessman described in Chapter I was noted as experiencing symptoms of acute depression; however, the clinical picture was more complicated. Additionally, the patient had been compulsive all of his adult life and had a history of marital difficulties for several years. The material presented in this chapter can now be applied to treatment planning for this patient. A thorough plan must consider the various uses of group modalities. The following discussion illustrates how this is done.

The first DSM-III diagnosis on Axis I is the major depressive episode. The brief clinical history does not describe any periods of euphoria or manic behavior, although the evaluation should try carefully to ascertain their presence or absence, particularly in view of the positive family history for psychiatric illness. Assuming that bipolar affective disorder can be ruled out and that the major depressive episode is the Axis I diagnosis, further consideration in treatment would be the use of medication, specifically antidepressants. The considerations involved in the use of medication are discussed elsewhere in this volume.

In addition to antidepressant medication, this patient, during the initial period of treatment and particularly during the acute and distressing phase of his depression, would need individual psychotherapy in order to help him to verbalize his disturbing thoughts and feelings and to gain the support of an individual relationship with a therapist. The type of individual psychotherapy that would be utilized is discussed elsewhere in this text.

Similarly, in a more extensive evaluation of the precipitating or aggravating factors in the patient's depression, a need for some form of marital therapy might become evident. Again, the factors in considering marital therapy are described elsewhere in this volume. A couples' group might be useful. Certainly, it could provide valuable diagnostic information as it would clarify the contribution of the marriage to the depressive episode. Should marital problems prove symptomatic of underlying personality problems, the couples' group may have limited therapeutic value.

These three treatment modalities—antidepressant medication, individual psychotherapy, and marital therapy—could be used either separately or together in the treatment of the depressive phase of this patient's illness. They would, alone or together, be helpful in lessening the patient's acute distress and helping him and his family work together to deal with the factors involved in his depression.

The second DSM-III diagnosis on Axis II is personality disorder, compulsive type. This is really the patient's major disability. The depressive episode, however severe and acute, and however much it currently may impair function, is simply an expression of an underlying difficulty related to the patient's personality characteristics or characterological traits. Even from the scanty description provided in the clinical vignette, it is clear that the patient's compulsive personality affects every aspect of his life: the need for perfection, the need for extreme control, the need for excessive commitment to work, and the inability to experience or express feelings all stem from his rigid attitudes. In the one important relationship in his life that is mentioned, his marriage, his personality has led to serious difficulties. One would suspect that this man has difficulties in other relationships, both socially and at work. What is even more important, his need for perfection would inevitably lead to frequent loss of self-esteem, making him prone to depressive episodes. Most important of all, an enormous amount of psychic energy would be devoted to maintaining his perfectionistic, rigid, compulsive attitudes at work and in social relations, leaving little energy for flexible adjustments to work, life situations, and personal relationships. This type of patient usually shows little or no understanding of underlying emotional factors, tensions, and conflicts.

Once the acute phase of the depression has subsided, this patient would be most effectively treated by a combination of individual and psychoanalytically-oriented group psychotherapy. In the individual therapy he would have time to discuss and explore and gain support in an individual relationship for his depressive and other painful symptoms. This type of patient, however, frequently has difficulty in the one-to-one relationship, not being used to intimacy or expression of feelings, and tolerating poorly relationships that focus on the expression of emotional conflicts.

In psychoanalytically-oriented group psychotherapy, all of these difficulties would be helped by the conditions existing in the group: the multiple identifications with the therapist and the other patients; the lessened intensity of one-to-one transference reactions through its deflection onto other members; and hearing other members express their emotional needs, conflicts, and difficulties. Supported by the other group members, the patient could learn to develop relationships with other patients in the group and could come to understand his emotional reactions. He would be confronted with and get feedback on the nature of the personality characteristics that lead to difficulties in his life, and would be able to share these insights with other group members. In a more realistic and effective way he would see the destructive manner in which his personality characteristics lead to feelings of disappointment, anger, and depression.

It is important to emphasize, for the purpose of this discussion, that whereas the acute presenting diagnostic category is the painful, depressive episode, the underlying psychopathology leads to the patient's difficulties in every sphere of his life, making him prone to the development of depression. Because of the pervasive influence of his personality disorder, a combination of individual and psychoanalytically-oriented group psychotherapy would be the best treatment following the alleviation of the depressive syndrome.

Conclusion

This chapter emphasizes the broad range of group therapies available in the current clinical arena. These therapies can be categorized into three levels: ancillary groups, homogeneous or specialized groups, and group psychotherapy proper, which is further divided into group counseling, supportive group psychotherapy, and psychoanalytically-oriented group psychotherapy. This profusion of group processes mandates careful assessment leading to discriminating treatment planning. Those variables that appear most useful in assessment and treatment planning have been emphasized in this presentation. It is hoped that its reading will make obvious that referral for "group therapy" is not something to be considered because it "might help," but rather involves the careful consideration of a wide range of crucial variables.

References

1. Pratt, J. H.: The Class Method of Treating Consumption in the Homes of the Poor, *Journal of the American Medical Association*, 49, 755-757, 1907.
2. Foulkes, S. H.: The Group as Matrix of the Individual's Mental Life, in L. R. Wolberg, and E. K. Schwartz, (eds.): *Group Therapy 1973*, New York: Intercontinental Medical Book Corporation, pp. 211-220, 1973.
3. Durkin, H. E.: *The Group in Depth*, New York: International Universities Press, 1964.

4. Stein, A.: The Nature and Significance of Interaction in Group Psychotherapy, *International Journal of Group Psychotherapy*, 20, 153-162, 1970.
5. Saravay, S. M.: A Psychoanalytic Theory of Group Development, *International Journal of Group Psychotherapy*, 28, 481-507, 1978.
6. Guidelines for the Training of Group Psychotherapists, Revised Edition, New York: *American Group Psychotherapy Association*, 1978.
7. Foulkes, S. H., and Anthony, E. J.: *Group Psychotherapy, Second Edition*, Baltimore: Penguin Books, 1973.
8. Stein, op.cit.
9. Yalom, I. D., and Lieberman, M. A.: A Study of Encounter Group Casualties, *Archives of General Psychiatry*, 25, 16-30, 1971.
10. Bion, W. R.: *Experiences in Groups*, London: Tavistock Publications, 1959.
11. Moreno, J. L.: Psychodrama and Group Therapy, *Sociometry*, 9, 249-253, 1946.
12. Berne, E: *Principles of Group Treatment*, New York: Oxford University Press, 1966.
13. Perls, F. S.: *Gestalt Therapy Verbatim*, Lafayette, California: Real People Press, 1969.
14. Ruitenbeek, H. M.: *Group Therapy Today*, New York: Atherton Press, 1969.
15. Furst, W.: Homogeneous Versus Heterogeneous Groups, *International Journal of Group Psychotherapy*, 1, 120-123, 1951.
16. Slavson, S. R.: Criteria for Selection and Rejection of Patients for Various Types of Group Psychotherapy, *International Journal of Group Psychotherapy*, 5, 3-30, 1955.
17. Stein, A.: Indications for Group Psychotherapy and the Selection of Patients, *Journal of the Hillside Hospital*, 12, 145-155, 1963.
18. Grunebaum, H., and Kates, W.: Whom to Refer for Group Psychotherapy, *American Journal of Psychiatry*, 134, 130-133, 1977.
19. Scheidlinger, S.: On the Concept of the "Mother Group," *International Journal of Group Psychotherapy*, 24, 417-428, 1974.
20. Freedman, M. B., and Sweet, B. C.: Some Specific Features of Group Psychotherapy and Their Implications for the Selection of Patients, *International Journal of Group Psychotherapy*, 4, 355-368, 1954.

Bibliography

Friedman, W. H.: *How To Do Groups*, New York: Jason Aronson, 1979.

Grotjahn, M: *The Art and Technique of Analytic Group Therapy*, New York: Jason Aronson, 1977.

Kadis, A. L., Krasner, J. D., Weiner, M. F., Winick, C. and Foulkes, S. H.: *A Practicum of Group Psychotherapy*, 2nd Edition, New York: Harper and Row, 1974.

Kaplan, H. I., and Sadock, B. J. (eds.): *Comprehensive Group Psychotherapy*, Baltimore: Williams and Wilkins, 1971.

Kibel, H. D.: A Schema for Understanding Resistances in Groups, *Group Process*, 7, 221-236, 1977.

Rabin, H. M.: Preparing Patients for Group Psychotherapy, *International Journal of Group Psychotherapy*, 20, 135-145, 1970.

Rosenbaum, M. (ed.): How to Begin a Psychotherapy Group: Six Approaches, *Group Process*, 7, 2-137, 1976.

Rosenbaum, M., and Berger, M. M. (eds.): *Group Psychotherapy and Group Function*, 2nd Edition, New York: Basic Books, 1975.

Stein, A.: Group Psychotherapy in the Treatment of Depression, Chapter II, in F. F. Flach, and S. Draghi, (eds.): *The Nature and Treatment of Depression*, New York: John Wiley & Son, 1975.

Stein, A.: Group Therapy, in E. S. Paykel (ed.), *Handbook of Affective Disorders*, Edinburgh: Churchill Livingstone, 1981

Shaffer, J. B. P., and Galinsky, M. O. *Methods of Group Therapy and Sensitivity Training*, Englewood Cliffs: Prentice-Hall, 1974.

Yalom, I. D.: *The Theory and Practice of Group Psychotherapy*, 2nd Edition, New York: Basic Books, 1975.

Chapter Three

The Biological Therapies

Judith G. Rabkin, Ph.D.
Donald F. Klein, M.D.

The authors would like to thank Drs. Max Fink, Rachel Gittelman, and Robert Spitzer for their assistance in preparation of this chapter.

Theoretical Premises

Chance and good fortune, rather than theoretically derived scientific research, led to the identification of the psychotropic drugs used today. Alert clinicians happened to notice that these drugs, each developed for other medical purposes, had positive effects on mood, activity level, or other manifestations of psychiatric disorder. In historical terms then, somatic therapies are the products of empirical discovery rather than of theoretical formulations. In a broader sense, however, a series of interlocking assumptions and beliefs underlie their application. In this brief overview, three of these assumptions have been selected for discussion.

PSYCHIATRIC DISORDER AS A PRODUCT OF PHYSIOLOGICAL DYSFUNCTION

Medical sociologists distinguished between the physiological, psychological, and social aspects of altered health states. The term disease is used to refer to a state of psychophysiological dysfunction regardless of whether it is recognized as such by the patient. Illness refers to subjective awareness of dysfunction, and sickness concerns the altered social role that may accompany illness and help-seeking behavior. All three components are ingredients of psychiatric disorder, although only the first is an essential characteristic.

According to this formulation, the definition of psychiatric disorder is not a value judgment or the product of social and cultural beliefs, but derives from a grasp of the evolutionary concept of real, distinct organismal functions and dysfunctions. For instance, among the functions of the digestive tract are processing and absorption of nutrients and discarding of wastes. If peristalsis stops, as in intestinal atony, these functions cannot be carried out. It is certainly no arbitrary statement, reflecting only social or individual values, if this lack of peristalsis is considered a dysfunctional state—a suboptimal deviation from evolutionary determined processes which should be considered the result of disease.

The objective reality of psychiatric disorder is corroborated by the finding of psychiatric epidemiologists that no society is free of the major forms of illness of which we know, although symptomatic manifestations and content may vary. While it is certainly true that the proportion of those who are treated or hospitalized by professionals of different kinds may differ widely between times and places, there is no convincing evidence that the "true" prevalence of major psychiatric disorders varies greatly.

The nominalist critique denies the possibility of objectively determining correct psychobiological function. No one will deny that this is difficult in practice. However, the stand that this cannot be accomplished, even in principle, is plainly false. As Aubrey Lewis states, "The concept of disease, then—and of health—has physiological and psychological components, but no essential social ones."[1]

No particular type of etiology is implicated in this conceptualization. Anything that affects the organism, whether it be symbolic interactions, affective relations, toxic agents, malfunctioning genes, or other pathogenic factors may conceivably result in dysfunction.

Research concerning the biological basis of psychiatric disorder has largely followed, rather than preceded, the appearance of somatic therapies and may indeed be considered a consequence of their development. Once the effects of psychotropic drugs were identified, scientists sought to find their underlying biological mechanisms. Not only would such research result in the development of better drugs with greater specificity of action and fewer side effects, but greater understanding of the etiology and pathophysiology of psychiatric disorders would be attained. At this time, structural anomalies or alterations have not yet been found to correspond to varieties of psychiatric disorder, although preliminary results of studies using computerized axial tomography suggest that they may exist in some instances. Neurochemical, neuroendocrinologic, and neurophysiologic studies are producing evidence of specific abnormalities in acutely ill patients, some of which are no longer evident upon remission, and of trait-type abnormalities that persist and may precede the manifest sickness. Cumulatively, the findings of biologic research have raised many questions, but also provide empirical evidence of altered physiological function in some illness states.

To summarize, the first assumption is that of a psychobiologic dysfunctional basis for psychiatric disorder. This is a somewhat narrower definition than those of others. It rules out varieties of subjective distress unrelated to biological dysfunction that may appear as clinically milder variants of the focus of our concerns, such as "garden variety unhappiness," which Freud also excluded from his conceptualization of illness and cure. We do not deny the reality of everyday psychological distress or the need for relief, but do not regard such problems as appropriate for psychiatric care.

TREATMENT GOALS AND SOCIAL VALUES

The second assumption underlying somatic therapies is that the goal of treatment is to either normalize dysfunction or compensate for the effects of the dysfunction. In this sense, effective treatment is objectively worthwhile, apart from any particular set of social values.

Useful therapeutic effects may well differ in terms of their depth and scope. Some address underlying causes and, therefore, may be thought of as etiologic, while others are symptomatic. Penicillin cures pneumococcal pneumonia, whereas aspirin symptomatically affects fever. There is a continuum with regard to the degree to which various treatments should be considered symptomatic. Diuretics are a good treatment for congestive heart failure because of their effects on secondary, exacerbating renal complications of the failing cardiac musculature. They clearly, however, are having a deeper effect than the benefit gained by propping the patient up in bed. A still deeper symptomatic treatment might help the heart muscle to contract without rooting out the basic cardiac dysfunction.

Is there any way to determine if a medication is acting in a symptomatic compensatory way or is having a deeper normalizing effect? One possibility is to consider whether the effects of the somatic treatment are similar in normals as in sick people. For instance, antacid agents lower stomach acidity both in normals and those with pathological hyperacidity. However, the normal gastric contents are made hypoacid whereas the hyperacid stomach contents are brought within the normal range. This is clearly a compensatory symptomatic intervention.

Psychiatric drugs such as the benzodiazepines, sedatives, and stimulants seem to be best considered this sort of agent in that they have quite similar effects on normals and most patients, although the normal may be made sedated whereas the hyperalert may be calmed.

On the other hand, there are agents whose effects on healthy individuals appear trivial and unrelated to the dramatic effects on the ill. For instance, aspirin does not lower the body temperature of the normal person but does bring down the fever of the ill person. The major psychotropic agents may fit this category. For instance, the tricyclic antidepressants do not raise the mood of the normal person but are profoundly antidepressant for those who have melancholia. It has been argued that this distinction is best conceptualized in cybernetic terms.

To sum up, just as mental illnesses are not myths but are due to real dysfunctions of the organism, so the beneficial effects of somatic therapy are not myths but are due either to the normalization of dysfunctional psychobiological processes or to compensation for these dysfunctions.

MEASUREMENT OF THERAPEUTIC EFFICACY

When the goals of somatic therapies are defined in these terms, they become measurable, and belief in the feasibility of assessing treatment outcome is one of the hallmarks of somatic therapists. Indeed, somatic therapy has led to the modern revolution in treatment evaluation, since it has demonstrated the necessity for and feasibility of adequately controlled comparative trials in the determination of treatment efficacy.

In short, then, the theoretical premises of somatic therapies include the assumptions that psychiatric disorders are the product of psychobiological dysfunctions; that the goal of somatic treatment is either to remedy or compensate for these dysfunctions; and that the effect of treatment can and should be assessed in order to identify those that are maximally efficient, quick, effective, and have the fewest undesirable side effects.

Range and Description of Specific Treatment Procedures

There are five broad categories of somatic treatment currently available in clinical practice, excluding surgical procedures, which are not considered in this chapter. The three therapies (lithium, antidepressant medication, and electroconvulsive therapy) used in the treatment of depressive disorders are reviewed first, followed by consideration of neuroleptics and anxiolytics. For each procedure we offer an overview of its development, associated risks and risk management, and treatment applications including indicators, pretreatment procedures, guidelines for prescribing, and choice within category where applicable.

In this chapter, routine procedures and standard practices will be noted. Prescription of medication, however, is an extraordinarily individualized undertaking, determined not only by the guidelines but by illness stage, severity, and spectacular biological variations in individual drug tolerance. For example, some patients can tolerate only 25 mg. a day of chlorpromazine while others can tolerate 10,000 mg. a day. The essential point is that drug dosage must be adjusted to individual needs, and that each patient should receive as much medication as is needed for clinical improvement as long as the side effects are manageable. Since nearly all psychotropic drugs, and indeed most active drugs of any kind, are likely to elicit some kind of side effect, the issue is not their appearance but their severity, duration, and reversibility. Caution should be used concerning the under-prescription of psychotropic drugs, both in dose and duration, that so often characterizes their use and which may stem in part from excessive reliance on general guidelines.

Both because of space constraints and the nature and goals of this book, our overview is selective rather than comprehensive without exploring unresolved issues in any detail or covering all facets of the material presented. Citations are also selective, and the reader is referred to several current basic texts listed at the chapter's end.

LITHIUM

History and Description

Lithium was identified by chance as an effective, specific chemical treatment for acute mania by the Australian psychiatrist John Cade in 1949. It was not approved by the U.S. Food and Drug Administration for treatment of acute manic episodes until 1970; maintenance use was approved in 1974. Consequently, lithium has become widely prescribed in the United States only in the past decade. Its early reputation as a dangerous and potentially lethal drug stems, in part, from its unfortunate use as a sodium substitute by cardiac patients in the 1940s. Subsequently, one of the few clear-cut contraindications for its use was found to be sodium depletion. At this time, clinical research supporting both the safety and efficacy of lithium in treatment of mania and prevention of recurrent episodes is considered "highly impressive."[2]

Lithium is usually marketed as lithium carbonate in 300 mg. tablets or capsules. Dosage is often about 1800 mg. daily in divided doses for acute episodes, and about 1200 mg. a day for maintenance therapy, but there is considerable variation. There is a six- to ten-day lag period before clinical effects occur. Maximum benefits may not be apparent for several weeks.[3] Because of lithium's potential toxicity, plasma concentrations must be measured frequently in the treatment of acutely manic patients and somewhat less often in continuation or maintenance usage. Once dosage is established and the acute phase subsides, monthly, bimonthly, or even more infrequent monitoring is sufficient.[3] Depending on the patient's age, weight, and renal status, optimal plasma concentrations are between 1.0 and 1.4 mEq per liter for acute treatment, and between 0.8 and 1.0 mEq per liter for prophylactic long-term use. Lower plasma concentrations fail to reach therapeutic levels; higher doses yield no apparent clinical advantage and increase the probability and severity of toxic side effects.

Lithium functions specifically as a mood-stabilizing agent. In acute mania, it restores normal sleep patterns and eradicates characteristic symptoms. Since it alleviates both manic and depressive symptoms, it is evidently neither a sedative nor stimulant, but is best conceptualized as a mood normalizer that affects deranged central regulating systems in psychopathologic states.

Risks and Risk Management

Common side effects include fatigue, muscle weakness, fine tremor, nausea, slurred speech, excessive thirst, and polyuria. Most of these mild side effects disappear after a week or so of continued treatment, but thirst, tremor, and increased urination tend to persist. When plasma concentrations exceed recommended levels, acute lithium intoxication may ensue, leading to central nervous system involvement, including impaired consciousness, coma, and even death. There is no specific antidote for lithium intoxication. In severe cases, dialysis should be considered.[2] In less extreme cases, if renal function is adequate, osmotic diuresis and intravenous bicarbonate solution can be used to accelerate excretion.

Treatment Applications

PRETREATMENT EVALUATION. Before lithium is prescribed, it is necessary to evaluate the patient's overall physical status and, in particular, sodium intake and thyroid, cardiac, and renal functioning. Total and differential white blood counts, hemoglobin estimate, and complete urinalysis are also indicated.[4] Ideally, lithium is prescribed for medically healthy adults or adolescents with normal sodium intake and normal cardiac, hepatic, and renal functioning, although exceptions are made when circumstances are sufficiently compelling.

USES OF LITHIUM. At least theoretically, there are five clinical contexts in which lithium treatment may be considered: for acute manic episodes, for acute depressive episodes in bipolar and unipolar illness, and for prophylactic management of both bipolar and unipolar forms of recurrent depressive disorder.

TREATMENT FOR ACUTE MANIA. Results of more than two dozen investigations, in addition to numerous clinical reports, cumulatively indicate that between seven and eight out of every ten manic patients respond well to lithium, regardless of age, sex, or response to other treatments.[5] Acute manic episodes constitute a serious problem; in most cases such patients require hospitalization both for their own protection and for medical management. The usual treatment of severely manic patients consists of large doses of a neuroleptic for five to ten days until the florid symptoms subside and food and fluid intake become stable. At that point, lithium is introduced and gradually replaces the neuroleptic medication.[2] Mildy hypomanic patients sometimes are treated with lithium alone on an outpatient basis if their behavior can be closely supervised, but this is relatively uncommon. As a rule, lithium is continued for six months after the patient becomes euthymic, even if long-term prophylaxis is not undertaken.[3]

TREATMENT FOR DEPRESSIVE EPISODES IN BIPOLAR ILLNESS. Lithium is also prescribed for the treatment of acute depressive episodes in bipolar illness.[3] It has not been shown to surpass tricyclic antidepressants in this context. Tricyclic antidepressants may, however, precipitate a sudden switch to mania or hypomania while lithium does not pose this risk.[2] On the other hand, the Food and Drug Administration (FDA) has not yet approved lithium for this use. It is not usually the first drug tried, but rather is prescribed when others fail or when the patient has responded well to lithium previously.

After patients recover from acute depressive episodes, standard practice is to continue medication at a lower level for another six months. Beyond that point, medication is generally considered as prophylactic rather than as continuation treatment. Because of the increased risk of mania from tricyclic antidepressants, it is sometimes recommended that lithium be used for continuation for all bipolar patients even if tricyclics were used to treat the acute episode.[3]

LITHIUM FOR UNIPOLAR DEPRESSIVE DISORDER. Lithium is not usually prescribed for patients with either phasic or chronic unipolar depressive illness, as it may not be as effective as other available therapies.[3] The available research evidence is, however, too sparse to draw firm conclusions. Design of studies of lithium's comparative efficacy for unipolar depressive disorder is complicated by the fact that 10% to 20% of such patients will have a subsequent manic episode and then will be reclassified as bipolar. In studies conducted to date, it seems likely that unipolar patients given lithium were suffering from severe recurrent episodes. Davis suggested that lithium might be effective "in a small group of frequently relapsing unipolar depressive patients, but much less effective in another subgroup of recurrent unipolar depressive patients who had relatively few relapses."[6] For unipolar patients with family histories of bipolar illness, and for those refractory to other antidepressants, lithium might be considered appropriate treatment.[2]

PROPHYLACTIC TREATMENT FOR BIPOLAR ILLNESS. The efficacy of lithium for preventing future episodes of bipolar illness has been established beyond reasonable doubt. Clinical questions to be considered are when to initiate lithium maintenance, at what dose level, and when to consider its termination. Treatment strategy following prophylaxis failure also requires consideration.

In view of the low therapeutic index for lithium, as well as some question of its nephrotoxic effects after prolonged use, maintenance regimens should not be recommended in all cases. Because most lithium maintenance studies have required that patients have several documented recurrent bipolar episodes within the few years prior to investigation, it is premature to generalize their findings to patients with different illness patterns. Consequently, no clinical guidelines are available regarding how much affective illness is sufficient to justify lithium prophylaxis. The clinician should consider factors such as duration and severity of illness, past frequency of episodes, and probable reliability of the patient with respect to taking medication regularly, reporting side effects, and coming for regular visits for clinical assessment and plasma level monitoring. The decision is best made in consultation with the patient (and family), after the advantages and drawbacks of lithium maintenance have been reviewed together.

In lithium maintenance, dose and plasma levels are somewhat lower than in acute treatment, as noted above. With respect to discontinuation after the patient has remained well for an extended period, there are currently no guidelines. Research data of Quitkin and colleagues suggest that after two or three years of euthymia, discontinuation of lithium may be warranted if the patient and his or her family are receptive to such a plan.[7] These investigators point out that this strategy is, at best, an educated clinical hunch and that further research is required to identify patients with a low risk of relapse following lithium discontinuation. Close, reliable surveillance may be an alternative to chronic lithium administration in suitable cases.

Some patients have depressive episodes on lithium maintenance. The question then becomes whether it is better to discontinue lithium and treat the depressive with tricyclic antidepressants, monoamine oxidase inhibitors, or ECT, or use one of these treatments in conjunction with continued lithium maintenance. Some authorities recommend simultaneous medication, which they regard as at least as effective as an antidepressant alone; after depressive symptoms subside, maintenance lithium can be continued.[6] There are, however, no standard procedures for management of this contingency; further research is indicated to identify optimal management.

Once established, lithium levels generally remain stable so that patients seldom develop adverse drug reactions during maintenance treatment; however, there are some problems to watch for over an extended period. To ascertain the effect of lithium on the kidneys, renal function should be evaluated at least semiannually in patients receiving chronic therapy. Plasma level monitoring is essential throughout. Routine assessment of thyroid function is also recommended by Davis, since lithium has been observed to lower protein bound iodine levels in prolonged treatment.[6] No known major adverse reactions have been reported even with treatment lasting ten to fifteen years; with sustained medical supervision, lithium is regarded as a safe maintenance medication.

LITHIUM PROPHYLAXIS FOR UNIPOLAR DEPRESSIVE DISORDER. Although some research has been conducted to compare the efficacy of lithium and tricyclics in preventing unipolar disorder, there is not yet enough evidence to decide which of the two prophylactic drugs is preferable.[8,6] Baldessarini suggests that lithium is effective in the "prevention of the emergence of recurrent depression," but its use in this context is not routine.[2] Indications include illness patterns with short cycles or infrequent but severe episodes associated with suicide attempts.[3]

ANTIDEPRESSANTS: I. TRICYCLIC ANTIDEPRESSANTS (TCAs)

History and Description

Antidepressants fall into two major categories: tricyclic antidepressants (TCAs) which are closely related to phenothiazines, and monoamine oxidase inhibitors, which will be discussed in the next section. Drugs in the TCA category are those most widely used for the treatment of depression.

The first TCA identified as having antidepressant properties was imipramine, whose efficacy has been equalled but never surpassed by any antidepressant subsequently developed. Imipramine was derived in the 1940s as a modification of chlorpromazine. In 1958, Kuhn (cited in 2) tested it with psychotic patients. Unlike the phenothiazines, imipramine had no effect on psychotic symptoms, but Kuhn noticed that it made depressed schizophrenic patients less depressed. He proceeded to study the drug with depressed patients and established it as an effective antidepressant. Today it remains the standard to which all newer drugs may be compared.

Since 1958, more than a dozen other antidepressants have been developed, and to date about half have been approved by the FDA for the treatment of depression. These include amitriptyline, desipramine, nortriptyline, protriptyline, trimipramine, amoxapine, and doxepin. All are considered interchangeable in terms of their efficacy for depression, although their side effects vary somewhat.

TCAs can be grouped in terms of chemical structure as having one methyl group or two. The former are referred to as secondary amines and include desipramine, nortriptyline, and protriptyline. Those with two methyl groups are referred to as tertiary amines and include imipramine, amitriptyline, doxepin, trimipramine, and clomipramine. The last of these is still classified as an investigational drug. These groups differ in their action on the metabolism of central nervous system neurotransmitters. Tertiary amines are metabolized into secondary amines.

All of the drugs in this category produce little effect other than sedation in people who are not depressed. The tertiary amines tend to have greater sedative properties than the secondary amines, and within this group, amitriptyline and doxepin more so than imipramine.

In addition to these approved drugs, a number of others are in various stages of development and testing. Investigators are trying to develop antidepressants with more rapid onset of action, greater biologic specificity, fewer side effects, and efficacy for patients refractory to available treatments. New and promising drugs include tetracyclic antidepressants such as maprotiline and mianserin, and serotonergic antidepressants such as fluoxetine, zimelidine, and others.[9]

Risks and Risk Management

Overdose of TCAs can be lethal, a major drawback for medication prescribed for depressed and possibly suicidal patients. Even when taken in prescribed doses, both minor and potentially serious medical complications may ensue. Common unpleasant side effects include dry mouth, fatigue, constipation, sweating, tremor, nausea, drowsiness, and insomina, among others. It is important to note, however, that all of these problems are also symptoms of depression, and may have been present before treatment or appear subsequently without being drug related. Nevertheless, TCAs do cause such anticholinergic effects. Extrapyramidal reactions apart from tremor are very rare. The range of side effects is wide, varies only slightly between TCAs, and often inconveniences the patient at least mildly.

More serious are potential cardiovascular effects associated with TCAs, particularly for older patients with pre-existing heart disease. TCAs slow conduction rate and may exacerbate cardiomyopathies and congestive heart failure. Nevertheless, as Kantor *et al.* has demonstrated, TCAs can be used safely for some cardiac patients with careful medical supervision and regular monitoring with serial electrocardiograms and may actually benefit dysrhythmias.[10] In therapeutic doses, TCAs are not associated with cardiac complications in healthy young and middle-aged patients.

TCAs interact with several widely used drugs including alcohol and antihypertensives. Their simultaneous use potentiates the effects (and side effects) of each, so that, for example, patients who use both TCAs and alcohol become intoxicated more quickly and TCA side effects are likely to be enhanced. TCAs alone sometimes induce orthostatic hypotension, so that their use in conjunction with antihypertensive medication can lead to excessive drop in blood pressure. The anticholingeric activity of TCAs makes it important to monitor functioning if they are used together with antiparkinsonian agents, phenothiazines, or other compounds that also have antimuscarinic effects. As a rule, combining antipsychotic and antidepressant drugs requires specific indications.

Finally, TCAs have been known to induce a switch to mania in bipolar patients (discussed elsewhere in relation to lithium treatment) and induce confusional states and delirium, especially in older patients. These drug-related symptoms are sometimes misinterpreted as being illness manifestations and so it is important to recognize their association with medication.

RISK MANAGEMENT. Suicide risk is reduced if only small amounts of medication are dispensed to acutely depressed patients. In cases of overdose, cardiac toxicity is the greatest hazard. Immediate admission to an intensive care unit with equipment for continuous cardiac monitoring, defibrillation, and resuscitation is indicated. With respect to confusional or delirious reactions, the best first step is to stop the antidepressant. Physostigmine salicylate can sometimes alleviate many of the antimuscarinic, cardiotoxic, and neurotoxic features associated with tricyclic overdose. This drug itself can be toxic, however, particularly when large doses are given rapidly, so that its administration by an experienced clinician is indicated. Negative drug interactions are minimized by getting a careful history of other medications and, if their use is necessary, maintaining medical surveillance. Administration of medication before bedtime reduces the discomfort of some of the minor but annoying side effects.

Treatment Applications

Based on cumulative evidence from more than 100 studies, the efficacy of TCAs for the treatment of depressive disorder has been decisively established. The research evidence shows that the response to placebo is between 20% and 40%, and to TCAs about 70%. In other words, about one-third of patients get better without medication, another third are effectively treated with antidepressants, and the remaining third do not respond to them.

TCAs are considered the pharmacologic treatment of choice for patients with major depressive disorders and for patients with approximately equivalent manifestations of anxiety and depression. Their utility has also been demonstrated for patients with panic disorder and agoraphobia. While a great deal remains to be learned about predicting medication response, it seems that patients with endogenous symptoms (e.g., nonreactivity of mood, insomnia, and appetite and weight loss) are most likely to respond to antidepressants, as are those more severely ill. Those who react with depression to life stressors, who have more "neurotic" symptoms and whose depression is chronic and nonphasic are less likely to benefit from TCA medication.

PRETREATMENT EVALUATION. Patients should be given a complete physical examination. A careful history should cover a review of other medications currently prescribed, evidence of substance abuse, prior treatment for depression, and cardiac status.

GUIDELINES FOR PRESCRIBING TCAs. As is true of other drugs, treatment failures are not uncommonly due to the use of insufficient doses for inadequate periods of time. Imipramine and amitriptyline are the two most commonly prescribed TCAs. Initial doses of 50 mg. in a single evening dose may be increased every four days to a maximum level of 300 mg. Dosage increments should be halted at the point of major improvement, even if this occurs at a lower dose level. These levels are higher than the maximum of 200 mg. a day of imipramine for outpatients listed in the Physicians' Desk Reference (PDR) or Goodman and Gilman, but there is no evidence to show that outpatients require lower doses.[11,2] Higher levels are often effective for patients who do not respond to lower doses.

ACUTE AND CONTINUATION TREATMENT. As a rule, treatment with TCAs consists of two phases: acute and continuation. In addition, prophylactic treatment sometimes is indicated. In the acute phase, when the patient is actively symptomatic, medication is prescribed in the doses cited for a minimum of five weeks before it is concluded that the drug is ineffective. Some evidence suggests that amitriptyline is a useful sedative and may be preferable for older, more severely ill patients. After substantial improvement is achieved, medication is usually continued for six months at about half the acute dose level. The rationale is that medication suppresses but does not cure the symptoms, and that the underlying pathophysiology lasts for about this length of time. Patients who are asymptomatic can be seen infrequently during this treatment phase. After six months, a continuation regimen is considered to become prophylactic. While we believe all patients should receive continuation treatment, prophylaxis is indicated only for those with a short cycle length, history of frequent relapse, or previous serious suicide attempts. For patients with bipolar illness, lithium rather than TCAs is usually used prophylactically.

The clinician must make a decision about hospitalization. In general, only patients who are a suicide risk require hospitalization. When uncertain about degree of risk, the absence of adequate family supervision, living alone, drinking, and a history of previous suicide attempts would increase probability of hospitalization. Although many severely ill patients have vague suicidal ideas, we are most concerned about specific plans or marked hopelessness. Otherwise, even severely depressed patients can be treated successfully as outpatients.

ANTIDEPRESSANTS: II. MONOAMINE OXIDASE INHIBITORS

Background and Description

Monoamine oxidase inhibitors (MAOIs) include a heterogeneous group of drugs having in common the ability to block oxidation of monoamines in the brain and various organs. Iproniazid was the first MAOI marketed for the treatment of depression. It was originally developed for the treatment of tuberculosis, and a mood-elevating effect was observed fortuitously. In the 1950s it was found to inhibit the enzyme MAO; in 1957 it was applied in psychiatry to treat depressed patients. Other MAOIs were developed but, because of their toxicity, several, including iproniazid, have been withdrawn from the market. At present, two are widely sold in the United States: phenelzine and tranylcypromine, and a third, isocarboxazid, is available. Pargyline is approved only as an antihypertensive.

There seem to be at least two types of MAO enzyme, and the three drugs in clinical use inhibit both of them. Several selective MAOIs, including deprenyl and clorgyline are investigational drugs now being assessed for clinical efficacy. They are not yet approved by the FDA for the treatment of depression. If safe and effective, they may be preferable to the nonselective MAOIs since they cause fewer side effects.

Since their introduction as antidepressants, MAOIs have been considered less safe and somewhat less effective than TCAs. In the past, they have been used only for patients who have failed to respond to TCAs. Recently, some evidence has been compiled to suggest that patients with a subtype of depressive disorder referred to as neurotic or atypical depression are more likely to respond to MAOIs than to TCAs.[12,13] Such patients do not have endogenous symptoms, but rather oversleep after initial insomnia, overeat, show reversed diurnal mood variation with mood worst in the evening, and have reactivity of mood. If these findings hold up, MAOIs will be increasingly common in clinical practice, since this group of atypical depressives has been estimated to comprise about 30% of depressed outpatients and are not notably responsive to TCAs.

Risks and Risk Management

Use of the first MAOI, iproniazid, was often complicated by liver toxicity and the drug was withdrawn from the market. Modifications were developed including phenelzine. The other widely used MAOI, tranylcypromine, initially was associated with several hypertensive fatalities and also was withdrawn. Once it was learned that dietary restrictions to avoid tyramine intake successfully prevent the development of hypertensive crises, the drug was reintroduced and is now considered safe as long as a tyramine-free diet is maintained. At present, all patients who take MAOIs must follow a tyramine-free diet throughout the duration of this treatment. In addition, they should be taught to recognize early signals of hypertensive crisis such as sudden onset of severe hypertension with palpitations, chest pain, sweating, headache, and related signs. Patients should be instructed to get immediate medical attention, at an emergency room if necessary, and to seek treatment with phentolamine with slow intravenous administration.

Apart from precipitation of hypertensive crises associated with dietary violations, which are best dealt with prophylactically, other side effects of MAOIs include dizziness, orthostatic hypertension, headache, and sometimes, impaired sexual function. Weight gain is a fairly common complaint.

MAOIs interfere with various enzymes in addition to monoamine oxidase, thereby intensifying the effects of other drugs taken simultaneously. This is particularly dangerous in relation to central depressants such as general anesthetics, sedatives, analgesics, antihistamines, and alcohol. Accordingly, patients treated with MAOIs must be warned against the use of any concomitant medication, including dental anesthesia, without explicit clearance by their treating physician. Patients who are not reliable, conscientious, or who for some other reason may not meticulously follow dietary, drug, and alcohol restrictions are not ideal candidates for MAOI treatment. In addition, some authorities do not recommend their use by patients with cardiac disease, hypotension, or who are over age 60, although the grounds for these judgments are not clear.[2]

Treatment Applications

PRETREATMENT EVALUATION. A complete physical examination and psychiatric and medical history are necessary. Patients currently receiving antihypertensive medication are not ideal candidates, nor are those with severe allergies for whom adrenalin may be required. Other criteria for exclusion on medical grounds follow from the drug interaction risks noted above.

PRESCRIPTION OF MAOIs. As noted, TCAs are regarded as the treatment of choice for depression by most practitioners, and MAOIs have been prescribed as the second step following nonresponse to TCAs. In the last several years, however, MAOIs have become more widely used in clinical practice as fears about adverse reactions have been allayed by cumulative favorable research and clinical reports. At this time, some clinicians are beginning to use MAOIs as drugs of choice for "neurotic" or atypical depressives, and those patients, sometimes referred to as hysteroid dysphorics, who abruptly become depressed in response to interpersonal rejection.

The usual starting dose of phenelzine is 15 mg. daily, gradually increasing every three or four days until a maximum of 90 mg. daily is reached, unless a therapeutic response is achieved or toxic side effects occur at a lower level. Some clinicians use a starting dose of 45 mg. daily. Tranylcypromine is prescribed in similar graduated fashion, beginning with 10 mg. daily and increasing to 40-60 mg. A six-week trial is considered adequate if maximum dose level has been given for at least ten days. The antidepressant effect may take two to three weeks to become apparent once a therapeutic dose level is reached.

CHOICE OF MAOI. Phenelzine is sometimes preferred since some clinical reports suggest it is less toxic. On the other hand, some anecdotal evidence suggests that phenelzine is more likely than tranylcypromine to cause weight gain and may thus be unacceptable to some patients. If a patient is taking one MAOI and a change to tranylcypromine is contemplated, a washout period of one week is recommended to prevent negative interactions.

CONTINUATION TREATMENT. The same rationale and procedures described with respect to TCAs apply here. Six months of continuation treatment is considered standard.

COMBINED TCA-MAOI TREATMENT. Although the PDR cautions against combined treatment because of safety considerations, numerous clinical reports suggest that the combination is both useful and feasible in limited situations with careful medical surveillance after nonresponse to other treatments. Apparently, the risk of dangerous adverse reactions, including convulsions, cerebral hemorrhage, and death, are greatest if a TCA is introduced after an MAOI already has been administered. For unknown reasons (perhaps the TCA blockade of tyramine uptake), simultaneous initiation beginning at very low doses of both TCA and MAOI after a drug-free interval lasting at least a week is considerably less hazardous. In such combinations, amitriptyline, imipramine, or doxepin are recommended.[14] As a rule, combined treatment is reserved for patients who fail to respond to either drug separately and for whom electroconvulsive therapy (ECT) is either unsuccessful or unacceptable. Clinicians with limited psychopharmacological experience may choose to refrain from undertaking this form of treatment.

ELECTROCONVULSIVE THERAPY (ECT)

History and Description

Convulsive therapy was first developed as a treatment for mental disorders in 1934 by the Hungarian, L. Mediena; it was modified to use electricity for induction by the Italians, Cerletti and Bini, and by 1939 was accepted in the United States. Initially used as a treatment for schizophrenia, its apparent efficacy led to trials with almost all types of psychiatric disorder. Over time, its effectiveness for depression became widely recognized, while for schizophrenia the results came to be seen as less compelling. At present, severe depressive disorder, almost regardless of subtype, is the principal indication for ECT.[19] As noted by Baldessarini in Goodman and Gilman, "ECT remains the most rapid and effective treatment for severe acute depression and is sometimes lifesaving for acutely suicidal patients."[2] Efficacy is believed to be greatest for patients with the most extreme depression and greatest number of symptoms, particularly those referred to as endogenous (non-responsivity of mood, insomnia, weight loss).

When first introduced, ECT was associated with many medical complications including fractures, cyanosis, panic, and cardiovascular problems. During the 1940s, refinements were introduced to ameliorate these effects. Barbiturate premedication, anesthesia, hyperoxygenation, and muscle relaxants greatly improved the safety of the procedure so that these complications are now very rare. The popularity and use of ECT declined with the introduction of psychotropic drugs in the 1950s, and many ECT facilities were closed. By the mid-1970s, however, as the limitations of antidepressants became recognized, interest in ECT revived.[15] At the same time, both public and professional concern about patient rights, safety, and efficacy led to the establishment of commissions, conferences, legislative regulation, and increased interest in well-designed research. Investigators are now seeking to assess the comparative efficacy of ECT and to develop procedural modifications and improved techniques to augment its safety and to clarify indications for its use.

Today's modified ECT consists of a series of treatments, usually scheduled two or three times a week for a total of six to ten treatments for depressed patients and 25 to 30 for schizophrenic patients.[16] In each treatment, a major seizure lasting at least 25 seconds is induced by passage of an electrical current between two electrodes situated either bilaterally (bitemporally) or, less commonly, both on the same side as the dominant hand. According to current safety standards, an anesthetic agent, muscle relaxant, and oxygen supplementation are introduced before seizure induction. To assure efficacy, muscle convulsive activity or EEG monitoring should be used to ascertain that a therapeutically adequate seizure has been induced.

During the course of treatment, patients may manifest an organic brain syndrome, are hesitant and slowed in response, and have problems in speech and memory. These are characteristic transient accompaniments to ECT that are seen even in optimal treatment conditions.

Risks and Risk Management

With the use of modified ECT, measurable long-term complications are relatively infrequent; adverse reactions are usually limited to transient impairment of memory and new learning ability. Deaths resulting from ECT are very rare and are far outnumbered by suicides among treatment-refractory or untreated depressed patients who do not receive ECT.[3] Minor side effects such as post-seizure confusion and headaches and skin burns at electrode sites are not uncommon.

A major source of risk in unanesthetized patients, now rare, is the phenomenon called a "missed" or "incomplete" seizure in which a current passes between the electrodes without inducing a seizure and its associated amnesia. Patients consequently experience pain, panic, fear, and are often unwilling to continue treatment. Use of anesthesia is an effective prophylactic for this complication. In anesthetized patients, a missed or imcomplete seizure may occur and may go unrecognized unless the seizure is monitored. When recognized, the treatment should be repeated.

Transient recent memory loss is a routine consequence of bilateral ECT, although far less common with right unilateral electrode placement. Those memories acquired during the days preceding a course of ECT may be lost permanently, but others are recovered, usually within a few weeks. Some patients complain about their memory, months and even years later, but pretreatment measures are not available to show that the ECT was the cause.[17] Although investigators have not observed permanent cognitive deficits following ECT, it is conceivable that subtle brain damage may occur, but it is impossible to prove a negative of this sort. Other physiological effects of ECT such as EEG changes, redundancy in speech, changes in language use, and performance on psychomotor tasks improve gradually after the last treatment and are substantially normal after six months.[16]

The risk for long-lasting or permanent impairment of memory and other cognitive functions increases with extended use of ECT. Patients who have received more than 50 treatments have been found to show long-term memory loss and other cognitive impairments. It is difficult to attribute these deficits to ECT, however, since these patients are ill for longer periods, are more severely ill than patients who did not get as much ECT, are refractory to other treatments, and in many cases have received cingulotomy as well as ECT.

Risk of memory loss can be reduced by use of unilateral ECT. Although controlled studies have not found significant differences in clinical response to unilateral and bilateral ECT, some authorities (e.g., Kalinowski) regard the unilateral procedure as less effective, and suggest that more treatments may be necessary to achieve equivalent clinical results.[18]

Spontaneous seizure activity following ECT occasionally has been reported, with an estimated prevalence of 0.5%; this is similar to that of the general population. It is difficult to reconcile the notion that ECT lowers the cerebral threshold for an epileptic focus with the observation that progressively more current is often needed to induce ECT seizures during the course of treatment. A causal relationship between ECT and subsequent seizures has not been demonstrated.

In general, risk management consists of keeping the number and length of treatments to the minimum necessary for clinical improvement. The American Psychiatric Association (APA) Task Force on ECT recommends that no more than fifteen ECT treatments be given to depressed patients in a given series, and that "care, judgment and restraint be exercised before prescribing a second course of ECT within a twelve-month period."[16] Another approach to risk management is the development of refined techniques such as use of pulsed rather than continuous current, and more controlled studies of the relations between treatment intensity, duration, and efficacy.

Informed Consent. ECT is widely known and often feared by members of the general public, including patients and their families. For clinical, ethical, and legal reasons, patients and their relatives should be told about the treatment course in some detail. This discussion should include the nature and severity of the patient's illness; a description of the procedure; the nature, degree, duration, and probability of side effects; reasonable alternative treatments, and why ECT is being recommended instead; the cost; and the right of the patient to refuse treatment or discontinue it at any time. The APA Task Force recommends that the patient and/or close relative or guardian sign a consent form for the procedure in which the duration of the treatment course is specified.

Treatment Applications

PRETREATMENT EVALUATION. Medical and psychiatric histories should be obtained and patients given a complete physical examination with laboratory tests as indicated. The histories should include previous response to anesthesia, orthopedic disease, head trauma, indications of organic brain syndrome, and prior ECT treatments (including the dates). The physical examination should include special attention to cardiovascular, neurologic and orthopedic disorders, and the presence of dentures. The major risk is cardiovascular, both from the anesthesia and the seizure itself. Laboratory procedures often include X-rays, which are useful in demonstrating radiographic abnormalities manifested prior to the proposed ECT.

GUIDELINES FOR PRESCRIPTION. ECT is considered by some the preferable treatment for severely ill, psychotic, and suicidal patients. For others with major depressive or bipolar disorder, ECT should be considered only after nonresponse to an adequate trial of antidepressant medication or lithium.

Neither age nor medical condition is necessarily a contraindication for ECT. It is, in fact, particularly useful for older patients without pre-existing organic impairment, whose cardiac status militates against use of tricyclic antidepressants. ECT may also be preferred to psychotropic drugs for depressed patients with cardiovascular disease, recent myocardial infarction, renal disease, or recent surgery.[19]

Patients with prominent "neurotic" and anxiety symptoms do not respond well to ECT. Diagnostic contraindications include the categories of anxiety, factitious, somatoform, dissociative and adjustment disorders, and those of impulse control. Patients with somatoform disorders are particularly unsuitable for ECT.

There is some disagreement with respect to the use of ECT for schizophrenia. Fink believes that patients with schizophrenia other than catatonic subtype should not be referred for ECT except as a last resort.[19] Kalinowksy, another major authority in the field, is more positive, but acknowledges that there are some schizophrenic patients for whom ECT does not work.[18] The APA Task Force, after reviewing the research evidence, concluded that findings to date are inconclusive, inconsistent, and methodologically flawed. It tentatively suggests that ECT, if used at all for schizophrenic patients, is most useful for those with catatonic or schizo-affective symptoms. In practice, according to a comprehensive survey of APA members, most American psychiatrists use ECT for schizophrenic patients only when they have failed to respond to other treatment modalities.[16]

Once a decision has been reached to use ECT, the major issues concern the choice of bilateral or unilateral electrode placement, number of treatments to administer, whether outpatient treatment should be undertaken, and subsequent management. Proponents of bilateral treatments, such as Abrams and Kalinowsky, argue that unilateral electrode placement is less effective and that more treatments may be required, which increase the dangers and cost.[18] The APA Task Force on ECT, on the other hand, favors the use of unilateral treatment as its members have been persuaded of its therapeutic equivalence to bilateral treatment and the clear advantages in causing far less memory loss and confusion. For most patients, other things equal, unilateral treatment is considered the preferable strategy. Further research is needed to resolve the question.

The number of treatments depends both on the patient's age and clinical response. The guidelines established by the APA Task Force, noted above, are recommended.[16] With respect to site of treatment, hospitalization is sometimes indicated, although for patients with available family members to look after them and a history of successful prior ECT, outpatient treatment is feasible.

Maintenance therapy with antidepressant medication to prevent recurrence of depression is usually prescribed for six months following ECT.[3] Some authorities regard this as a reason not to use ECT for any but medication-refractory patients. Otherwise, it may be argued, the patient will be getting two treatments with different sets of potentially serious side effects which doubles their exposure to risk. Other authorities do not regard this as a valid reason to withhold ECT, especially for severely depressed and delusional patients.

ANTIPSYCHOTIC DRUGS

History and Description

Although lithium was identified earlier as a psychotropic agent, chlorpromazine was the first drug to become widely used for the treatment of mental disorders. After development in the 19th century by the dye industry, it was initially applied in a medical context around 1950 as a potentiator for anesthetic action in surgery. Its sedative and relaxant properties led to clinical use with mental patients and then to its widespread adoption for psychiatric purposes in the mid-1950s. Today chlorpromazine, a member of the phenothiazine chemical class, remains the prototype drug of its kind, equalled but never surpassed by any of the more than 30 antipsychotic drugs subsequently developed.

Antipsychotic drugs, originally called ataractics or major tranquilizers, are also known as neuroleptics. Those currently marketed are all approximately equal in efficacy and vary chiefly in terms of their side effects, which consequently constitute the basis for selecting which one to use in a given case.

Classification of antipsychotic drugs can be based on their chemical structure or on level of potency, which is measured by dose size needed to achieve therapeutic efficacy. FDA-approved antipsychotics belong to five chemical classes: phenothiazines, thioxanthenes, butyrophenones, hydroxyindolones, and dibenzoxazepines. The phenothiazines are further subclassified as aliphatics, paperazines, and piperidyls. Investigational drugs now under development belong to other chemical classes. As noted by Baldessarini in Goodman and Gilman, "The United States has been particularly slow to accept many psychotropic agents that are in common use in Europe."[2]

For practical purposes, categorization by chemical class has proved less useful than grouping based on level of potency with respect to identifying characteristic side effects. Low potency drugs are defined as having a minimum daily dose approximating 300 mg.; high potency drugs are in the 10 mg. to 15 mg. per day minimum range. It has been found that two drugs of the same potency range are more alike in their side effects than are two drugs in the same chemical class. To put it another way, there is as much variation in drug side effects within chemical class as between classes, while for potency groups, between-group differences are greater than within-group differences.

When drugs are classified by potency level, two major clusters of central nervous system side effects are easily identifiable. Low potency drugs such as chlorpromazine, thioridazine (both phenothiazines), and chlorprothixene (a thioxanthene) are more likely to cause sedation and are less likely to induce extrapyramidal effects, while the converse is true for high potency drugs such as haloperidol (a butyprophenone), flupenazine and trifluoperazine (phenothiazines), and thiothixene (thioxanthene). Of the available antipsychotic drugs, thioridazine probably is least likely to induce extrapyramidal effects.

Risks and Risk Management

Antipsychotic drugs induce both central nervous system and peripheral adverse reactions. The CNS effects, alluded to above, include sedation, lowered threshold for seizures, and extrapyramidal side effects such as Parkinson's syndrome, dystonia (uncoördinated, spasmodic body movements, and oculogyric crises), and akathisia (involuntary motor restlessness and pacing). Akinesia is also a common side effect and is frequently unrecognized. In addition, all antipsychotic drugs, regardless of chemical class or potency level, are associated with tardive dyskinesia, which is discussed later in this chapter. Sedation cannot be managed directly, but over a period of days or weeks tolerance develops and the problem diminishes. If there is a known risk for seizures, a high potency drug can be used safely with concomitant anticonvulsant therapy if moderate doses with gradual increments are employed.[2]

With the occasional exception of akathisias, extrapyramidal symptoms are usually controllable with antiparkinson medication such as procyclidine. Accordingly, some clinicians routinely prescribe an antiparkinson agent to all patients on antipsychotics without waiting for symptoms to appear; others do not recommend this procedure until overt symptoms are manifested.[3] If such drugs are prescribed, gradual reduction is often feasible since tolerance for extrapyramidal symptoms commonly develops after about three months.[2] If symptoms prove refractory to antiparkinson medication, dose reduction or switching to another antipsychotic drug is often effective.

In addition to CNS effects, antipsychotic drugs may induce autonomic nervous system reactions such as orthostatic hypotension and annoying symptoms such as dry mouth, nasal congestion, dizziness, nausea, constipation, blurred vision, weight gain, and others. In addition, skin, cardiovascular, ophthalmologic, and other effects may be induced. All of these symptoms are distressing and annoying but are seldom serious.

TARDIVE DYSKINESIA. This neurological syndrome, associated with every class of antipsychotic in current use, is characterized by stereotyped involuntary movements especially of the lips, tongue, and jaw. Its symptoms may be scarcely noticeable or grossly disfiguring. It occurs gradually, can be masked by antipsychotic medication, and persists for varying lengths of time after drug discontinuation. Little is known about its pathophysiology; histological examinations on postmortem reveal no consistent lesion nor is the neurochemistry understood. The syndrome is thought to occur in anywhere from 10% to 40% of patients given antipsychotics for more than one year, but no useful predictors of risk have been identified on the individual level.[20] Analyses of aggregate data show that older age and prolonged drug administration increase risk, but cases of tardive dyskinesia have been described in young people after a few months of treatment. Although rare, cases in children have been reported.[21] Spontaneous remission occurs sooner or later in some cases, but for others (perhaps the majority) the condition is not reversible.[20].

In view of its iatrogenic nature, clinically significant prevalence, occasionally great severity, and lack of satisfactory treatment, tardive dyskinesia constitutes a difficult problem for clinicians and their patients. At present, prevention is the most feasible approach to risk management. This entails conservative prescription with optimal doses that achieve efficacy for the shortest time. This does not rule out high dose prescriptions; indeed, high dose treatment may ultimately reduce risk of tardive dyskinesia by facilitating earlier remission and smaller cumulative dosage.[22] Since schizophrenia is, unfortunately, an illness with recurrent exacerbations, maintenance therapy with antipsychotics is often clinically warranted. Nevertheless, reduced dose levels, drug holidays, use only for patients who clearly respond, and other strategies intended to minimize drug exposure seem reasonable approaches in risk reduction. Drug-free periods, even if only a few days, may reveal early indications of tardive dyskinesia and so facilitate early diagnosis.[4] Special caution is indicated in prolonged use of antipsychotics for patients over age 50.

INFORMED CONSENT. In view of the unavoidable risk of tardive dyskinesia and other side effects, many clinicians believe it advisable to discuss the risks and benefits of antipsychotic drugs with patients and relatives in some detail. Always in research settings and sometimes in private practice, written consent is sought to document the informed consent procedure. After ECT, this is the situation in psychiatric practice that most clearly warrants detailed discussion with patients and family members. This may not be feasible during the acute stage of the illness but is clearly appropriate once maintenance treatment becomes indicated.

DRUG INTERACTIONS. Chlorpromazine was once used to potentiate central depressants; it and other low potency antipsychotics also potentiate sedatives and analgesics, antihistamines, alcohol, and related drugs. This group also blocks the effects of several antihypertensive medications, at the same time directly inducing hypotension so that the combination can cause unpredictable results. Use of more than one antipsychotic at a time is not recommended; increased efficacy has not been demonstrated, the patient is exposed to twice the risk entailed by one drug, and it becomes impossible to identify to which drug the patient is or is not responding.

Treatment Applications

INDICATIONS. Antipsychotics are used primarily for treatment of schizophrenia in incipient, acute, and residual stages; for mania and for other acute psychoses; and for neuropsychiatric disorders including Gilles de la Tourette's syndrome and Huntington's chorea. Multiple controlled clinical trials have established their efficacy for these conditions when used in adequate doses for sufficient periods. Antipsychotics are also preferable to the non-antipsychotic barbiturates because they are rarely lethal even in overdose, are nonaddictive, and because abuse by patients is controlled by the emergence of side effects. They are much more effective than ECT or benzodiazepines for acutely psychotic patients.

Good treatment response is difficult to predict in the individual case. Characteristics often associated with favorable response include good premorbid adjustment and relatively acute illness of brief duration. Schizophrenic patients with a history of childhood associality tend not to improve. Nevertheless, since no other treatment is demonstrably effective with such patients, an antipsychotic drug trial is warranted.

PRETREATMENT EXAMINATION. The usual physical examination and medical and psychiatric history are indicated. For patients with a history of cardiovascular disease, seizures, orthostatic hypotension, or impaired hepatic function, high potency drugs seem preferable.

PRESCRIPTION: ACUTE TREATMENT. The usual strategy in treating acute psychoses is to initiate high-dose medication at frequent intervals in order to rapidly control symptoms of activation disorder. Intramuscular medication is often administered as frequently as hourly in doses of 25 mg. to 100 mg. of a phenothiazine or 5 mg. of haloperidol (or the equivalent of other drugs) until acute symptoms subside. Response within 48 hours is not uncommon, although psychotic signs may persist. Medication is then given orally once a day at lower levels equivalent to at least 300 mg. to 800 mg. of chlorpromazine for the duration of the episode, unless toxicity or clear improvement occurs at lower levels. However, if satisfactory clinical response has not been elicited at the usual ceiling, further dose increases are indicated unless toxicity occurs. This may result in seemingly high doses, but underdose is far more common than overdose and more harmful in the long run. The time course for major response is usually about six to twelve weeks, although incremental improvements may occur for up to six months.[2]

CONTINUATION TREATMENT. Studies have shown repeatedly that among those who respond to antipsychotic drugs, most relapse within six months to a year if treatment is not continued. Consequently, at least six months of maintenance medication is common clinical practice at the lowest dose required to preserve therapeutic gains. At present, one cannot identify those patients who do not need maintenance treatment; it is clearly inappropriate only for patients who showed minimal or no clinical response. Most patients do require maintenance antipsychotic drugs. At the same time, it is recognized that adverse reactions are common, and the risk for tardive dyskinesia mounts with prolonged drug use, especially beyond one year.

CHOICE OF DRUG. High potency drugs are recommended as the treatment of choice for patients with incipient, acute, and chronic schizophrenia.[3] They are preferred by the patient who dislikes sedation, and in many cases, larger equivalent doses can be given before reaching unacceptable levels of side effects. Low potency drugs may be used either when the others fail to elicit a response, when they induce extrapyramidal side effects refractory to antiparkinson drugs, or when insomnia is a significant problem.

ANXIOLYTIC DRUGS

History and Description

Alcohol is perhaps the oldest anxiolytic. In the 19th century, barbiturates and bromides were introduced, but their addictive or toxic side effects led to development of chemical analogs and derivatives such as meprobamate, first marketed in this country in the early 1950s. By the end of the decade, chlordiazepoxide was discovered, and since then a half dozen additional benzodiazepine congeners, including diazepam and flurazepam have been marketed.

Anxiolytics belong to a dozen chemical classes including antihistamines, barbiturates, and alcohol. Because the most effective, safe, and popular drugs in current use belong to the benzodiazepine class, this is the group we focus on.

Anxiolytic drugs are extraordinary in terms of their popularity. In the United States, diazepam has been the single drug most often prescribed for each of the last dozen years and, indeed, is the most widely used prescription drug in the history of medicine.[23] In an international survey of the United States and nine western European countries, from 10% to 17% of adults in each country reported using an antianxiety drug during the preceding year. The figure for the United States is about 15%. Despite concerns about overprescription, use peaked in 1972 and since then has declined by about 20%. The popularity of diazepam continues to far outstrip that of all other anxiolytics.

All benzodiazepines have antianxiety, sedative, and hypnotic properties and, therefore, are sometimes referred to as ASH drugs. They are similar to each other in their neuropharmacologic properties, but vary in the rate at which they are metabolized. For short-acting drugs with rapid metabolism, such as oxazepam, a therapeutic dose is reached in two or three days, and after drug discontinuation it takes about two days for complete washout.

Longer-acting drugs, such as diazepam, take about a week to either accumulate to steady state or dissipate after discontinuation.

Evaluation of the efficacy of anxiolytics is more difficult than that of antipsychotics and antidepressants because anxiolytics are prescribed for a much less well defined patient population, including many with minor illnesses. Disorders for which anxiolytics are prescribed are less clearly defined, regardless of severity, so that amelioration or remission is also hard to define. Nevertheless, cumulative data from over 100 studies make it very clear that the benzodiazepines and related compounds are effective short-term antianxiety agents and are demonstrably superior to placebos, although the size of the difference is not dramatic. According to Rickels, data from controlled studies indicate a level of efficacy of about 35% for placebo, 50% for barbiturates, and 70% for benzodiazepines.[24] Among benzodiazepines, no one has been shown more effective than the others, either in magnitude of effect or spectrum of application. The difference in efficacy between barbiturates and benzodiazepines is probably not clinically significant, but the latter are overwhelmingly safer, being far less addictive and having a much larger ratio of therapeutic to lethal dose. In contrast to the barbiturates, suicide is almost never accomplished with uncomplicated benzodiazepine overdose.

Still experimental, a new chemical class of anxiolytics known as beta blockers (e.g., propranolol) shows promise in attenuating the somatic symptoms that often accompany anxiety. In dose appropriate to the treatment of anxiety, their effect seems attributable to a peripheral rather than central mechanism, affecting the heart rather than the brain. As a result, these drugs relieve difficulties such as palpitations and sweating, but do not decrease worry or tension, which are helped by centrally acting drugs like the benzodiazepines. At higher doses, beta blockers may have clear-cut central nervous system effects and toxic reactions.

Risks and Risk Management

The major risks of antianxiety drugs are associated with their sedative properties. Psychomotor coordination and alertness are reduced to varying degrees; central nervous system effects such as drowsiness, blurred vision, slurred speech, tremor, and hypotension may develop. These reactions are best controlled by careful monitoring of patient reactions and dose adjustment as indicated.

Experts disagree on the question of whether tolerance and addiction develop with anxiolytics. For example, Shapiro reports that they often do; Ayd disagrees; both cite supporting data.[25,26] It does seem that physiological tolerance occurs with high doses for extended periods, and a withdrawal syndrome may develop following abrupt drug discontinuation, although these problems are far less pronounced with benzodiazepines than with barbiturates.[3] In any case, sudden termination of antianxiety drugs is not recommended. Gradual tapering of medication circumvents the emergence of whatever withdrawal symptoms might develop. In the rare instance when they do appear, they are best treated by reinstitution of medication and its slow withdrawal in a supervised setting.

DRUG INTERACTIONS. The sedative property of anxiolytics is potentiated by alcohol and other CNS depressants. The combination can cause severe intoxication and even death, so that patients must be warned of the possible synergism of alcohol or other sedatives while taking anxiolytics. Otherwise, benzodiazepines may be combined with many other medications and are safely used with medically ill and cardiac patients.[2] It is likely that their compatability with so many other medications contributes to their widespread use by nonpsychiatric physicians, which far exceeds their use by psychiatrists.

The benzodiazepines, meprobamate, and phenobarbital are classified as Schedule IV agents under the Federal Comprehensive Drug Abuse Prevention and Control Act of 1970. Prescriptions may be refilled up to five times within six months and must be written by a registered physician who must keep records for at least two years.

Treatment Application

PRETREATMENT EXAMINATION. Apart from the standard physical examination, no special tests are usually indicated prior to prescription of anxiolytics. Patients with impaired liver function should be given small doses; those with severe pulmonary insufficiency should be supervised with care if these drugs are prescribed. A history of substance abuse should alert the practitioner to a greater-than-usual risk of dependence on and possible abuse of anxiolytic drugs.

CLINICAL INDICATIONS. Antianxiety drugs are not intended to alleviate the stresses of everyday living. They should be prescribed only when anxiety is severe enough to interfere with functioning—occupational, family, or interpersonal.

Studies of predictors of response to antianxiety drugs show that the more somatic complaints and anxiety the patient expresses and the sicker he or she is, the greater the improvement.[24] Patients with anticipatory anxiety also respond well. In contrast, the more depressed an anxious patient is, the poorer will be the response. Patients who seem to be equally anxious and depressed generally respond more favorably to antidepressants than to anxiolytics.

Patients with incipient, acute, or resolving psychotic states should not be given anxiolytics since their effects may further erode an already impaired self-control. Their use for chronically anxious patients may be helpful, but no longitudinal data are available to show incremental risk of tolerance over time. Anxiolytics are not indicated as the sole treatment of panic disorder; imipramine is the drug of choice, although the adjunctive use of anxiolytics and psychotherapy is sometimes helpful. Efficacy has not been established in treatment of simple or social phobias; obsessive-compulsive reactions do not respond to anxiolytics.

PRESCRIPTION. Because patients vary widely in their rate of metabolism of anxiolytic drugs, it is best to initiate treatment with a low dose and build up over three or four days. While dosage varies with the individual patient's illness, genetics, and metabolism, the usual therapeutic daily dose of diazepam is 10 mg. to 40 mg. (or the equivalent for other drugs), given in divided doses two to four times a day.

While clinical effect cannot be predicted accurately before treatment is initiated, the probability of final outcome is accurately indicated by degree of improvement obtained after one week of treatment. Rickels has reported that nearly 90% of patients who improve during the first week on anxiolytics show improvement after six weeks, while early nonresponders seldom do well later.[27] In addition, maximum improvement is reached within four to six weeks. In practical terms, if the patient shows no response to an antianxiety drug in the first week, or if level of improvement attained after six weeks is not considered adequate, another treatment modality should be tried.

CONTINUATION TREATMENT. Anxiolytics are usually prescribed for single episodes or intermittent use in accordance with fluctuations in the intensity of anxiety. Some patients, however, may require prolonged medication.[4]

CONCLUDING REMARKS REGARDING SPECIFIC TREATMENT PROCEDURES

The sedative-benzodiazepine-stimulant group of drugs seems to relate primarily to the patient's position on the sedation-vigilance axis. When too vigilant, the patient may also develop insomnia. When too fatigued, the patient may develop difficulties with attention and alertness. This axis cuts across the general diagnostic system, and patients vary within each of the diagnoses. They may be at various times either over-vigilant and anxious, or fatigued with difficulty in attending. Each patient requires review with regard to his or her position on this continuum. For patients in a chronic state of marked anticipatory anxiety, the use of benzodiazepine agents is often useful. Therefore, these data must be gathered as a supplement to the diagnostic considerations. Similarly, information about insomnia is necessary for all diagnostic categories. Transient states of fatigue and exhaustion are usually best treated by rest rather than stimulants.

The major psychotropic agents seem to work primarily upon states of activation and affective dysregulation. It follows that conditions not characterized by this defect should be refractory to these drugs, and this is largely accurate. These drugs are of no value in simple senile and presenile dementias, substance-induced intoxications, factitious disorders, somatization disorder, conversion disorder, dissociative disorders, psychosexual disorders, mental retardation, specific developmental disorders, conduct disorders, eating disorders, speech disorders, and adjustment disorders.

There is considerable doubt whether they are effective in states characterized primarily by anticipatory anxiety, such as social phobia, simple phobia, obsessive-compulsive disorder, generalized anxiety disorder, and their analogues in children.

With regard to personality disorders, there is little substantial information, but those personality disorders that are not characterized by marked emotional lability, rejection sensitivity, or disorders related to separation anxiety seem refractory to the major psychotropic agents.

Information Other Than Diagnosis Needed for Treatment Planning

In this section we focus on the data required for the practitioner to arrive at a sensible treatment plan during his or her initial investigation of the patient's difficulties. Although we will not discuss the practitioner's ongoing review and modification of treatment plans as more about the patient and his or her response to therapy is learned, that is understood to be a core part of the treatment process.

We shall emphasize the specific data particularly relevant to somatic therapy, recognizing that much of what is necessary for the proper treatment planning of somatic therapy is also needed for the proper treatment planning of any sort of therapy, so there is apt to be redundancy with other chapters in this volume.

As a rule, there is no direct correspondence between a DSM-III diagnosis and a specific somatic treatment, although, in general, antipsychotics are considered for schizophrenic disorders; lithium, antidepressants, and ECT for affective disorders; and anxiolytics for anxiety disorders. The fit between standard diagnoses and response to somatic treatment is sufficiently imprecise to warrant the compilation and analysis of several sets of supplementary information. Such data may be considered as moderator variables, operating between diagnosis on the one hand and treatment on the other, and can increase substantially the probability of therapeutic efficacy.

The areas that seem particularly important to review are the following: current symptomatology apart from formal diagnosis, medical history and status, clinical and treatment history, family history, and sociodemographic characteristics and social setting. Each area will be reviewed in turn.

CURRENT SYMPTOMATOLOGY

Even within DSM-III diagnostic categories, symptoms may differ considerably, both in type and severity. For example, some patients with a diagnosis of major depressive episode may have insomnia, while others sleep excessively; some display psychomotor agitation, while others show retardation. The presence of suicidal ideation or an expressed sense of helplessness, regardless of diagnostic category, must be taken into account in treatment planning. Such variations in clinical picture may influence choice of drug class, type of drug within class, mode of administration, dose of medication, and treatment site. Illustrations of each of these clinical issues are presented in turn.

CHOICE OF DRUG CLASS. At the onset of an acute manic episode, patients may be treated effectively with lithium, chlorpromazine, or heloperidol, none of which is clearly superior to the others in terms of the available research evidence. The diagnosis does not automatically lead to use of one or the other drug; the decision is determined by degree of the patient's agitation, excitement, belligerence, sleep disruption, and disturbance of food and liquid intake. If the patient is not sleeping and not eating, lithium treatment should be deferred until biological processes (e.g., electrolyte balance, sodium level) are stabilized.

Another example is seen in the treatment of patients who are both anxious and depressed. This is a common combination, and is often seen by nonpsychiatric physicians in patients with medical illnesses or impending surgery. Although there has been a tendency to first try benzodiazepines for such patients, it is now recognized that for those who seem equally anxious and depressed, or in whom depressive symptoms predominate, tricyclic antidepressants are the treatment of choice.[27]

CHOICE OF DRUG WITHIN CLASS. In most instances, choice of drug class is fairly straightforward. Within class, even when efficacy is equivalent (which is usually the case), side effects and sedative properties tend to vary and thus serve as determinants of drug choice. An example is seen in the choice of antipsychotic neuroleptic for patients with a DSM-III diagnosis of schizophrenia. High-potency drugs, such as haloperidol, are less soporific and are, therefore, often preferred by patients who object to sedation. Low-potency drugs, such as thioridazine, are indicated when high-potency drugs induce extrapyramidal side effects refractory to antiparkinson treatment. Refractory insomnia is also an indication for chlorpromazine or another antipsychotic with sedative properties.

A similar option exists in selecting antidepressants. Patients with insomnia may fare better with tertiary amine tricyclics, among which amitriptyline and doxepin have greater sedative properties than imipramine.

ROUTE OF ADMINISTRATION. Although, particularly in Europe, some antidepressants have been given intramuscularly, in the United States this mode of administration is almost exclusively confined to anti-psychotics. Injectable medication should be used only when there are clear-cut indications, because there is somewhat greater risk of hypotension. Intravenous administration is more hazardous than intramuscular because of the risk of periphlebitis and severe hypotension, and, therefore, is not generally used.[25]

Injectable medication may consist either of the standard dose, in which case only the route of administration differs, or it may be long-acting, as in the case of fluphenazine decanoate or enanthate. Standard dose injectable medication is preferred in crisis situations (e.g., mania or acute schizophrenia) when rapid pharmacological response is sought. Depot medication is recommended for long-term maintenance treatment when there is a question about patient compliance with daily oral doses. Injectable medication is also appropriate for delusional patients who believe that the medicine is "poison," or for those with nausea, vomiting, catatonia, or other conditions precluding oral administration.

DOSAGE. Initial dose, rate and size of dose increment, and maximum dose level depend not so much on diagnosis as stage and severity of illness. Maintenance doses, prescribed after at least partial symptom amelioration, are usually half or less the dosages given during acute illness.

In an effort to improve response rates of schizophrenic patients to antipsychotic drugs, some doctors have used extremely high doses of these drugs with both acute and chronic patients. For example, instead of the usual dose of 300 mg. to 800 mg. daily of chlorpromazine, megadoses up to 2,000 mg. daily have been given to chronic schizophrenic patients with remarkably good tolerance but mixed therapeutic results.[2] Large doses, frequently administered, seem more clearly useful for the rapid control of agitated psychotic episodes. It is not yet established whether such treatment more rapidly reverses delusional states or simply provides rapid symptomatic relief without altering the time to cognitive recovery.

HOSPITALIZATION. Except for acute mania, there are no diagnostic classifications that almost always mandate hospitalization. The three major clinical justifications for inpatient care are to protect the patient (e.g., the suicidal), to protect others (e.g., the belligerently assaultive psychotic patient), or to provide necessary medical supervision and care (e.g., the elderly, depressed patient with cardiovascular disease). These indications cut across diagnostic categories and may include patients with schizophrenia, schizo-affective and affective disorders, as well as acute organic and other conditions.

In addition to these clinical indications, the decision to hospitalize is often influenced by social contingencies (e.g., geographical proximity to a hospital or nature of insurance coverage) and treatment considerations (e.g., use of investigational drugs or drug combinations). These issues are considered elsewhere in the chapter.

Hospitalization has the advantages of providing maximal protection and medical supervision. Its drawbacks include the possibility of stigma for the discharged patient who seeks to resume a normal life in the community, and discontinuities of psychiatric care and clinical supervision, which is not uncommon after discharge.

MEDICAL HISTORY AND MEDICAL STATUS

All psychiatric patients, whether or not they are to receive somatic treatment, should have a detailed medical workup with appropriate laboratory investigation of any detected abnormalities. If prescription of psychotropic medication or ECT is contemplated, such an evaluation becomes essential in view of the many reported negative interactions with medical conditions and drugs prescribed to treat them. The presence of such conditions does not automatically rule out somatic treatment, but requires careful assessment of the risk-benefit ratio and closely supervised care if such treatment is undertaken.

Psychiatric and behavioral symptoms may reflect dysfunction of brain mechanisms and may arise from causes either external to the brain (as in toxic states, infections, anoxia) or central to it (head trauma, organic brain syndromes such as Alzheimer's Disease). In this context, a detailed history of physical illnesses and trauma is extremely useful. When there is a question or evidence of organic impairment, neurological consultation and psychological testing for presence and extent of brain dysfunction are indicated.

In patients who may receive somatic treatments, special consideration should be given to those conditions that may affect the safety of treatment; cardiovascular, renal, hematological, hepatic, and metabolic functions warrant particular attention. Considering the range of toxic effects of neuroleptics, TCAs, and MAOIs, the examining physician should consider the presence of cardiac decompensation, arrhythmia, conduction defects, hypertension or hypotension, renal disease, and any metabolic disorders which may affect speed of drug clearance.

For patients who may be considered for ECT, additional questions must be answered in anticipation of the use of anesthesia. These include the history of porphyria (intolerance of barbiturates), genetic cholinesterase deficiency, severe liver dysfunction or malnutrition (inability to metabolize succinylcholine), and glaucoma (ocular hypertension with atropine).

Because of the possibility of negative interactions with other medications and medical conditions, a complete enumeration of current medications should be elicited from the patient and, if possible, any treating physician. Psychotropic drugs can interact with those prescribed for medical conditions with potentially grave consequences. For example, if patients are treated pharmacologically for both depression and hypertension and neither physician is aware of the other's treatment, the medication prescribed for each may cause orthostatic hypotension and their cumulative effect can be dangerous. Another example is the interaction found between cimetidine and diazepam. Even brief use of cimetidine significantly decreases the total clearance of diazepam leading to higher plasma concentrations, thus increasing the intensity of side effects.[28]

Psychotropic medications may also aggravate existing medical conditions apart from the medications used to treat them. Both TCAs and phenothiazines lower the threshold for major convulsions and, therefore, epileptic patients so treated require particularly close supervision. Both of these drug classes also may exacerbate preexisting glaucoma because of their anticholinergic effects, so again, close monitoring and appropriate consultation are indicated.

Overall, for both therapeutic and legal reasons, a meticulous medical workup, backed up where possible with medical records from other physicians and institutions, is a prerequisite to the initiation of somatic treatment for psychiatric disorder.

CLINICAL HISTORY

This area of inquiry is a key determinant in treatment planning, providing guidelines in the setting of reasonable therapeutic goals as well as effective means of achieving them. Issues included here are developmental history, premorbid social adjustment, prior psychiatric illnesses, and previous treatment experiences.

In general, it is helpful to use a structured form or checklist to cover these areas. Without systematic procedures it is too easy to miss large areas of potential relevance. A specific checklist for note-taking is an aid to the novice and a useful reminder to the experienced clinician. Such an outline need not be gone through in any mechanical order, but by the end of the assessment, all areas should have been covered.

Developmental History

A developmental history should cover childhood behavioral patterns, rate of growth and maturation, school performance, and family and social relationships. Inquiries should be made regarding developmental variables sometimes referred to as "behavioral soft signs" that are thought to have diagnostic and prognostic implications. They include low birth weight, difficult birth history, delay in reaching developmental milestones, speech peculiarities, childhood hyperactivity, clumsiness, inability to develop simple athletic skills, learning problems, and temper tantrums. While the presence of one or two of these variables is not necessarily significant, their cumulative presence may suggest a substratum of neurological impairment that would influence the formulation of treatment goals and methods.

Several patterns of childhood behavior have been related to adult psychopathology, and their identification may have prognostic and, therefore, treatment implications. Clinging, demanding, fearful, and separation-anxious behavior has been noted as a precursor of panic disorder. Impulsive, destructive, hyperactive, and antisocial behavior manifested before the age of fifteen is required for a diagnosis of antisocial personality disorder.

Childhood behavior is also a necessary component of diagnosis of a subtype of schizophrenic disorder known as Schizophrenia with Premorbid Asociality (SPA), which is not specified in DSM-III, but which is regarded by Quitkin, Klein, and their colleagues as a separate subtype with distinctive etiologic and prognostic features.[39,7] Diagnosis rests on the presence of grossly impaired social functioning in childhood, together with the presence of a cluster of behavioral soft signs indicative of mild neurological deficit. As children, SPA patients utterly fail to establish friendships of any kind with other children, are not only isolated but characteristically are actively rejected and scapegoated by their peers. They usually attend regular schools and are not given psychiatric treatment in childhood, but become manifestly psychotic in late adolescence or early adulthood. In this subtype, childhood history is an essential component in diagnosis, which modulates expectations of both therapist and family.

Premorbid Adjustment

In the foregoing example, impaired childhood social adjustment is a necessary feature in the diagnosis of SPA. More generally, premorbid adjustment has been regarded as a crucial dimension in diagnosis and treatment, particularly for schizophrenic disorders. In fact, one of the earlier and more widely accepted approaches to the subtyping of schizophrenia was based on the distinction between good and poor premorbid functioning, which overlaps with the process-reactive distinction. Both of these classifications are primarily concerned with predicting course and outcome and, indeed, level of premorbid functioning is one of the strongest predictors of future functioning yet identified. Among these measures, that of premorbid social adjustment "appears to be the most powerful predictor of outcome."[29] More specifically, the best predictor of future work function is premorbid work function, and degree of social recovery is related to the level achieved before illness onset.

Effective somatic therapies restore patients to the level of functioning preceding the particular illness episode for which they are being treated. Acuteness of onset may obscure the chronicity of the psychopathology. In such instances, restoration to former level of functioning is not equivalent to cure. This perspective is essential for adequate treatment planning concerning aftercare and provision of ancillary therapeutic, training, or support services.

Some information about premorbid adjustment is furnished by Axis V of the DSM-III multiaxial classification, which provides an assessment of highest level of adaptive functioning during the past year. This is intended to be a composite rating of three areas: social relations, occupational functioning, and use of leisure time. The composite score is expressed as one of six possible levels of overall functioning. For patients who were functioning effectively and whose current illness began during the year being evaluated, this rating provides the necessary information. For others whose current episode has lasted longer than one year, the Axis V rating does not describe premorbid functioning. In these cases, additional information from the patient or family members will be necessary.

Psychiatric History

Meticulous elucidation of previous psychiatric difficulties and illness episodes, both untreated and treated, is essential for treatment planning. While some information of this nature must be gathered in order to make certain DSM-III diagnoses to begin with (e.g., bipolar disorders), a more detailed history is indicated for treatment planning. It is useful to learn about the nature of onset, course, and resolution of previous episodes, as well as related circumstances and coping mechanisms used by the patient and his or her family. Also of interest are the symptoms previously manifested and the order of their appearance.

The importance of knowing the sequence of symptom manifestations is illustrated by patients who abuse or are dependent on alcohol and may have a history of untreated psychiatric illness. For example, it has been reported that up to one-third of patients at alcoholism treatment facilities may have experienced panic attacks or disabling phobias that they self-medicated with alcohol. Apparently, it is not uncommon for patients who experience acute anxiety or panic attacks to use alcohol, hoping to alleviate both the attacks themselves and the anticipatory anxiety that develops in relation to fears of their recurrence. The alcohol may be useful in alleviating the anticipatory anxiety but is utterly ineffective for the panic attacks. In a futile effort to get relief, they drink more and eventually the signs and symptoms of alcohol abuse become more obvious clinically than those of the panic disorder which, in this context, may be misdiagnosed as alcohol withdrawal signs.

A similar progression has been reported with respect to posttraumatic stress disorder (PTSD) and alcoholism. Drinking initially relieves the symptoms of PTSD (especially the recurrent nightmares, which are a core feature) since alcohol usually suppresses dreaming sleep, but tolerance develops, leading to increased alcohol use. Attempts to reduce drinking can lead to withdrawal symptoms that resemble and even exacerbate the initial PTSD symptoms, culminating in resumption of alcohol use and abuse. One must note the sequence of symptoms in order to unravel the clinical picture and to select primary treatment targets. In the former example, one might choose to treat the panic disorder with imipramine as an initial strategy before addressing the alcoholism. In the latter, pharmacologic or other treatment of the PTSD may lead to spontaneous reduction in alcohol use or abuse. Although there currently are no established pharmacological indications for PTSD, some preliminary data suggest that MAOIs may be useful, particularly if spontaneous panics occur.

It is useful to inquire about possible precipitants associated with the onset of current and past illness episodes and coping mechanisms and solutions attempted outside of formal treatment. Some data about precipitants are furnished by Axis IV of DSM-III, which provides an assessment of overall severity of psychosocial stress experienced in the year preceding diagnosis. Axis IV provides a seven-point rating scale and also gives the clinician an opportunity to note the specific stressor experienced. As noted in DSM-III, the rationale for Axis IV is that if the stressors are still present, treatment planning must help the patient change them or adjust to them. In addition, prognosis is sometimes seen as more favorable if illness develops as a consequence of marked stress, although clear-cut evidence on this point has not been established.

The relationship between stressors and psychiatric illness remains elusive despite the efforts of many investigators. It is generally agreed that life events experienced in the course of ordinary living may play some role as precipitants of illness onset, especially in the case of affective disorders. There is some evidence to suggest that stressful life events may also influence the course and outcome of illness even if they do not have an etiological role. It also seems established that stressors do not alone cause psychiatric illness in otherwise intact people, unless they are of catastrophic intensity or duration, such as concentration camp or prisoner of war experiences. There seems rather to be a reciprocal relation between stress and vulnerability; milder stressors precipitate illness more readily in those with greater genetic or other predispositions to illness.[30] The only syndromes in DSM-III in which a causal relationship is assumed between stress and illness are that of PTSD, which in DSM-II had been classified under "transient situational disturbances," and Brief Reactive Psychosis. The DSM-III definition of precipitant for both syndromes refers to a "traumatic event that is generally outside the range of usual human experience," thus excluding such life events as bereavement, going away to school, or job loss.

The patient's previous efforts to cope with illness, either in the current episode or an earlier one, are of interest in treatment planning. It is seldom the case that someone goes directly to a psychiatrist without first attempting other solutions. Even if these efforts were ultimately unsuccessful, as is evidently the case at least for the current episode, they may provide leads regarding potentially available ancillary resources.

Treatment History

Perhaps the most immediately useful material the patient can supply is a detailed description of previous treatment, including nature of response or lack of response. In addition to the patient's report, records of all previous care should be obtained, if possible. Reactions to somatic therapies are of particular interest. As a rule, medication that was previously successful for a comparable illness episode is the treatment of choice for the current episode. The same reasoning applies to ECT. Patients usually respond to successive courses of ECT as they did earlier (barring changes in cerebral function), both in type of response, number of treatments, and stability. Patients with good responses to prior courses of ECT should be considered for ECT, unlike those who failed previously to respond to a complete course of treatment.

While a report of past positive drug response is generally valid and can be accepted at face value, reports of negative outcome do not necessarily mean that the medication previously used should be disqualified from consideration in the current episode. While previous negative experiences may actually indicate that the medication is not useful for a particular patient, it is also possible that the drug was prescribed incorrectly or the patient's compliance was inadequate. Unfortunately, it is not uncommon to find that presumably appropriate medication fails because it was prescribed at levels high enough to elicit side effects but insufficient to attain a therapeutic level, or else the trial was too brief to assess the drug's efficacy. A third possibility is that the wrong medication was chosen as, for example, the prescription of benzodiazepines for panic disorder or for patients who are equally anxious and depressed.

If the correct drug was prescribed at appropriate dose levels for a sufficient period of time and the patient failed to respond, it is possible that he or she did not take the medication as directed. In this context, both the patient and family members must be interviewed in order to assess the degree of the patient's cooperation with taking prescribed medication. Often patients do not accurately report what happened. Simply asking the patient whether he or she took the medication regularly will not suffice; patients may say they took their medication regularly and by this mean only once a week. One should ask specific questions such as how many pills were taken how many times a day. Further, patients often report that they had bad reactions to certain drugs or were allergic to them. This is often an inaccurate representation of the facts and detailed reviews are necessary to avoid discarding potentially useful interventions. It is also possible that adverse drug reactions did occur that could be modified with suitable ancillary treatment. For example, acute extrapyramidal reactions in response to antipsychotics can be offset by simultaneous prescription of anticholinergic agents.

If the correct drug was prescribed at suitable doses, and the patient followed the regimen correctly, had a diagnosis compatible with a specific drug benefit but reported a reliable history of refractoriness, one other consideration may be relevant. The diagnosis must then be reviewed with particular emphasis on the possibility of histrionic personality disorder or malingering.

Finally, one should determine the nature of the patient's past experience with drugs having addictive potential as well as any history of drug dependence and alcoholism. Anxiolytics should be used cautiously, if at all, in patients with such a history.[25]

In summary, identification of previously effective treatment for a similar illness episode would indicate its use in the present. On the other hand, prescription of medication of a similar class to medications that have already failed is only occasionally useful. Apart from probable lack of efficacy and delay in relieving the patient's symptoms, there is the problem of further demoralization and loss of hope by the patient who experiences multiple ineffective therapeutic trials.

Family History

In view of increasingly persuasive evidence of familial or genetic patterns of illness, a family history of psychiatric disorder is often useful. Diagnostic and prognostically relevant information may be generated by a knowledge of illness in relatives and the nature of their clinical response to specific somatic therapies if they were treated.

Family histories are usually sought for first degree relatives: parents, siblings, and offspring. Illness in more distant relatives is also of interest, but has not been obtained systematically in most genetic research to date. The easiest way to find out about family illness is to ask the patient and one biologic relative. Since this leads to errors in the direction of underreporting, more accurate data are obtained from individual interviews with all available family members. Because of problems of patient and relative consent, cost and time, this is not a feasible strategy for clinical purposes and can be difficult even in a research setting. As a rule, the patient's report, if backed up by that of a relative, usually yields enough information to be useful.

Schizophrenia was the first major psychiatric syndrome in which a genetic component was convincingly established. Twin and adoption studies, conducted since the late 1960s, have been able to separate the effects of heredity and environment. It is now believed that risk for schizophrenia is about 50% to 60% if one has an identical twin with schizophrenia, about 40% if both parents are schizophrenic, and about 15% if one parent is so diagnosed.

In view of these distributions, investigators do not hypothesize that there is a schizophrenia gene, but rather an inherited vulnerability or predisposition that presumably interacts with psychosocial or other environmental factors to produce illness in some individuals. Quite certainly, if nearly half of all twin pairs studied have been found discordant for schizophrenia, factors other than genetic transmissions are implicated.

Another syndrome widely regarded as having a clear-cut familial or genetic component is bipolar disorder, as noted in DSM-III. Even if a patient's only illness is depression, a bipolar diagnosis may be suspected if there is a family history of bipolar illness. The biological substratum of this syndrome is suggested not only by the nature of the symptoms themselves, but by the remarkable success of lithium in its treatment.

Other syndromes and symptoms that run in families and seem to be either genetically or socially transmitted include alcoholism, antisocial personality, and suicide. A family history of suicide has specific and immediate implications for patient care, especially if the current episode is one of depression. Preliminary evidence suggests that some subtypes of anxiety disorder such as agoraphobia may also be more common in relatives of patients than in the general population, but further evidence is required on this point.

With the possible exception of bipolar disorder, family history is not customarily considered in arriving at a diagnosis. One group of investigators, however, has developed a classification of depressive subtypes based entirely on such data. Schlesser and his colleagues have delineated three subtypes of unipolar depressive disorder based on the presence and type of psychiatric disorder found among first degree relatives.[31] Based on small samples, these investigators have tentatively identified differential responses to medical and variations in neuroendocrine characteristics. If these findings are substantiated, then family history will prove to have major significance in treatment planning beyond that already recognized.

Family histories can provide an additional dimension with respect to the patient's and relatives' assets as well as their individual and collective pathology. Patients interviewed when ill may be unable to appraise realistically their abilities and strengths when well, while relatives can provide this perspective. They can also present their own positive strengths, their attempts to cope with the patient and help him deal with the illness.

SOCIODEMOGRAPHIC CHARACTERISTICS AND SOCIAL SETTING

Age; sex; marital status; family composition; educational, occupational and social status; personal and familial resources; and current life circumstances together provide a picture of the patient and his or her world that is indispensable in the selection of treatment strategies. While no evidence has been provided to show that drugs or ECT act differentially in a biologic sense for patients with varying sociodemographic and family characteristics, with the possible exception of age, such variables should influence formulation of treatment goals and methods.

Sociodemographic Characteristics

Age alone is not considered an automatic contraindication for any somatic treatment, especially for adults in the 18-65 range. As a rule, however, clinicians tend to be more conservative in their use of ECT at the lower end of the range, and the cardiovascular effects of antidepressant medications require more rigorous preliminary medical checks and closer medical supervision for older patients. Recent evidence shows a nonlinear association between age and risk for tardive dyskinesia among patients taking neuroleptic drugs. Up to, but not beyond, age 70 there is a strong correlation between older age and both the prevalence and severity of tardive dyskinesia, as well as reduced likelihood of spontaneous remission. Caution, therefore, is indicated in the prolonged use of neuroleptics in patients over age 50. In addition, there are some tentative indications of differential efficacy in relation to age within certain drug classes. For example, amitriptyline seems more effective than imipramine for older patients, independent of illness severity, although this remains to be substantiated.

Studies of predictors of drug efficacy suggest that women, older patients, and those with higher educational and social status and greater personal and family resources show greater improvement. These factors may actually only predict patient cooperation in following drug regimens which, of course, is an essential aspect of efficacy.

Social and Financial Resources

These resources govern access to different treatment options. It has long been acknowledged that in the United States there are two distinct and largely nonoverlapping mental health systems—for those with less and those with more. As a rule, patients with fewer resources go to public facilities and are treated by less experienced and less trained staff. While such a system at first seems quite unjust, there is, in fact, no decisive evidence that these factors substantially influence treatment outcome and future health status. Indeed, a college student who makes a serious suicide attempt may be hospitalized for one or two years at a private mental hospital where he or she is treated with intensive psychotherapy alone after the first month of recuperation. In contrast, another student whose family cannot afford to pay $100,000 annually (few insurance companies cover as much as this) may be treated with medication as an outpatient after medical recovery from the suicide attempt, thereby facilitating earlier resumption of social ties and educational career. There are no data to show that the first patient is less likely to make another suicide attempt than the second. There are, however, data to show that prolonged interruptions of schooling and friendships can create massive psychosocial problems so that long-term hospitalization is seldom seen as the strategy of choice.[32, 33] In such a case, social advantage may not constitute a health advantage.

Another example is access to ECT. In the past, among patients with psychotic depressions, the rich were more likely to be offered psychoanalysis and the poor given ECT. Civil libertarians were effective in changing legal and administrative procedures to restrict the use of ECT in public institutions at the same time that scientists were showing its efficacy in severely depressed patients refractory to medication. Now we have the curious reversal where ECT is largely available to the rich and is withheld from the poor.

While social and financial resources are not necessarily always a guarantee of access to the best available treatment, it is certainly clear that they govern the options available for treatment planning. Consequently, knowledge of the patient's finances and insurance coverage are necessary for realistic strategies regarding the feasibility of private care, hospitalization, length of stay, and choice of practitioner. Higher fees are charged by psychiatrists than other mental health professionals, and in the case of psychotropic medication, nonmedical personnel cannot deliver equal services since they cannot prescribe. On the other hand, since somatic treatments may require far fewer visits for shorter periods of time, the total cost is lower in most cases than for psychotherapy. These factors must be considered before effective and economical treatment recommendations can be made.

Current Life Circumstances

Family composition, marital status, occupation, organizational affiliations, and social and financial resources affect treatment planning in the sense that they reflect the patient's current living arrangements, life style, and social network. Especially with more seriously ill patients, the entire design of treatment may be contingent on the availability of sympathetic relatives or friends to support the patient before medication becomes effective, to supervise medication compliance and doctor visits, to report adverse drug reactions or illness exacerbations, and to provide supervision and guidance during acute episodes. Except for frankly suicidal or acutely manic patients for whom hospitalization is nearly always indicated, the presence or absence of close relatives, friends, religious advisors, or other competent, caring people may be the determining factor in making custodial arrangements. Close, continuous observation and companionship are necessary for the patient's morale and protection during the customary two- to three-week drug lag, and become critical when either drug reactions or illness symptoms may impair the patient's judgment. For example, one of the early signs of lithium toxicity is clouding of consciousness so that the patient may not be able to recognize the need to seek immediate medical care. On the other hand, patients entering a manic episode see no reason to get psychiatric treatment, and such a determination becomes the responsibility of concerned others.

Knowledge of a patient's job and the significance of income for the family's functioning may influence decisions not only about hospitalization, but sometimes other treatment strategies. For example, ECT often requires time off from work, while antidepressant medication usually does not. The decision to discontinue lithium after a period of well-being would also be influenced by the degree of disruption, both financial and social, that might ensue if an illness episode were thus precipitated.

In general, life circumstances, social supports, and family composition influence the clinician's willingness to treat patients on an outpatient basis, to use medications that entail risk of major adverse reactions, or, in the case of treatment refractory patients, to use unusual medication or treatment combinations that have higher probabilities of benefits as well as greater risks.

Procedures Used to Obtain Data

INTERVIEWS

In the preceding section, the clinical, family, and social data regarded as useful in treatment planning were briefly outlined. This material comes from three sources: medical and psychiatric records, interviews with patients and relatives, and laboratory data. Although occasionally unavailable, medical records and patient and family interviews are highly valuable. Every effort should be made to include them in gathering information to formulate a treatment plan, particularly when the patient is acutely ill. Laboratory tests as they presently exist are useful to the practitioner in circumscribed areas to address particular questions, rather than as blanket prerequisites.

PATIENT INTERVIEW. The patient can often provide extensive information about his or her past life, history of prior illness and treatment, circumstances associated with the onset of the current episode, and the reasons for seeking psychiatric help. Gathering this detailed information should be considered a step preliminary to the actual start of therapy; the practitioner should not be dissuaded from inquiries that the patient might think unrelated to the presenting complaint. In fact, patients often regard a thorough historical interview as a reflection of professionalism on the doctor's part. More than one session may be required to cover all the material; where feasible, a single two- to three-hour intake evaluation may provide enough time and has the advantage of not delaying the start of treatment.

Relative Interviews. Patients may not accurately portray either their current illness or previous level of functioning, errors that relatives usually can correct. For example, patients who are currently depressed may recall nothing but a life of unremitting pain and misery, whereas relatives may recall years of intact functioning and report strengths and abilities useful in long-term planning. Patients may either exaggerate or minimize their assets so that external corroboration is helpful.

Often the patient is unable to describe what is good about his or her family and their past efforts to help the patient cope with the illness. Interviewing relatives also may illuminate the patient's long-term family role and the extent to which he or she resembles other family members. Inquiries regarding relatives' reasons for having the patient seek treatment and the treatment goals they seek are also useful. Sometimes they differ considerably from what the patient or therapist have in mind, and these discrepancies are best dealt with early.

Relatives are valuable reporters and offer helpful aids regarding the patient's current illness and response to treatment over time. After their initial interviews, relatives should be contacted regularly for additional information and exchange during the acute illness episode. The option of seeing relatives together with the patient, rather than separately, should be considered as a frequently useful strategy.

BIOLOGIC TESTS

Plasma Drug Levels. After medication has been initiated, the practitioner may wish to consider the utility of monitoring drug levels that presumably are related to treatment effect. With the exception of lithium treatment, in which plasma levels must be measured because of the small difference between therapeutic and toxic doses, this is not done routinely because the nature of the correspondence between blood level, drug dose, and clinical response requires further study. With respect to antipsychotics, the available evidence does not indicate a systematic relationship between plasma levels and response. Measures of plasma level of MAOIs are still being developed and do not yet have clinical utility.

More of a case can be made for measuring levels of TCAs and anxiolytics, although here, too, the evidence of a correlation between plasma level and clinical outcome is inconclusive. In view of these considerations, regular monitoring of plasma drug level is not indicated, but a plasma level determination may be useful for the depressed or anxious patient who fails to respond to high doses of medication during a trial of adequate duration.[3] In elderly patients or those with pre-existing heart disease, monitoring of the TCA plasma level may increase the safety of drug treatment and, thus, extend its benefits to higher-risk patients who might otherwise not be considered eligible for such treatment.[34]

NEUROENDOCRINE TESTS FOR DEPRESSION. Exciting leads have been generated by the identification of specific deviant neuroendocrine responses in patients during illness episodes. For example, eighteen hours after administration of an oral dose of the synthetic steroid dexamethasone, investigators have discovered that a sizeable number of patients with endogenous depressive disorder (melancholia) have higher plasma cortisol levels than normals, whose cortisol levels are "suppressed" by the ingestion of dexamethasone. This abnormality is related to changes in circadian cortisol secretion in depressed patients, and both are manifestations of abnormal hypothalamic-pituitary-adrenal regulation in depressed patients.[35] The dexamethasone suppression test identifies very few "false positives" in the sense that almost all nonsuppressors are indeed depressives; however, many depressed patients are "false negatives" in that they do not fail to suppress cortisol output after dexamethasone administration.[36]

Another provocative finding is that depressed patients may show an abnormal response to the hormone TRH (thyrotropin-releasing hormone), which ordinarily stimulates secretion of the hormone TSH (thyroid-stimulating hormone). In some depressed patients, the TSH response is diminished. These and other tests may some day provide laboratory measures of specific forms of psychopathology in the same way that urine tests can signify the presence of diabetes. At the present time, these tests are not clinically useful in routine practice and their application in treatment planning is not indicated. Nevertheless, this is a rapidly developing area, and the potential for such objective diagnostic tests is great.

Clinical Vignette

ASSESSMENT

The authors of chapters on each of the major treatment modalities were requested to address the question of how they would evaluate the specific patient presented in the clinical vignette in the introductory chapter by the editors. The vignette was made brief in order to provide them flexibility in demonstrating the specific type of information required for their evaluation and treatment planning. Of course, well-trained clinicians, regardless of therapeutic specialty, should show many more similarities than differences in these processes. Simply because one is an expert in a particular treatment modality does not mean that procedures used for patient evaluation must differ significantly from those of an expert in another area of treatment specialization. Presumably all who use DSM-III's multiaxial design are concerned with the patient's present clinical status, medical history and status, prior illness and treatment history, family history and current social setting, recent stressors, and premorbid functioning. Well-trained clinicians will draw upon the available auxiliary sources of information such as medical records, relatives' reports, and feedback from previous therapists when available. Finally, we would expect clinicians of any persuasion to integrate such information, arrive at a diagnosis, and formulate a treatment plan consistent with the patient's illness and the patient's resources.

Axis I: Current Clinical Status

The Axis I diagnosis signifies a first episode of major depressive disorder. Areas we would seek to clarify include:

1) timing of illness onset
2) presence of psychosis
3) manifestations of suicidal thoughts, hopelessness, and demoralization
4) elaboration of clinical symptoms

The brief clinical vignette did not clearly state when the patient first became depressed. The clinician would need to learn whether or not there had been previous milder periods of depression that triggered subsequent events, rather than being reactive to them. For example, the patient indicated that his marriage had been "worsening for several years." Possibly previous mild depressive intervals rendered him emotionally unavailable to his wife, which, in turn, may have provoked her angry self-distancing. It would be important to learn whether or not this is indeed a first episode or a recurrent affective disorder; the latter would subsequently raise the issue of prophylactic medication.

The thorough diagnostician would require substantiation of some of the patient's statements. A good example would be the conclusion that there was an absence of psychotic features. Psychotic features are frequently denied or minimized by patients, and often can only be evaluated on the basis of interviews with informed relatives and associates. Without this supplemental material, it would be premature to conclude that there were no psychotic features. Similarly, suicidal ideation might be denied by the patient even when present.

Suicidal preoccupations, feelings of hopelessness, and demoralization are important issues to assess in treatment planning for depressed patients. There is increasing evidence that hopelessness rather than depressed mood is a reliable predictor of suicidal behavior. Since hopelessness often appears with depression, the latter traditionally has been regarded as an index of suicide risk, but when the variable of hopelessness is controlled, this relationship is no longer significant. It is, therefore, necessary to separately assess the patient's sense of hopelessness—the feeling that his situation is irremediable and will never improve.

It is stated that the patient has "recurrent thoughts of death without, however, suicidal ideation"; details of these recurrent thoughts are crucial. Are they thoughts such as, "My wife would be better off without me. I will always be an intolerable burden to her"? Such thoughts are not specifically suicidal but entail both hopelessness and a potential for self destruction.

Demoralization is another frequent accompaniment of depression, but unlike suicidal thoughts and hopelessness, it is not largely restricted to depressive illness. It is not itself a manifestation of mood disorder, but a secondary reaction provoked by the sense of helplessness and hopelessness that are depressive features. As Jerome Frank noted years ago, it is probably demoralization rather than specific symptomatology that leads people to seek psychiatric treatment.

When demoralization is pervasive and severe, the patient may be unlikely to comply with any treatment plan, so that the clinician must be prepared to address this problem at the outset of any therapeutic efforts. Further, demoralization is not alleviated by tricyclics, as are core depressive symptoms, and must be addressed separately.

Feelings of hopelessness and suicidal ideation generally signify the need for hospitalization for the patient's protection. To some degree, this decision depends upon the extent of supervision that can be provided by the family. The wife in this case is described as helpless under stress and, therefore, is unlikely to be a useful resource in patient management. Again, it is important to ascertain whether this is the patient's description of his wife or whether it has been validated by direct evaluation. Depressed patients are not the most reliable informants with regard to their own or other peoples' level of competency. Therefore, the decision to hospitalize in this context is best reached after consultation with the wife, as well as more detailed assessment of risk.

More details about symptomatic features would have to be secured to establish the diagnosis of Melancholia (a fifth digit indication of the presence of a typically severe form of depression, elsewhere referred to as "endogenous" or "endogenomorphic"). In making the diagnosis of Melancholia, the essential feature is autonomy of mood (lack of responsivity to pleasant events). Associated features include terminal insomnia, weight loss, diurnal mood variation with mood worst in the morning, distinct quality of mood, psychomotor agitation or retardation, and excessive guilt. For purposes of treatment planning, identification of this characteristic symptom configuration is significant since, as noted in DSM-III, melancholia "is particularly responsible to somatic therapy" (p. 205).

Axis II: Personality Disorders

A diagnosis of compulsive personality disorder is provided. As noted earlier, depressed patients frequently are poor reporters. They may exaggerate and magnify aspects of their personality in a self-derogatory way. If depressed patients report that in their usual state they are unable to express warm and tender emotions, are insensitive to the feelings of others, are controlling, demanding, and unpleasant to deal with—all this may be true. On the other hand, it may be a depressive exaggeration of a moderate degree of emotional reserve. Once more, information from other informants is needed.

An important aspect of compulsive personality disorder is the quality of indecisiveness. This is described in DSM-III as avoidance, postponement, or protracted efforts at decision-making due to fear of making a mistake, and is listed as an essential feature of the disorder. The diagnostician assesses this type of behavior both to confirm the Axis II diagnosis and to modify the treatment plan.

Axis III: Medical Disorders

It is stated that physical, laboratory, and neurological studies were negative, but it is necessary to know the specific studies that were performed. Without knowing this, it is difficult to rule out various possibilities. For example, what was the degree and kind of thyroid workup? It is not unusual for patients with subclinical hypothyroidism to develop major depressive episodes. The list of medical illnesses that can generate depressive episodes is quite lengthy (see Table 1), and none can be ruled out without knowing that an appropriate test had been conducted. With the information provided, we simply have to assume that the statement regarding Axis III is correct.

In addition to the utility of medical tests for diagnostic purposes, detailed information about cardiovascular, pulmonary, renal, and hepatic functioning is needed to assess the feasibility of planning a course of treatment that includes drugs. As indicated earlier in our review of specific drugs, medical illnesses seldom constitute absolute contraindications for psychotropic drugs, but there are clear hazards in certain contexts that then require careful determination of risks and benefits and close medical surveillance, possibly in an inpatient setting, if pharmacotherapy is initiated in such cases.

Axis IV: Stressors

The marital difficulties described in the vignette are seen as constituting "moderate" psychosocial stress on Axis IV. As we speculated earlier, these difficulties may have been a response to rather than precipitant of the patient's depressive illness if, in fact, it had its onset more than six weeks prior. In the literature on stress and

TABLE 1
MEDICAL ILLNESSES THAT FREQUENTLY INDUCE DEPRESSION[37]

Pernicious anemia	Hyperaldosteronism
Folic acid deficiency	Addison's disease
Multiple sclerosis	Hyperparathyroidism
Influenza	Hypoparathyroidism
Viral hepatitis	Hyperthyroidism
Cirrhosis	Hypothyrodism
Uremia	Acromegaly
Disseminated carcinomatosis	Systemic lupus erythematosus
Oat-cell carcinoma of the lung	Ulcerative colitis
Lymphomas	Regional enteritis
Chronic myelogenous leukemia	Whipple's disease
Carcinoma of the pancreas	Amyloidosis
Cushing's disease	

illness, it has long been recognized that marital and other problems are as likely to be consequences of illness as factors contributing to its onset. Other possible sources of stress in the patient's recent experiences also warrant review; areas often considered in this context include role entrances and exits, changes in employment, health and family relations, legal and financial events, and so forth. The cumulative impact of concurrent stressors is often greater than their effects, if temporally separated, so that enumeration and timing of occurrences are worth noting. In addition, available social supports warrant assessment, since such resources may modify the impact of potential stressors.

In general, Axis IV constitutes an area of inquiry that needs considerable additional elucidation beyond that provided by the vignette, both to better understand precipitating factors and to formulate an effective treatment plan.

Axis V: Adaptive Functioning

The patient's highest level of adaptive functioning in the previous year is described as "fair." This rating is defined as signifying "moderate impairment in either social relations or occupational functioning or some impairment in both" (DSM-III, p. 29). For this rating, the clinician would require details indicating some impairment in either of these areas. Even if one accepts the Axis II diagnosis of Compulsive Personality Disorder, this does not necessarily signify social or occupational impairment unless it is shown how the compulsive personality interferes with adaptive functioning.

The comparatively poor level of functioning in an episode of only six weeks duration reported for this patient might point to the probability that the present illness is not the first one of this nature. Additional past history might support our conjecture that he has a recurrent affective disorder.

This estimation of functioning is useful in structuring goals when the treatment plan consists of somatic therapy since such treatment is expected only to restore the patient to his former level of functioning rather than to elevate his behavior to a level of competence not previously attained. Given this rating, one's expectations would be relatively modest.

TREATMENT PLAN

If we accept the multiaxial diagnostic classification provided in the vignette, we consider the treatments of choice to be antidepressant drugs or ECT. If the subtype of Melancholia is established, there would be no question. Even with Major Depressive Disorders, we prefer this approach to psychotherapy, because the superiority of psychotherapy of any variety over psychotropic medication for patients with Major Depressive Disorder has not been shown (Smith, Glass, & Miller, 1980), and superior efficiency in terms of treatment duration and cost of drugs over psychotherapy is demonstrable.[38]

In view of these considerations, we would refer the patient either to a private practitioner experienced in psychopharmacology or, if he can't afford private treatment, to an appropriate clinic where drug treatment is offered.

As noted earlier in the chapter, there are many antidepressant drugs and little evidence for the superiority of any particular one. The class of MAOIs is generally considered to be less effective or, at least, no more effective than tricyclic medications for patients with this type of symptomatology (including weight loss, insomnia, and generalized loss of interest in usual activities). MAOIs are also more difficult to use because of the dietary restriction they require, so that a TCA should be tried first. (Recently several new antidepressants such as maprotiline and trazodone, which technically are not tricyclic drugs, have been released, but their relative advantages and disadvantages have not yet been clearly established.)

When treatment involves medication, the patient and his or her relatives require education regarding the prognosis and probable complete reversibility of the condition, the need for adequate dosage, the time lag of several weeks until medication becomes effective, common side effects and their anticipated duration, and the need for regular contact with the doctor to assure proper monitoring of the patient's clinical condition and medication management. In the case at hand, this information should be shared with both the patient and his wife, and the wife's aid enlisted in assuring that her husband complies with the treatment regimen. After these issues are thoroughly clarified and a medication plan is formulated, ongoing contact usually can be maintained by weekly visits, with telephone calls as needed. The need for psychotherapy is best assessed after the mood disorder has improved.

If the patient does not respond positively to medication after four weeks at an adequate dose level, determination of drug plasma level may be useful, especially if imipramine has been prescribed, since for this drug a therapeutic minimum has been established for patients with endogenous depressive disorder (Melancholia). If the patient's plasma level falls below this minimum, dosage should be increased. If the level falls within the therapeutic range, treatment with another class of antidepressant drugs is indicated.*

A second, and on rare occasion, third class of antidepressant drugs may have to be tried before improvement is established. Once accomplished, we recommend drug maintenance until full clinical remission, and then treatment for another six months at a reduced dose (often half that prescribed during the acute illness phase). This strategy is based on the premise that medication controls symptoms

*Other biological tests and family history are of interest but are not treatment determining since false negatives frequently occur. Even if all available biological tests were negative, as was the family history, one would still treat as indicated above.

but does not alter the underlying phasic course, which typically lasts about six months.

ECT is also a safe and effective form of treatment. It is, however, common practice to defer the use of ECT until it has been shown that the patient is refractory to an adequate course of antidepressant medication. This treatment sequence is especially reasonable if the patient does *not* manifest psychotic or suicidal tendencies.

References

1. Lewis, A.: *The State of Psychiatry*, New York: Science House, 1976.
2. Baldessarini, R. J.: Drugs and the Treatment of Psychiatric Disorders, in L. S. Goodman, and A. Gilman (eds.), *The Pharmacological Basis of Therapeutics*, 6th edition, New York: Macmillan, 1980, pp. 391-447.
3. Klein, D. F., Gittelman, R., Quitkin, F., and Rifkin, A.: *Diagnosis and Drug Treatment of Psychiatric Disorders*, 2nd edition, Baltimore: Williams & Wilkins, 1980.
4. *AMA Drug Evaluations*, 3rd edition, Littleton, Mass.: Publishing Sciences Group, Inc., 1977.
5. National Institute of Mental Health, *Lithium in the Treatment of Mood Disorders*, DHEW Publication No. (ADM) 77-73, Washington, D.C.: Government Printing Office, 1977.
6. Davis, J.: Overview: Maintenance Therapy in Psychiatry: II. Affective Disorders, *American Journal of Psychiatry*, 133:1-13, 1976, p. 6
7. Quitkin, F., Kane, J., and Rifkin, A.: Prophylactic Lithium With and Without Imipramine for Bipolar Patients: A Double-blind Study, *Archives of General Psychiatry*, in press.
8. Quitkin, F., Rifkin, A., and Kane, J.: The Prophylactic Effect of Lithium and Imipramine in Bipolar II and Unipolar Patients: A Preliminary Report, *Psychopharmacology Bulletin*, 15:35-39, 1979.
9. Feighner, J. P.: Pharmacology: New Antidepressants, *Psychiatric Annals*, 10:388-394, September, 1980.
10. Kantor, S., Glassman, A., Bigger, J., Perel, J., and Giardena, E.: The Cardiac Effects of Therapeutic Plasma Concentrations of Imipramine, *American Journal of Psychiatry*, 135:534-537, 1978.
11. *Physicians' Desk Reference*, 34th edition, Oradell, New Jersey: Medical Economics Co., 1980.
12. Quitkin, F., Rifkin, A., and Klein, D.: Monoamine Oxidase Inhibitors: A Review of Antidepressant Effectiveness, *Archives of General Psychiatry*, 36:749-760, 1979.

13. Quitkin, F.: Comparison of Monoamine Oxidase Inhibitors and Tricyclic Antidepressants in the Treatment of Atypical Depressive Disorder. Paper presented at Psychiatric Research Society, Boston, September, 1980.
14. White, K., and Simpson, G.: *Combined MAOI-Tricyclic Antidepressant Treatment: A Reevaluation*, Report to the American College of Neuropsychopharmacology, October, 1980.
15. Comeback for Shock Therapy? *Time*, November 19, 1979, p. 76.
16. American Psychiatric Association Task Force on Electroconvulsive Therapy, *Electroconvulsive Therapy*, Task Force Report 14, Washington: American Psychiatric Association, September, 1978.
17. Freeman, C. P., and Kendell, R. E.: ECT: I. Patient's Experiences and Attitudes, *British Journal of Psychiatry*, 137:8-16, 1981.
18. McDonald, M.: ECT: Lothar Kalinowsky Remembers, *Psychiatric News*, 13:1, 8-11, May 5, 1978.
19. Fink, M.: *Convulsive Therapy: Theory and Practice*, New York: Raven Press, 1979.
20. American Psychiatric Association, *Task Force Report on Late Neurological Effects of Antipsychotic Drugs*, Washington, D.C.: American Psychiatric Association, 1980.
21. Petty, L. K., and Spar, C. J.: Haloperiodol-Induced Tardive Dyskinesia in a 10-Year-Old Girl, *American Journal of Psychiatry*, 137:745-746, 1980.
22. Davis, John M.: Overview: Maintenance Therapy in Psychiatry: I. Schizophrenia, *American Journal of Psychiatry*, 132:1237-1245, 1975.
23. Hollister, L. E.: A Look at the Issues. Benzodiazepines 1980: Current Update, *Psychosomatics*, 21 (supplement):4-8, 1980.
24. Rickels, K.: Clinical Comparisons, Benzodiazepines 1980: Current Update, *Psychosomatics*, 21 (supplement): 15-20, 1980.
25. Shapiro, A. K.: Psychochemotherapy, in G. Grenell, and S. Gabay, (eds.), *Biological Foundations of Psychiatry*, New York: Raven, 1976, pp. 793-835.
26. Ayd, F. J.: Social Issues: Misuse and Abuse, Benzodiazepines 1980: Current Update, *Psychosomatics*, 21 (supplement):21-25, 1980.
27. Rickels, D.: Benzodiazepines: Use and Misuse, in D. F. Klein, and J. G. Rabkin, (eds.), *Anxiety: New Research and Changing Conceptions*, New York: Raven Press, in press 1981.
28. Klotz, U., and Reimann, I.: Delayed Clearance of Diazepam Due to Cimetidine, *New England Journal of Medicine*, 302:1012-14, 1980.
29. Carpenter, W., and Stephens, J. H.: Attempted Integration of Information Relevant to Schizophrenic Subtypes, *Schizophrenia Bulletin*, 5(3):490-508, 1979.
30. Rabkin, J. G., and Struening, E. L.: Life Events, Stress and Illness, *Science*, 194:1013-1020, 1976.
31. Schlesser, M., Winokur, G., and Sherman, B.: Hypothalamic-Pituitary-Adrenal Axis Activity in Depressive Illness, *Archives of General Psychiatry*, 37:737-743, 1980.
32. Glick, I., and Hargreaves, W.: *Psychiatric Hospital Treatment for the 1980s*, Lexington, Mass.: Heath and Co., 1979.

33. Bachrach, L.: *Deinstitutionalization: An Analytic Review and Sociological Perspective*, DHEW Public. No. (ADM) 76-351, Washington, D.C.: Government Printing Office, 1976.
34. Smith, R., Chojnacki, M., Hu, R., and Mann, E.: Cardiovascular Effects of Therapeutic Doses of Tricyclic Antidepressants: Importance of Blood Level Monitoring, *Journal of Clinical Psychiatry*, 41:57-63, 1980.
35. Frazer, A.: Biological Aspects of Mania and Depression, in A. Frazer, and A. Winokur, (eds.), *Biological Bases of Psychiatric Disorders*. New York: Spectrum, p. 219, 1977.
36. Carroll, B. J.: Clinical Applications of the Dexamethasone Suppression Test, *International Drug Therapy Newsletter*, 16:1-4, January, 1981.
37. Hall, R. C., Ed.: *Psychiatric Presentations of Medical Illness*, New York: SP Medical and Scientific Books, p. 38, 1980.
38. Smith, M., Glass, G., and Miller, T.: *The Benefits of Psychotherapy*, Baltimore: Johns Hopkins University Press, 1980.
39. Quitkin, F. M., Rifkin, A., and Klein, D. F.: Neurologic Soft Signs in Schizophrenia and Character Disorders, *Archives of General Psychiatry*, 33:845-853, 1976.

Chapter Four

Treatment Evaluation and Behavior Therapy

C. Barr Taylor, M.D.
Robert P. Liberman, M.D.
W. Stewart Agras, M.D.
David H. Barlow, Ph.D.
George E. Bigelow, Ph.D.
Donna M. Gelfand, Ph.D.
A. John Rush, M.D.
Linda C. Sobell, Ph.D.
Mark B. Sobell, Ph.D.

Introduction and Theoretical Premises

Behavior therapy is best conceptualized as an emergent, applied, clinical science standing on a theoretical and operational foundation that clarifies the interrelationships between the environment and various dimensions of biology and behavior.

Assessment and treatment are inextricably interwoven in the practice of behavior therapy. First and foremost, behavior therapy is an empirical approach to the understanding and treatment of clinical problems. Accordingly, a firm and systematic adherence to specification and measurement is the distinguishing characteristic of behavioral practitioners. Behavior therapy is not a cookbook filled with treatment recipes. With regular assessment of the various levels and modes of human behavior, a self-correcting feedback loop generates new and improved methods for helping individual patients and populations of patients with designated disorders. Behavior therapists encourage their patients to take an active role in modifying their environments and cognitive processes. Behavior, biology, and the environment influence each other in reciprocal ways; hence, the individual functions as both an agent and the target of behavior change.

While there are numerous historical influences and antecedents, the origins of contemporary behavior therapy and the growth of operant conditioning in the United States can be traced to three researchers in the early 1950s: Wolpe's introduction of important therapy techniques, Eysenck's proposal of learning-based treatment methods as an empirical alternative to psychotherapy, and Skinner's demonstrations of experimental control and prediction by principles of operant conditioning and their extension to personal and social problems.[1,2] Skinner's *Science and Human Behavior* reconceptualized emotional problems and psychotherapy in behavioral terms.[3] He considered psychotherapy an educative process and recognized behavior as important in its own right, instead of merely reflecting more basic, underlying processes. Since Skinner and his associates had demonstrated in many elegant animal experiments that behavior could be controlled by environmental influences, extrapolating these environmental-behavioral relationships to humans was logical.

But operant conditioning, as developed by Skinner, represents only one set of learning mechanisms. In 1959, Eysenck defined behavior therapy as the application of modern learning theory to treat psychiatric disorders, basing his formulation on four modern learning theorists—Pavlov, Hull, Mowrer, and Skinner.[4,5,6,7,3] He criticized psychotherapy as unsuccessful and lacking proof of efficacy and considered that symptoms were learned through empirically verifiable processes and did not require abstract constructs such as unconscious motives to explain them.

At the same time, Wolpe introduced systematic desensitization, a technique applicable to many other behavioral procedures and still in use today.[8] He demonstrated that principles derived from learning theory could be translated into specific clinical techniques that were effective for many anxiety disorders. Adherents of the various "schools" of learning theories may have differed in assumptions about how learning occurs, but all shared a commitment to experimental methods and stressed the importance of evaluating the therapeutic outcome of their methods.

In the following two decades, behavior therapy expanded in many directions, embracing a variety of techniques and theories. Four major trends are clear: applied behavioral analysis, social learning theory, cognitive behavior therapy, and behavioral medicine.

The first trend, applied behavioral analysis, arose as a systematic method of applying and studying the clinical and social effects of operant techniques. It assumes that behavior is a function of its antecedents and consequences and utilizes a variety of innovative methods. One example is the experimental study of single cases wherein patients serve as their own controls to demonstrate the effectiveness of techniques based on reinforcement, extinction, punishment, stimulus control, and other learning techniques to modify certain behaviors.

In social learning theory, a second direction in modern behavior therapy, Bandura describes interactive regulatory systems that affect responses.[9] These systems include behavioral, cognitive, and environmental ones. Social learning theory focuses on the person as the agent of change. Cognitive processes are used to explain how learning experiences have lasting effects and serve to activate future actions. An individual's perceived self-efficacy to perform a given task is viewed as the critical variable for future performance. The individual's self-efficacy judgments are based on four sources of information: performance accomplishments, verbal persuasion and allied types of social influence, vicarious experiences of observing the performance of others, and states of physiological arousal. Bandura maintains that the first of these, performance accomplishments, is usually the most influential source of efficacy information: successes raise, and failures lower, efficacy appraisals. Vicarious experience is another important source of efficacy judgments. Many individuals judge their ability to perform a task based on watching others. Verbal persuasion is a primary characteristic of traditional psychotherapy and placebo responses. Finally, individuals may use emotional arousal to assess their capabilities in a particular situation. One therapeutic technique that has been derived from social learning theory is participant modeling.

Cognitive behavior therapy is a third direction that behavior therapy has taken in recent years. These therapeutic techniques attempt to identify cognitive processes that influence behavior and serve as intervening variables between environmental stimuli and responses of the individual. Cognitive behavior therapy approaches derive in part from Ellis, Lazarus, Eysenck, and Wolpe, who include "private events" such as thoughts, sensations, imagery, and other covert processes within the proper domain of learning theory.[10,11,4,8] Cognitive behavior therapy assumes that clinical disorders are the result of maladaptive or faulty thought patterns. The task of therapy is to identify these thought patterns and replace them with more adaptive ones, assuming that it is not behavior per se that determines future behavior, but the person's perception of that behavior. A variety of techniques have been developed to change cognitive processes. These include cognitive restructuring as developed by Ellis, which aims to confront and alter the patient's irrational ideas that contribute to dysfunction, and self-instructional training, as expounded by Meichenbaum, in which individuals learn to verbalize self-instructions of a more adaptive nature.[12] Another technique is cognitive therapy for depression, as developed by Beck, which includes a variety of therapist maneuvers and behavioral tasks designed to restructure or reinforce new thought patterns.[13]

The fourth direction behavior therapy has taken is behavioral medicine, defined as the interdisciplinary field concerned with the development and integration of behavioral and biomedical sciences, knowledge and techniques relevant to the understanding of health and illness, and the application of this knowledge and these techniques to prevention, diagnosis, treatment, and rehabilitation.[14]

A broad scope of problems has been addressed by behavioral medicine. The field includes studies on changing the pathophysiology of organic illnesses, reorganizing psychosomatic wards to include token economy principles, increasing percentage of clinic visits kept, humanizing treatment facilities, and changing entire communities through media combined with limited face-to-face intervention.

THEORETICAL PREMISES

Despite the diversity of views and broad range of procedures included under the umbrella of modern behavior therapy, a common core of assumptions is identifiable. The basic tenets of behavior therapy include the concept that behavioral disorders are determined by current events in the social and personal environment to a much larger extent than formerly believed. Thus, while the historical development of a psychiatric problem is of interest to the behaviorally-oriented clinician, the major focus in evaluation is upon the definition of the presenting problem and the current interpersonal and intrapersonal influences on that problem.

A precise definition of the presenting problem is important, since the aims of therapy are thereby clarified and its outcome can be monitored. The presenting problem needs to be defined operationally so it can be observed or monitored by the patient and others. Once the problem has been defined, the events surrounding and contributing to it can be investigated. Careful investigation, including direct observations of the problem behaviors, either *in vivo* or in a clinical laboratory setting, is often required to understand the subtle determinants of a given behavior. Cognitive events influencing the behavior of interest should also be carefully defined and taken into account when planning treatment.

Some of the major assumptions underlying behavior therapy are outlined in the following summary:[1]

1) Abnormal behavior that is not a result of specific brain dysfunction or biochemical disturbance is assumed to be governed by the same principles that regulate normal behavior. Even deviant behavior stemming from biological disturbances can be affected by environmental influences.

2) Many types of abnormal behavior formerly regarded as illnesses in themselves or as signs and symptoms of illness are better construed as nonpathological "problems" of living (examples include neurotic reactions, various forms of sexual deviance, and conduct disorders).

3) Most abnormal behavior is assumed to be acquired and maintained in the same manner as normal behavior and can be treated through the application of behavioral procedures.

4) Behavioral assessment focuses on the current determinants of behavior rather than the post hoc analysis of possible historical antecedents.

5) Specificity is the hallmark of behavioral assessment and treatment, and it is assumed that the person is best understood and described by what he or she does in a particular situation.

6) Treatment requires a fine-grain analysis of the problem into components or subparts and is targeted at these components specifically and systematically.

7) Treatment strategies are individually tailored to different problems in different individuals.

8) Understanding the development of a psychological problem is not essential for producing behavior change; conversely, success in changing a problem behavior does not imply knowledge about its etiology.

9) Since behavior change occurs in a specific social context, therapeutic interventions may result in side effects, i.e., changes in behaviors that were not the focus of treatment. These are not necessarily deleterious effects or a product of "symptom substitution." More often than not, these broader treatment effects are positive outcomes.

10) Behavior therapy involves a commitment to an applied science approach. This includes the following characteristics:

- an explicit, testable conceptual framework
- treatment that is either derived from, or at least consistent with, the content and method of experimental-clinical psychology
- therapeutic techniques that can be described with sufficient precision to be measured objectively and be replicated
- the experimental evaluation of treatment methods and concepts

Specific Behavioral Procedures

Specific treatment techniques used in behavior therapy derive from experimentally validated principles that describe how people learn and how human behavior changes. Other techniques have developed through serendipity, creative experimentation, trial-and-error tinkering, and "packaging" a group of techniques. Whether derived from existing learning theories or "synthesized" more inductively, the emphasis and criterion for developing new techniques has been on their demonstrated effectiveness. Thus, the term "technical eclecticism" has been used to describe the practice of behavior therapists.[11,15]

Before describing some of the commonly used behavioral procedures, it should be noted that newer and more effective or efficient behavior techniques are continuously being developed. While systematic desensitization and aversion therapy were two principal techniques used by behavior therapists a decade ago, they are now overshadowed by newer methods such as exposure *in vivo*, overcorrection, contingency, contracting, covert sensitization, anxiety management training, social skills training, and biofeedback. Behavioral techniques can be organized into those aimed at increasing the frequency of or strengthening adaptive, appropriate, and "healthy" behavioral repertoires and those aimed at reducing the frequency of or weakening maladaptive, symptomatic, and deviant behaviors. Most clinical problems and disorders are treated with a combination or "package" of techniques. For example, deficits in social competence and skills are treated or trained with instructions, modeling, reinforcement, shaping, and behavioral rehearsal. Sexual dysfunction is treated by instructions, counterconditioning, relaxation, graded *in vivo* assignments with reinforced practice, and desensitization.

One way to classify the multitude of behavioral techniques and interventions is to place them in temporal context with the problem behavior or clinical syndrome. Some interventions are introduced before the problem behavior occurs and some are applied afterward. Therapeutic instructions, relaxation, and modeling are offered before the patient engages in the problem behavior, while reinforcement, biofeedback, and covert sensitization are given after the behavior of interest has occurred. Table 1 lists some of the more common behavior procedures.

BEHAVIORAL ANTECEDENTS

Respondent or classical conditioning refers to the process in which learning occurs by repeated associations of an environmental event and a behavior, usually visceral or autonomic. Extinction of a con-

TABLE 1
GENERAL BEHAVIOR THERAPY PROCEDURES

Behavioral Antecedents
Respondent conditioning
Stimulus control
Fading
Therapeutic instructions
Self-instructions
Modeling
Behavioral Consequences
Positive reinforcement
Negative reinforcement
Shaping
Self-reinforcement
Reinforcement of autonomic responses
Extinction
Aversive procedures
Information feedback
Self-monitoring
Therapist feedback
Biofeedback

ditioned response occurs if the conditioned stimulus is presented a number of times without being followed by the unconditioned stimulus. Many conditioned responses may be alleviated when the unconditioned stimulus is changed. For instance, improved interpersonal communication may result in less blood pressure reactivity in hypertensive subjects. Conditioning techniques are, however, more often used to produce a new response.

Since behavior is controlled by a variety of antecedents, therapists may use a variety of discriminative stimuli to change behavior. Problem behaviors can be altered by a procedure known as "fading," where one discriminative stimulus is slowly eliminated as another is introduced. This has been done in training pedophiles to prefer mature, adult sexual partners.

Therapeutic instructions and the rationale the therapist gives to the patient about the therapy can be viewed as a set of discriminative stimuli. Therapeutic instructions, including patient expectation, treatment credibility, and other so-called nonspecific effects, have major impact on behavior change. Self-instruction or what people say to themselves is also an important source of behavior change.

Finally, many people learn by imitation (or modeling). Modeling is one of the techniques most frequently used to induce behavior change. Subjects can observe both a modeled behavior and its consequences, describe it verbally, or practice the behavior, which then comes under the control of its consequences.

BEHAVIORAL CONSEQUENCES

Positive reinforcement refers to both a procedure and an effect in which the behavior of interest leads to an environmental consequence and is thereby more likely to occur in the future. Attention and concern from significant others is the most common form of positive reinforcement that maintains symptomatic behavior. While in traditional psychiatric parlance, attention and solicitude have been termed "secondary gain," these reinforcers are primary and potent from the behavior therapist's point of view. Negative behavior occurs when the behavior of interest enables the individual to escape from or avoid some noxious environmental consequence. Hence, the phobic's fear and avoidance and the obsessive's compulsive rituals are all negatively reinforced by virtue of a symptomatic behavior being successful in temporarily reducing anxiety and discomfort. The term "reinforcement," whether positive or negative, always refers to a learning or maintenance situation where the behavior of interest is being increased in frequency or strengthened in form by the contingent environmental consequences. Social reinforcement, or attention from others, is most often the reason for symptomatic behavior being maintained, even when it is ego-dystonic and burdensome.

Punishment reduces the likelihood of a behavior on which it is contingent occurring in the future. Thus, an individual's fledgling efforts at expressing feelings may be stifled by criticism or ridicule coming from a relative, friend, or boss. Unassertive people with a constricted range of emotional expression often have histories of being "punished" for incipient attempts at self-affirmation; however, they may also have failed to develop assertiveness by growing up in a household where relatives were unassertive and reserved. Many sexual inhibitions and problems, now being treated at sex therapy clinics, are the result of past and present punishment. Punishment is not defined by the perceived quality of the environmental event as it is in the vernacular. Rather, it is defined by the suppressant effects it has on the associated behavior. Many negative emotional responses issued by significant others—such as anger, arguments, or spankings—actually may have the paradoxical effect of strengthening the behavior on which they are contingent. Hence, such negative emotional responses are serving as positive reinforcers.

Extinction is again both a procedure and an effect by which consequences of a behavior reduce the behavior's future occurrence. In this case, the reduction of future behavior occurs because few or no consequences accrue from the individual's behavioral response. The response is weakened because no reinforcement is forthcoming.

Shaping refers to the process of building up desired behavior by applying selective positive reinforcement. Subjects must exhibit some initial behavior, which is then built up by reinforcing closer and closer approximation to the desired final response.

Self-reinforcement simply refers to the individual reinforcing herself or himself, for instance, with tokens or money or a social consequence such as attention or praise for a behavior he or she wishes to increase.

Informational feedback is another behavioral procedure employing consequences. In this procedure, behavior not only produces positively valued reinforcing consequences but also provides information as to the extent of action. Self-monitoring, therapist feedback, and biofeedback are all forms of information feedback used to change behavior.

Finally, many behavioral techniques have been developed to the point of being considered therapies in their own right, e.g., systematic desensitization, cognitive behavior therapy, participant modeling, and social skills or assertiveness training. Relaxation therapy, which was used in behavior therapy initially as a component of systematic desensitization, now is used to treat problems independently, such as essential hypertension. Implosion-flooding, rational emotive therapy, and even paradoxical intention are not considered behavioral therapies. Token economies have also achieved wide use as complete therapies in settings where the contingencies for behavioral change are carefully described and programmed.

In addition to the theoretical aspects and assumptions of behavior therapy and many of the commonly used procedures, there are other assumptions of behavior therapy that relate to its clinical practice. These include:

1) The patient is always "right," with the therapist responsible for developing the patient's "motivation" for change.
2) The therapist must be self-critical and explore reasons for patients' successes or failures.
3) Behavioral methods can be specified, taught, and learned by paraprofessionals and patients.
4) Contrary to stereotypes, behavior therapy is "happiness enhancing" since positive reinforcement is emphasized and potentially "fulfilling" since human repertoires are expanded. Aversive procedures are used sparingly, focally, and only when paired with skill building.
5) Behavior therapy, as with other therapies, must be embedded in the therapeutic alliance and relationship for maximum effectiveness.

Clinical Data Necessary For Treatment Planning

A general framework for behavioral assessment, presented in Table 2 (found in the Appendix to this chapter), guides the clinician in carrying out a systematic and comprehensive evaluation prior to selecting and using behavior therapy techniques. It is important to note, however, that these assessment processes are not sequentially linear; they are overlapping, reciprocal, and recur in a cyclical manner during the course of treatment. Behavioral assessment and therapy are inextricably linked in clinical decision making, intervention, and evaluation. Figure 1 depicts the way in which assessment and treatment interlock.

PROBLEM IDENTIFICATION

Since behavior is multidimensional, behavioral assessment must encompass all of the levels of behavior that contribute to clinical symptoms, role impairments, and treatment outcome. Instrumental behavior, social interaction, imagery, sensory experiences, cognition, affect, and biological processes need to be assessed during both the initial evaluation and the course of therapy.

Thus, it should be clear that a behavioral assessment includes all modalities of human expression and experience. If a phenomenon can be discriminated, counted, directly or indirectly observed, reported, or measured in any way, then the clinical problem is relevant to behavioral assessment. From the point of view of the clinician, behavioral specification and measurement need not be confined to treatment methods subsumed under the rubric of behavioral therapy. For example, the clinical and research strategies utilized by behavior therapists—specification of discrete behavior problems and goals, repeated measurements of the behavior of interest, using patients as their own controls by sequentially introducing and withdrawing treatment interventions until desired effects are produced—can also be allied to psychopharmacology.[15] In this manner, the confounding effects of interindividual differences in dose-response can be resolved by monitoring individual patients' clinical

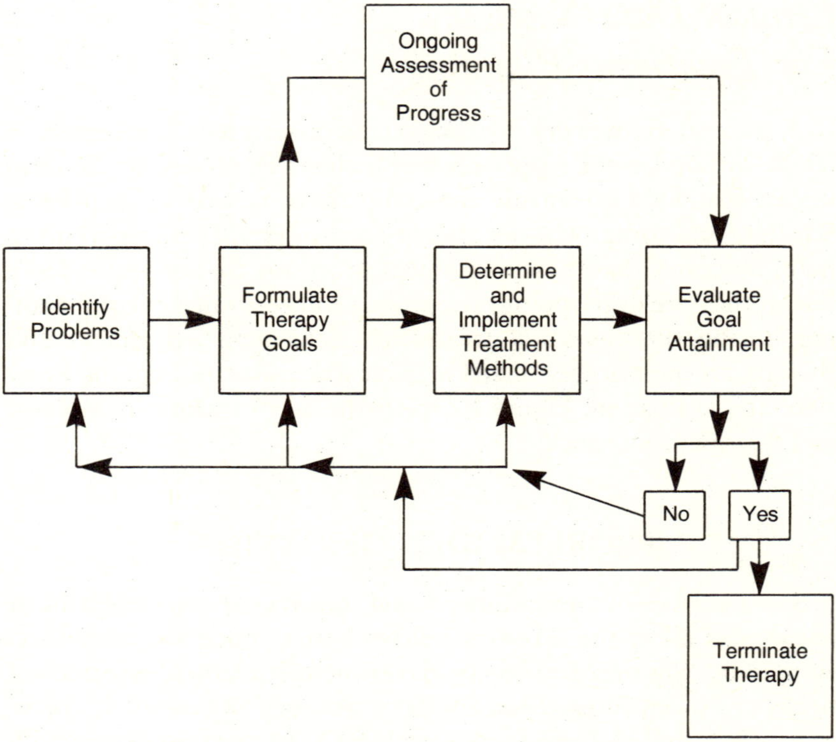

FIGURE 1

FLOW CHART OF THE EMPIRICAL APPROACH TO THE TREATMENT OF CLINICAL PROBLEMS

When clinical goals are attained, therapist and patient consider termination or working on additional problems and goals.

behavior intensively as each is exposed to several dosage levels of a drug in sequence. This clinical and research strategy, capitalizing on the widely known fact of the uniqueness of each individual's response to medication, allows an assessment of latency, peak potency, duration of effects, and the interactions between drug and psychosocial modes of therapy.

The behavior therapist is interested in the dynamic interplay between behavior and environment as well as between different modes or levels of behavior. The individual who suffers a loss and feels low, apathetic, or anxious may begin to use a "script" that leads to talking to himself or herself in ways such as, "I am helpless," "The world is grim," "I can't do anything anymore," and "I am worthless." These negative self-statements, in turn, may produce more dysphoria, anxiety, and even vegetative symptoms.[16] Thus, the behavior therapist working with a depressed individual will also attempt to correct such cognitive distortions. In a similar fashion, the phobic patient will be taught to make coping self-statements such as, "I can 'hang-in' until the anxiety diminishes," or "By facing my fears, I will find out that nothing catastrophic will happen." Changes in one behavioral mode may produce desirable changes in another mode only after a latency or time delay; thus, improvements occur in socializing and task completions. Muscular activity and skin temperature increases—induced by biofeedback or relaxation training—generally precede reductions in essential hypertension and headaches.[17,18]

Behavioral assessment begins with an operational description of the topography of the target behavior. A list of positive examples describing the behavior is usually sufficient. Having done this, one has clarified the patient's reason for seeking treatment and specified the behaviors that will be monitored throughout therapy in order to assess the progress or lack of progress as a result of treatment. A firm and systematic adherence to specification and measurement of multimodal levels of human behavior are the distinguishing characteristics of behavioral practitioners. It is essential to help the patient translate vague and general complaints into more concrete terms before therapy can proceed. Examples of operationalizing problems can be noted in Table 3.

If patients are not easily able to translate their vague complaints into behavioral terms, the diagnostic task becomes the identification of events and behaviors associated with the unpleasant thought, feeling, or problem. For example, feelings of "depression" may be associated with excessive free time or lack of social interaction; "anxiety" may be associated with a difficult performance or receiving criticism.

Sometimes the patient may merely be reticent to disclose a specific undesirable behavior, e.g., exhibitionism or paranoid thoughts, and the assessment task is to help the patient feel comfortable enough to

TABLE 3
OPERATIONALIZATION OF GENERAL AND VAGUE PROBLEMS INTO SPECIFIC BEHAVIORS

Vague Problem	Behavioral Translation
Paranoid	Believes others are always speaking about him/her; believes someone is out to kill him/her
Agitation	Tremulousness; dizziness; faints often; cries frequently
Immature	Cannot plan ahead well; whines and complains when needs are not immediately met; lacks basic survival skills for community life
Low self-esteem	Critical of himself/herself; feels he/she will not do well in school; feels no one likes to talk to him/her
Narcissistic	In conversation, does not let anyone else finish a sentence; frequently interrupts others; talks often about self; does not ask questions about others' feelings
Withdrawn	Does not initiate conversation; does not eat meals with others; spends most of time alone
Anxiety	Palpitations; sweating; apprehensive that something catastrophic may occur; muscles tense; fearful of losing control of self

talk about the problem. More often, the patient finds difficulty in associating some general dysphoria with any specific behavior. Alternatively, the problem may be a deficiency of some desirable behavior that reduces the amount of positive reinforcement received from the environment, and thus is responsible for malaise and dysphoria.

During the initial evaluation interview(s), it is important for the clinician to understand the problems from the patient's point of view, adopting a "consumer approach" in which the patient describes his or her concerns and reasons for seeking help. After discussing the patient's view of the problems, the clinician encourages the patient to translate the feelings and problems into operational terms, focusing on what the patient is *doing*, *feeling*, and *thinking*. The goal is to determine which behaviors, in the multimodal spectrum, need to be modified, i.e., which specific behavior patterns require change in their frequency of occurrence, their intensity, their duration, or in the conditions under which they occur. At this point in behavioral assessment, the clinician should determine if the problems consist of an excess of maladaptive behaviors and/or a deficit of adaptive behaviors. Behavioral excesses are problems that occur too often, with too great intensity, last too long, or occur at the wrong time or place. Clinical examples of behavioral excesses are compulsive rituals, palpitations and sweating linked with anxiety, antisocial behaviors of children, enuresis and encopresis, and complaints of helplessness and worthlessness by a depressed person. Behavioral deficits are defined as problems because desirable, adaptive behavior is not occurring frequently or long enough, in sufficient magnitude, or at the right time and place. Clinical examples of deficits are unassertiveness, impotence, mutism, procrastination, phobic avoidance, and inadequate grooming. Making the distinction between behavioral excesses and deficits has implications for the choice of treatment strategies, since some methods are useful for increasing the strength and frequency of behaviors while other methods are useful for suppressing undesirable behaviors. In most clinical situations, a combination of excesses and deficits coexists.

Once the problems are identified in specific terms of excesses and deficits, the next task is to determine the scope of the problems. Problem behaviors can be categorized along the dimensions of frequency, intensity or magnitude, duration, latency, and appropriateness.

During an initial evaluation, patients will often overestimate the frequency of self-reported problems. Depressed persons might spontaneously report that they feel miserable, hopeless, and pessimistic "all of the time" when, in fact, they may be able to elaborate periods of feeling "OK" when questioned more specifically. Direct, clear questions about the *frequency* of the occurrence of a problem help to elicit more reliable information. Structured interview guides and questionnaires are available to assist the clinician in the task of obtaining reliable information on the frequency of a problem during an evaluation for adults and children.[19,20,21,22,23,24]

Another approach to obtaining a reliable picture of the frequency of the patient's problems is to assign the patient homework to count the episodes when the problem occurs. This can be done through a daily diary or log, with a wrist counter or the inexpensive counter used to tabulate grocery prices, or by making checkmarks on a piece of paper. Self-observation and recording promote commitment by the patient to the evaluation and treatment effort and provide more detailed information to either substantiate or qualify initial complaints.

The *intensity* or *magnitude* of a problem is another key dimension of behavior. Some problems are not easily counted, but are more suited to estimates of intensity. Thus, a Target Complaint Scale is a simple 12-point "thermometer-like" scale that can be used by patients to report how much particular problems are bothering them during a defined period of time.[25] The evaluation of a desensitization treatment program for a patient with four separate phobias was conducted by means of a weekly Target Complaint Scale. As can be seen in Figure 2, the patient initially reported intensity levels of "very severe" or "couldn't be worse"; as the desensitization was introduced for each phobia in turn, the intensity levels dropped to "a little" or "not at all."[26]

The *duration* of a problem behavior is relevant for situations such as temper tantrums, rage reactions, panic attacks, suicidal ruminations, obsessional preoccupations, and catatonic immobility. A patient, nursing staff member, or psychiatrist can use a watch or timer to monitor the duration of a problem behavior. The complement of duration is latency of a response, e.g., a therapist can measure the time elapsed between the start of a therapeutic session and the onset of some problem behavior. Figure 3 shows the use of latency as a measure of baseline assessment and then improvement in four chronic schizophrenic patients with hard-core, paranoid delusions. In this case, the nursing staff, during four daily interviews, monitored the time elapsed between the start of the interview and the first sign of delusional speech. The treatment that produced the improvement (up to 600% increases in the latency for delusional speech or, for a complementary point of view, increases in duration for rational speech) was contingent attention and conversation for rational speech and immediate cessation of the interview at the first sign of delusional speech.[27]

The *situational context* of a particular behavior can also determine whether or not it is a problem. A person is not considered an exhibitionist if he walks nude around his home, a nudist colony, or

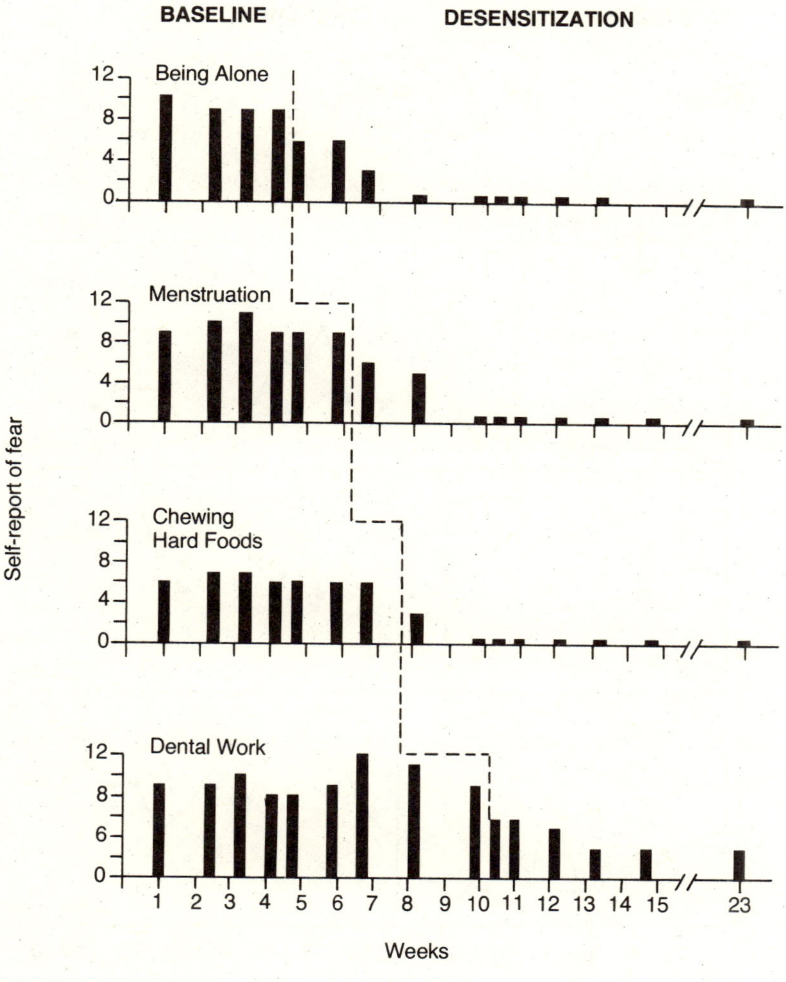

FIGURE 2

Severity of Target Complaints of Anxiety Used to Assess Efficacy of Systematic Desensitization Treatment of a Woman with Four Phobias

Note how the record of progress indicates that the anxiety symptoms markedly improve only after the treatment has been introduced for each specific phobia in turn (Liberman and Smith, 1972). Reprinted from Behavior Therapy.

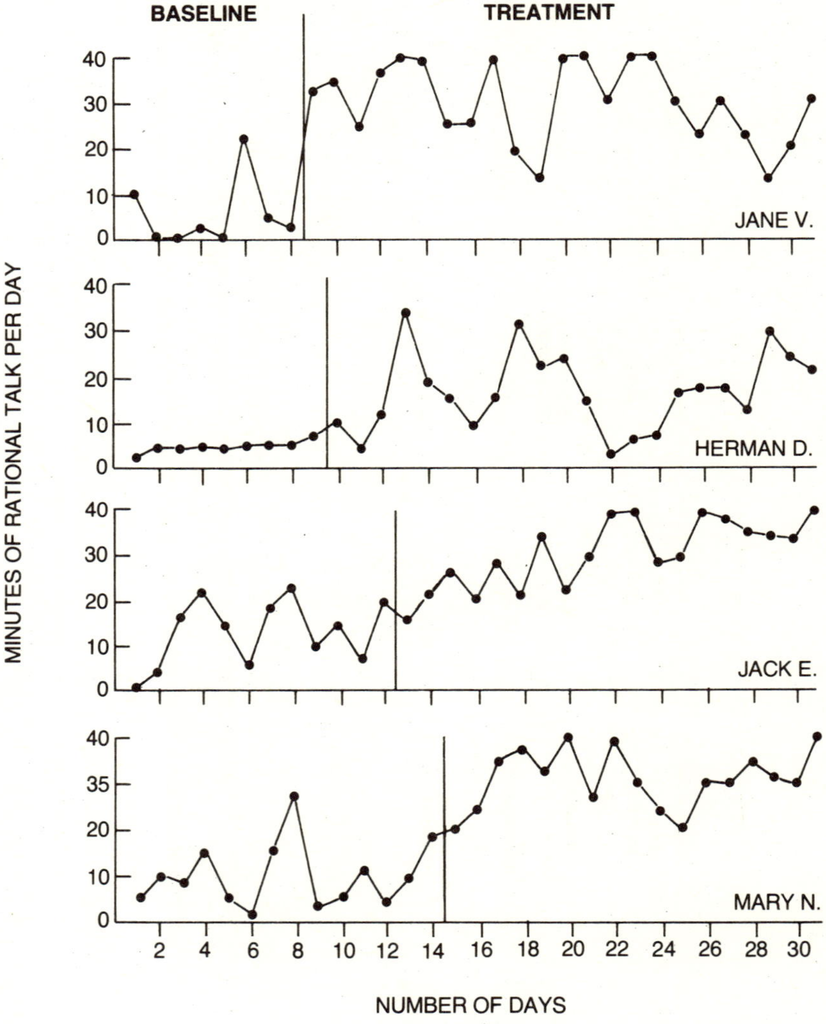

FIGURE 3

USE OF DURATION RECORDING TO ASSESS IMPACT OF REINFORCEMENT THERAPY ON RATIONAL SPEECH IN CHRONIC, DELUSIONAL SCHIZOPHRENICS

The record reflects the duration of rational speech before the onset of delusions in four, ten-minute, daily interviews. Treatment consisted of an informal evening chat (social reinforcement) with a staff member contingent upon rational speech in the daytime interviews (Liberman et al., 1973). Reprinted from Journal of Applied Behavior Analysis.

deserted beach. A man is not considered to have poor self-care skills if he fails to shave and shower on his day off at home. Even schizophrenic persons with frequent delusional thinking can "pass" for normal if they do not openly verbalize the delusions or act them out. Thus, the frequency, duration, latency, and intensity of a behavior have to be placed in the perspective of social norms and situational expectancies. The dimension of contextual appropriateness often affects the labeling of behavior as a "problem."

There are many scientifically reliable and clinically feasible ways to observe and record the frequency, intensity, and duration of problem behaviors. These methods have been described in volumes on behavioral assessment.[28,29,30]

SETTING GOALS AND PRIORITIES

The clinical utility of a clear and unambiguous statement of the patient's problem lies in its serving as a stepping stone for a specific formulation of goals toward which to direct therapeutic change. The task of developing treatment goals can be described succinctly in a question for both patient and clinician: "How will you know when treatment has been successful and can be terminated?" The following advantages accrue from clear and specific goal setting:

1) The therapist will know what is being worked toward and can more effectively plan the sequence of the treatment program.
2) The patient knows better what must be changed and can, therefore, make plans and subgoals more effectively.
3) Awareness of goals helps both patient and therapist to measure progress as therapy proceeds and to secure positive reinforcement as approximations are made.

It is important to move quickly to goal setting, since dwelling on problems inadvertently reinforces them through the attention they receive from the patient and therapist. The goals of therapy need to be stated as specific changes in one or more of the multimodal levels of behavior shown or experienced by the patient. Setting explicit goals is a critical process, particularly with patients who get "stuck" in focusing on their problems. For example, patients might insist that they do not know what they want from therapy, but just that they feel miserable and depressed. The clinician's responsibility is to assist the patient in making goal statements. This can be done by asking the patient, "How would you like your life to be different from the way it is now?"; "What limitations do your symptoms place on you that you would most like to change?"; or "How would you know when you were no longer feeling depressed and miserable?"

There are a number of phases in goal setting. While there are many ways to attain the end result of a set of goals, it is more efficient to proceed in a structured manner, actively coaching the patient to choose treatment objectives. It is so much easier for both patient and therapist to remain at the nondirective, general level of discourse that behavior therapists underscore the importance of a systematic pursuit of goals.

The following phases of goal setting are recommended only as guidelines; each clinician will find ways of individualizing the phases. The clinician and patient:

1) review identified problems and potential goals that may lead to the resolution of the problems
2) develop additional goals based on changes seen as desirable
3) specify the goals in behavioral terms
4) generate alternative ways of achieving the same goal
5) evaluate alternatives by examining their likely consequences, i.e., the pros and cons of each alternative goal's pathway
6) select preferred alternatives for each of the goals

Since it is rarely possible to pursue all goals at once, priorities need to be arranged. The patient can be aided in this activity by the clinician asking, "Which outcomes would you like to attain first?" or "Which problems and goals are of greatest concern to you now?" In selecting goals, it is better to err on the side of having too few than too many; an overburdened patient may quickly become demoralized, and the treatment process put in jeopardy. A variety of criteria can be employed when helping the patient to set priorities on working toward goals. For example:

1) How functional is the goal in the patient's everyday life?
2) How easy will it be to attain the goal?
3) How frequently does the behavioral goal or problem occur?
4) How accessible is the goal?
5) How salient and important is the goal to the patient?
6) How dangerous is the problem?

7) Are there treatment techniques available to reach the goal?
8) Is the goal congruent with the clinician's value system?
9) How costly will it be to reach the goal?
10) How likely will the goals be maintained in the post-treatment period when they will need support from the natural environment?

The last-mentioned criterion is especially important for programs in institutional settings, where behaviors selected for change are often those that make life easier for the staff rather than the residents. A hierarchy of subgoals should be elaborated when the longer-term goal requires several weeks or months to reach.

INVENTORY OF ASSETS

It is expedient to build treatment goals on the individual's assets, since this gives both therapist and patient a "running start" with already existing behavioral repertoires. In many clinical cases, the therapist is well advised to give priority to goals that are not directly linked to symptoms, but are based upon the patient's strengths. A paranoid schizophrenic's delusions may be impenetrable through direct treatment efforts, but might interfere less with daily living if social interaction and work performance are improved. An obese individual may be extremely resistant to efforts aimed at changing eating habits directly, but might eat less if alternative social and recreational activities are engaged in, especially at times of peak hunger. A person with a somatoform disorder might respond better clinically to interventions aimed at the goal of improving communication in marriage rather than at the symptoms per se, particularly if the symptoms serve the function of gaining concern and reinforcement from the spouse. In other words, goals that strengthen the assets and strengths of the individual on various levels of existence often indirectly reduce psychopathology and symptomatology.

Development of an inventory of assets is of use, of course, in determining Axis V of DSM-III, the patient's highest level of adaptive psychosocial functioning in the past year. The clinician should obtain from the patient and significant others, as well as from records of performance, answers to questions such as:

1) What are the areas in which the patient functions well, now or in the past?
2) What are the patient's interpersonal resources and social support networks?
3) What agencies and helping professionals can be mobilized for participation in a treatment plan?
4) How aversive is the current impairment to the patient?
5) How responsive is the patient to the therapeutic alliance and setting?

As in identifying problems and formulating goals, assets should be inventoried from a multimodal perspective. While levels of functioning vary from one patient to another, each patient does have a unique set of assets in areas of affect, cognition, instrumental role behavior, interpersonal relations, and biological endowment. These assets can be matched against those skills and changes needed for the patient to attain chosen goals. Steps toward reaching long-term goals can build on patients' resources in a way that facilitates gradual and comfortable change, taking advantage of already existing and developing assets.

FUNCTIONAL BEHAVIORAL ANALYSIS

When a beginning has been made in cataloging the patient's problems, goals, and assets, the clinician can turn to analyzing the antecedents and consequences in the patient's present and past environments that may be responsible for the initiation and maintenance of the problems. A delineation of both antecedents and consequences can be viewed as contributing to the rating on Axis IV of DSM-III, severity of psychosocial stressors.

Antecedents

Events, situations, and other people, as well as physical stimuli, all serve to influence the subsequent behavior of an exposed individual. These may be considered as cues, prompts, signals, or instructions to behave in a certain way. One example of antecedent events is that persons with obsessive-compulsive disorders will have words, colors, furniture, dirt, stove knobs, doorlocks, and light switches serving as cues that elicit unwanted thoughts and, possibly, undoing rituals. Another example is that a phobic patient will find certain situations anxiety-provoking, e.g., driving on busy streets or visiting crowded stores and theaters, and will actively avoid them. These antecedents should be identified with specific details so that they can be used in developing treatment procedures. Antecedents usually occur in combination across all levels of experience. As an example, antecedents may contribute to a depressed person withdrawing from a social event because of anticipating awkwardness and rejection (cognitive), feeling especially low that day (affect), observing a person in the setting who had been critical and rude in the past (interpersonal), fantasizing humiliation (imagery), entering a room that had been the scene of an unpleasant experience (situational), and not sleeping well the night before (biological).

Some situations spontaneously elicit maladaptive behavior because in the past the behavior has been reinforced in that situation. For example, a child's crying and tantrums when put to bed might be prompted by contact with the bed that, in turn, has been associated with parental nurturance, reassurance, and attentiveness. Other situations can affect physiological responses, as when work stressors increase the secretion of gastric acid or muscle tension in the neck and head. Behavioral clinicians, as clinicians from other persuasions, view major life events and losses as important precipitants to many psychiatric disorders, given an individual with the predisposition and vulnerability to stressors.

Modeling, or being influenced by observing the behavior of others, is a particularly powerful antecedent in determining behavioral responses. Models include parents and relatives, friends, entertainment and television figures, and subjects in advertisements. The process of acquiring attributes through "identification" occurs essentially through modeling. Most complex skills and symptoms are learned on a vicarious basis by observing other persons' behavior and its consequences for them. Thus, for example, a patient with hypochondriasis may have initially acquired the sick role and somatic complaints through observing another person with similar complaints. Similarly, "epidemics" of conversion symptoms quickly spread among individuals who are in close proximity to each other through seeing or hearing graphic accounts of those afflicted.

Cognitive responses are a special class of antecedents that can function as mediating steps in maintaining or exacerbating clinical problems. The labeling given to emotional states, self-perceptions, and self-instructions can perpetuate maladaptive behavior. For example, a schizophrenic who says to himself or herself, "I am a loser and can't work," may increase anticipatory anxiety to the degree that his or her work performance may decline.

Consequences

While most mental health professionals are sensitive to the antecedents or precipitants of emotional problems, less attention is given to the consequences of the problems; these consequences may strongly determine the status of the problems. Consequences can either strengthen and increase or weaken and decrease the frequency, duration, and intensity of the behaviors that precede them.

Reinforcers are environmental consequences that increase the probability that a preceding behavior will occur in the future. When consequences of a behavior decrease the likelihood of future occurrences of that behavior, the processes of punishment or extinction are in play.

The contingency that defines the temporal relationship between the occurrence of a behavior and the environmental consequence is very important in determining whether or not a particular consequence will affect preceding behavior. For example, consequences occurring immediately after a problem behavior are more likely to influence the future status of the problem than are delayed consequences.

How does the clinician evaluate the pertinent antecedents and consequences of the patient's problems to determine their salience and potential contribution to treatment planning? Information on the environmental antecedents and consequences can be obtained from the patient through comprehensive interviewing and questionnaires. The Fear Survey Schedule developed by Wolpe, for example, can be filled out by the patient and indicates how much fear of discomfort each of 87 items or situations produces.[31] As mentioned, there are a variety of reinforcement surveys that elicit reports by the patient of things, people, events, and activities that are viewed as desirable and pleasant, and thus presumed to be reinforcing. The clinician is not limited, however, to the patient as a source of information. In fact, because behavioral assessment requires knowing the antecedents and consequences of behaviors, it may be necessary to interview significant others or observe directly the patient in the situations where the troublesome behaviors take place.

There may be significant discrepancies between what the patient reports as being critical antecedents and consequences and those that are actually observed as critical. Reasons for discrepancies include retrospective distortion, social desirability, lying, and poor self-observation. When such discrepancies occur, the behavioral clinician gives greater credence to what the patient *does* rather than what the patient *says he or she does*. While it is not always convenient or possible to conduct direct observations of the patient, it is the most reliable means of determining the factors in the environment that are maintaining the problems. The behavioral-environmental interrelationships observed on an inpatient unit, in a day hospital, and even during an outpatient therapy session, provide useful information in making a functional analysis. Home visits and community outings, perhaps conducted by a nurse or paraprofessional, can also improve the scope and quality of the behavioral assessment.

THE USE OF REINFORCEMENT

Locating reinforcers that can be employed in behavior therapy is an essential step in behavioral assessment. To the extent that a patient is bereft of reinforcers, that individual's responsiveness to therapy will be diminished. Gambrill outlines the types of reinforcers, mediators, settings, and punishers that can be identified and then utilized in treatment plans.[32]

In all therapy programs, reinforcers serve as the motivation for change. Reinforcers can be found in the patient (e.g., relief from dysphoric symptoms), in the therapeutic relationship (e.g., positive feedback from the therapist), in tangible items (e.g., food, money, tokens), and in the natural environment (e.g., attention and recognition from family members). The emphasis in behavior therapy on strengthening prosocial and adaptive behaviors requires a search for effective reinforcers. This search may involve trial and error over time since a reinforcer is determined only by virtue of its impact on the behavior of concern. Reinforcers can be considered to fall on a hierarchy, depending upon the level of functioning and sophistication of the patient. The hierarchy runs from primary biological reinforcers to symbolic reinforcers; examples are provided in Table 4.

TABLE 4
REINFORCEMENT HIERARCHY CAN BE USED TO GUIDE THE CLINICIAN IN IDENTIFYING WAYS TO BUILD MOTIVATION FOR CHANGE IN A PATIENT. THE CHOICE AND USE OF A SPECIFIC REINFORCER MUST REMAIN AN EMPIRICAL PROCESS.

Type of Reinforcer	Examples
Primary/biological	Candy, food, cigarettes
Immediate tangible	Money, tokens
High frequency behavior	Physical activity, conversation, TV watching
Immediate symbolic or informational feedback	Checkmarks, points, biofeedback
Delayed symbolic	Academic grades, prizes
Social	Approval, attention, sympathy
Self-reinforcement	Positive self-statements
Cognitive	Mastering a challenge

One good rule of thumb in locating a reinforcer is to observe the individual to determine high frequency or preferred activities. Behaviors that are engaged in frequently or preferentially are usually effective when employed as reinforcers in building up the strength of other behaviors that are weaker or occur infrequently. Thus, since persons with anorexia nervosa have a high activity level, access to walking and exercising can be used as a reinforcer to increase food intake and weight.

One can find reinforcers through a variety of means:

1) Observation of the patient's behavior—this may reveal high probability behaviors that can be used to reinforce low probability behaviors.

2) Self-report by the patient—patients can be administered questionnaires that tap reinforcers or simply asked what foods they consume, which people they spend time with, what places they visit, and in which activities they engage.[33] One useful questionnaire is the Pleasant Events Schedule, containing 302 activities, situations, and events for which the patient reports the fre-

quency and pleasure of involvement.[34] Self-report, however, may be unreliable and require validation by others or through direct observation.

3) Reports by significant others—these should point to potentially useful reinforcers in the patient's natural environment.

4) States of deprivation of the patient—for patients who are deprived of sexual activity because of inadequacy, gradual exposure to sexual pleasure, and reinforcement of sexual performance. Likewise, patients who are socially isolated may find interaction with others (including the therapist) highly reinforcing.

Mediators

While the therapist and the patient are in the best position to evaluate change occurring in treatment, others, through talking with the patient, can serve as mediators in the assessment process. Thus, parents are important assessors of change in their children and are relied upon to collect initial baseline data on which interventions are planned and to monitor changes over time. Teachers can serve the assessment function when a child's problems occur in the classroom. Other examples of mediators who can collaborate with the clinician in the assessment procedure are probation and parole officers, social workers and caseworkers, recreation directors, volunteers in agencies and institutions, houseparents, residential care operators, police, and peers.

Settings

The effectiveness of reinforcers in a therapy program can be amplified if an appropriate treatment setting is used. For example, in dealing with a child diagnosed as having an aggressive, undersocialized conduct disorder, the appropriate social and tangible reinforcers will be facilitated if they are dispensed in the setting in which the problem behavior occurs—namely, in the home and classroom. Furthermore, linking the patient's classmates with the therapy as peer counselors may facilitate the treatment through more relevant modeling and positive feedback. It makes little sense, therefore, to offer individual therapy in a clinic office to a child whose problems are occurring in a place remote in time and distance from that office.

Similarly, teaching a withdrawn schizophrenic adult social skills at parties, lounges, dances, restaurants, and stores is likely to be more effective than doing the training in a hospital or clinic setting. The challenge to clinicians at the time of assessment is to identify settings that can be employed later in attaining the goals of treatment.

Punishers

While behavior therapists stress increasing adaptive behavior through modeling, prompting, and reinforcement procedures, it is sometimes necessary to employ punishment or response cost contingencies as well. In response cost, the maladaptive behavior "costs" the patient something of value, (e.g., an oppositional adolescent who persistently breaks curfew may lose three hours of a weekend, late-night privilege, or hyperactive children might lose fifteen minutes of recess time if they got out of their seats more than twice during the preceding class period). Combining punishment with positive reinforcement will bring about behavior change more quickly, a matter of great importance when serious or life-endangering problems are involved. Thus, with a severely self-injurious autistic child, the combined use of candy and praise for prosocial behavior plus overcorrection for self-abusive behavior may prevent tissue damage and permanent disability. The clinician's assessment task is to identify potential punishers and response costs in case they are needed.

MONITORING PROGRESS IN THERAPY

What distinguishes behavior therapy from other therapeutic approaches is its fundamental adherence to measuring and monitoring clinical change. Assessment is a continuing process that begins when the patient undergoes an initial evaluation. The behavioral model, depicted in Figure 1, highlights the importance of ongoing assessment of progress in the clinical process. With repeated and regular assessment information, the behavior therapist can collaborate with the patient in making decisions about terminating, continuing, or changing the goals and methods of treatment.

There are many ways for the clinician to obtain information on the patient's progress. Information can be collected by the therapist, the patient, other observers, and significant others. The levels of clinical information can include subjective self-report, observations of overt behavior, and physiological indicators. Interviews, questionnaires and surveys, and direct observational procedures are all useful in monitoring progress with each source of information complementing and supplementing the others. While it is important to know whether the agoraphobic is now entering previously avoided social situations (overt behavioral level), it is also important to know how the patient feels about the changes (subjective self-report level) and whether physiologic indices (such as heart rate or muscle tension) have changed. Termination of therapy should rest ideally on improvements in each level of behavior.

Thus, an indispensable feature of behavior therapy is the extension of assessment procedures into the process of treatment, using assessment data in clinical decision making. There are three major tasks in assessing the ongoing process of therapy:

1) fidelity of application of the treatment methods
2) monitoring the effectiveness of the methods
3) modifying the treatment program[30]

Fidelity of application

It is first necessary to assess whether or not the treatment methods are being applied properly. Since so much of behavioral treatment relies on instructions and homework assignments, it is critical to determine if the patient is complying with the program. Compliance is as common a problem with behavioral interventions as with medication regimens. For example, without regular home practice, the learning of the relaxation response for systematic desensitization or for treatment of essential hypertension will not occur. Regular practice is also required for effective implementation of sexual therapy. Early detection of noncompliance allows the therapist to take extra steps to ensure compliance (e.g., daily phone call reminders) or to select a treatment approach that does not depend upon home practice.

Another example of checking on treatment compliance occurs in the fidelity of ward staff in token economies where it is essential to monitor the timing and interaction surrounding the dispensing of tokens. If the nursing staff delay too long before rewarding appropriate behavior, and if they fail to praise the patient's behavior while giving the tokens, the tokens will have much less reinforcement potency. Because of the neglect of immediate token and social contingencies for reinforcement, many token economies are "token" efforts and are ineffective in changing behavior.

Still another example of treatment fidelity is questioning the patient directly at the therapy session about homework assignments or, alternatively, the patient can be asked to fill out checklists or diaries that describe the completion of assignments. Finally, direct observations can be made in the home, on the ward, and in the community by the therapist, aides, or significant others.

Monitoring treatment effectiveness

The same techniques used to assess the patient's baseline behavior are also appropriate for monitoring treatment progress. While behavior therapists are inclined to favor frequency counts obtained through event recording or time sampling, a goal attainment method for record keeping may be more appropriate for a busy clinical setting. Counting the frequency of positive self-statements by a depressed individual during a therapy session, for example, may be a less valid measure of change than whether or not the patient spent an afternoon with a friend in a recreational activity. Thus, completion of an important all-or-none activity or assignment may be a better indicator of therapeutic progress than carrying out an elaborate time sampling of less important behavior.

Assessment guides treatment

The ultimate value of ongoing behavioral assessment is its serving as a guide for the therapy process. Much like a navigator using instruments to chart directions, the behavioral clinician uses assessment data to modify the goals and tactics of treatment. If progress is smooth, then the therapist may wish to maintain the treatment program. If progress slows or stops, the therapist must examine, together with the patient, the following questions:

1) *Have inappropriate goals been chosen?* Are the goals too difficult, too large, of only lip-service value, too vague, or not functional for the patient?

2) *Is the behavioral analysis of the environmental determinants of the problems incomplete?* Have the antecedents and consequences of the problems been incorrectly analyzed? For example, has there been a failure to locate a major source of reinforcement that is sustaining the problems, as in the case of some "secondary gains"?
3) *Are the treatment techniques not being applied properly?* Does the patient fail to complete homework assignments? For example, in the case of a phobic patient, does the patient remain exposed *in vivo* to the feared situations long enough for the anxiety to diminish?
4) *Are the techniques lacking in effectiveness for this particular patient?* Does the intervention approach simply need readjustment, or is it time to try a different treatment method?

The monitoring of ongoing therapy permits periodic re-evaluation and changes to be made in the choice of goals or treatment methods. Adherence to a treatment method, without repeated validation from ongoing assessment that the method is producing desired changes in the patient's behavior, is to be avoided. However, some long-term problems that have been overlearned, overpracticed, and sustained by intermittent reinforcement are not quickly responsive to therapeutic intervention. Obviously a balance is needed between prematurely discarding an intervention strategy and keeping one in operation too long.

A commitment to ongoing behavioral assessment at the multiple levels of human functioning and experience outlined above, provides the practitioner with helpful information for dealing with each clinical case and also for dealing with similar cases in future practice.

Treatment Planning in Behavior Therapy

The following case example of a schizophrenic patient serves as a vehicle for understanding the kinds of data and procedures for conducting behavioral analysis and treatment with severely psychotic patients.

> *Al graduated from high school as a straight A student, intending to pursue a career in science, which was his special area of interest. His father, an engineer, and his mother, a lawyer, both encouraged him to develop his intellectual skills. They were concerned, though,*

that Al didn't pay enough attention to his social life. While he had a few casual friends, he didn't chum around and had not gone out on a date. He enrolled at a nearby state university and for two semesters commuted daily to class from home. While he passed his courses, he found it increasingly difficult to concentrate and complete homework assignments. He and his parents were puzzled by his decline in academic performance, but they did not think of seeking medical or psychiatric consultation.

Instead of returning to college the next fall, Al decided to work instead, and he tried a succession of jobs from file clerk to busboy. He withdrew from his few acquaintances and family, preferring to spend long hours listening to music in his room. He told his parents that he was tense and fearful, but they thought it was because of pressures at work and suggested that he quit his job. Now spending all of his time at home, Al became more isolated and fatigued. He had trouble falling asleep and had several frightening nightmares. His mind wandered to strange thoughts, such as a belief that he had leprosy and might be dying. Frequently, while lying in bed alone he heard two male voices commenting on his indolence and referring to him as a "failure" and a "loser."

He refused to eat, stayed in bed and stopped caring for his personal appearance. He told his father one night that he thought his actions were being controlled by a force from outer space. He went on to say that by remaining perfectly still, he could prevent this external control. His father shrugged off these fantastic ideas and reassured Al that no one was controlling him. The next day, Al fretfully told his mother that he discovered that he could broadcast his thoughts and was afraid that the neighbors would hear what he was thinking.

After several weeks of increasing indolence, Al stopped talking. He stared into space, urinated in his pants, sat immobile, and failed to respond to questions. He could be physically prompted to change positions, but it was as though he had no volition and was as passive as a lump of clay. Finally, Al's parents, weary of waiting for him to "snap out of his daze," brought him to a mental health center where he was admitted for inpatient treatment.

Al was treated with a neuroleptic drug and showed gradual improvement in his appearance and behavior. He resumed speaking, first in a whisper and only in response to questions. His confusion and disorientation cleared. He took a shower and brushed his hair, albeit with some prompting. His eating improved and, after five days of hospitalization, he began smiling and looking at people. He avoided interacting with fellow patients or staff, however, and secluded himself in his room or in remote corners of the ward whenever possible. The medication appeared to improve his self-care skills and cognitive abilities, but he remained socially withdrawn and passive. He appeared to be returning to his premorbid personality–shy, quiet, and a loner.

PROBLEM IDENTIFICATION

As in the case with many schizophrenic patients, Al presents with severe and disabling problems in almost every sphere of functioning. Pinpointing these problems in operational and behavioral terms is the first step toward setting goals and instituting treatment. In fact, the decision to use neuroleptic medication at the time of his hospital admission was prompted by clinical observations of his catatonic immobility, mutism, incontinence, and by the specific history of characteristic delusions and hallucinations provided by his parents. The psychiatric evaluation of Al proceeded along multiple dimensions and is outlined in Table 5. A problem list was formulated with specific objectives, treatment plans, and a data base.

It can be readily seen that the information required for a comprehensive assessment of a schizophrenic patient comes from interviews of the patient and family, checklists and questionnaires filled out by the patient and family, and direct observations made by professional and nursing staff of the patient's spontaneous behavior on the ward, in the home, or in community settings. Using these assessment modes, the clinician can generate relevant information from the patient's self-report, relatives' descriptions, and staff's direct observations.

With an acutely and floridly psychotic patient such as Al, behavior therapy is aimed at cognitive and behavioral reconstitution so that more comprehensive assessment and treatment planning can be carried out with a reasonably attentive and socially responsive patient. The therapeutic environment, with proper programming, can lead to improvements in floridly symptomatic schizophrenics. Along with neuroleptic medication, the treatment team responsible for reducing Al's level of symptomatology also arranged for him to:

TABLE 5
PROBLEMS OF A SCHIZOPHRENIC AND METHODS FOR ASSESSMENT—THE CASE OF "AL"

Level of Behavior	Specification of Problem	Methods of Assessment
Cognitive	Delusions of hypochondriasis Delusions of control Thought broadcast Reduced span of attention and concentration	Mental status interview of patient (e.g., Present State Examination or Schedule for Affective Diseases and Schizophrenia); family interview; on-ward observations
Affective	Tension, fear	Interviews, on-ward observations, checklists, and questionnaires (e.g., Fear Survey Schedule)
Social	Isolation, withdrawal, poverty of speech, and mutism	Interviews, on-ward observations, family interviews, questionnaires
Instrumental behavior including self-care	Immobile, requires prompting and manual guidance, incontinent, failure to eat, does not respond to instructions, unable to work, groom, and dress self	On-ward observations (e.g., Behavioral Performance Tests); family interviews
Sensory	Auditory hallucinations with depreciatory content—voices talking about him	Patient interview
Imagery	Fantasies of body being distorted with leprosy	Patient interview, drawings by patient

1) be removed, at least temporarily, from a possibly stressful family environment
2) receive clear and concise messages from the staff regarding daily needs
3) spend time in a quiet, unstimulating part of the ward

4) receive "prompts", for making small movements with positive feedback for any sign of awareness, communication, or self-care

Once Al's catatonic symptoms subsided, efforts were made to measure his remaining problems; establish a priority of his goals; inventory his assets; locate reinforcers; conduct a functional analysis of his problems; monitor his progress; and determine when treatment techniques and settings could be changed.

In reviewing Al's problem list, the staff operationalized his problems so that an assessment could be made of their severity in an ongoing manner. Gauging the severity of the problems enabled the staff to establish goal priorities and to monitor progress.

Cognitive problems and psychopathology

On a weekly basis, Al was interviewed by the unit psychiatrist who rated him on twelve dimensions of psychopathology using the Brief Psychiatric Rating Scale (BPRS). The BPRS and a host of other convenient and valid rating scales can be found in the Assessment Manual for Psychopharmacology.[35] To supplement the ratings of delusions and hallucinations, the psychiatrist also used a measure of response latency during the weekly interviews, measuring the elapsed time between his question and Al's response. Initially there were pauses of up to 30 seconds, but as Al reconstituted, the latency was reduced to five seconds or less.

During daily sessions of social skills training, therapists kept a record of the number of correct and incorrect responses made by Al to questions probing his ability to solve interpersonal problems. For example, after a family or peer interaction situation was role-played, Al was asked such questions as "Who were you talking with?"; "What did the other person want?"; "How was the other person feeling?"; "What was your short-term goal in the situation?"; and "What alternatives could you have used to deal with the situation?" Al's ability to perceive and process accurately the information inherent in the role-playing gradually improved, with his error rate declining to zero, reflecting his growing attentional and cognitive abilities.

Affective problems

Each day, Al checked off (on a Target Complaint Scale) the magnitude of his tension, fear, dysphoria, and discomfort. This was graphed by the late-night shift on the inpatient unit and revealed a decrease from "Couldn't be worse" to variable levels between "A little" and "Pretty much." It is of interest that a similar type of global rating of dysphoria, after "test doses" of neuroleptics, has been shown to accurately predict a schizophrenic patient's ultimate clinical response to the neuroleptic.[36] Thus, early and systematic assessment of the affective domain may not only reflect stress levels, but also may enable clinicians to predict effectiveness of neuroleptic treatment.

Social-interpersonal problems

Using a Social Interaction Schedule, the nursing staff unobtrusively observed Al on the ward four times daily and recorded his level of activity, interaction, and inappropriate behavior. During his first week, Al was noted to be isolated and inactive for 90% of the nursing staff's observations. He showed several inappropriate behaviors such as posturing, rocking, and grimacing. When initially approached for two- to three-minute conversations at these four daily Social Interaction Schedule sessions, Al actively moved away and would close his eyes. As time went on, observations revealed his more active engagement with the environment, although he was still isolated from others. By the third week of hospitalization, Al was interacting with other patients and staff about 40% of the time and was responsive in conversations with staff.

During the social skills training sessions, which began after a week of drug treatment, Al was rated on the adequacy of his performance in role-played scenes. He was rated as satisfactory on eye contact and voice volume but needed improvement in voice tone, fluency, and facial expression, which reflected his blunted affect. He also filled out an assertiveness inventory prior to starting the training and again at the end of training.[37] The inventory showed an increase of fifteen points, moving Al up into the near normal range by the time his one-month hospitalization was over.

Instrumental behavior

Al's self-care and work skills were evaluated by the nursing staff numerous times each day within the context of a credit incentive system, a type of token economy. The number of prompts that were required to get Al to satisfactorily wash himself, shower, brush his teeth, comb his hair, and dress himself in appropriate attire were recorded. Full credits were given for satisfactory completion of these tasks without prompts; half credits were given for satisfactory completion after one prompting. Varying amounts of credits were also given for room maintenance and ward chores depending upon the quality of the performance and the number of prompts required to instigate their completion. Thus, Al's credit earnings reflected his role performance on the unit and served as an ongoing assessment of his progress.

Sensory problems

The severity of Al's hallucinatory experiences was rated weekly on the BPRS by the psychiatrist. The frequency of auditory hallucinations was self-monitored by Al by activating a wrist counter for each occurrence during the day. By the time of discharge, hallucinations were no longer occurring.

Imagery

Al's fantasies and hypochondriacal delusions were followed during weekly recreational therapy sessions by his drawing a picture of himself. The first few drawings revealed distorted body shapes and numerous sores placed on the figure's hands and face. Subsequently, the drawings showed a figure isolated from others, but with coherent outlines and no sign of lesions.

Inventory of assets

Al's premorbid history indicated that he had good academic skills and was conscientious and reliable in meeting his commitments. He had a concerned, albeit overinvolved and critical family, who were willing to be involved in the treatment process. These assets were duly noted by Al's treatment team who individually tailored and set goals and monitored his progress through the inpatient unit's credit incentive system, social skills training sessions, and family therapy. The fact that Al had completed a year of college and had held, although briefly, jobs in the competitive marketplace, were also viewed as assets to be built upon for after-care goals.

Goal setting

Initial goals, such as reducing Al's catatonic, delusional, and hallucinatory symptoms, were set primarily by his psychiatrist and the treatment team. Once neuroleptic medication and the consistent and optimally structured hospital environment effected behavioral and cognitive recompensation, Al began to participate in setting goals for himself. This was done with his psychiatrist, at biweekly "rap" sessions, or patient-staff planning meetings. Al worked out a series of problem situations that he wanted to work on in social skills training—starting conversations with strangers, maintaining a friendship, asking for a job, making small talk with co-workers, and communicating his concerns about medication side effects with his doctor. He also indicated when he felt ready to start family therapy and suggested a number of family scenes in which he needed improved communication skills. These included telling his parents that he was annoyed and embarrassed by their discussing his illness with neighbors and requesting time and space to be alone when he felt under stress.

Priorities for treatment goals were guided by the principle of "shaping"—reinforcing small steps or approximations to the desired level of functioning in each of Al's social and behavioral deficits. For example, before working on maintaining friendships in the social skills training, Al first had to learn more rudimentary conversational skills such as asking open-ended questions, giving "free" information about a topic, judging the appropriate level of self-disclosure to use, and sensing when it is time to end a conversation. Similarly, in the credit incentive system, initial goals of improving his grooming and room maintenance with immediate feedback from staff members preceded more complicated work tasks and autonomous self-evaluation of his personal hygiene.

The goal setting enterprise is paced by the patient's progress and, hence, ongoing assessment of change is critical for decisions about goals. In Al's case, the monitoring of his progress in the multiple dimensions listed above enabled the patient, his family, and his therapists to rank order treatment objectives in an orderly and efficacious sequence.

Functional analysis of problems

What were the influential environmental antecedents and consequences in the development and sustaining of Al's clinical problems? Axis IV in DSM-III prompts clinicians to assess antecedent stressors that may have a role in the development of psychopathology. Without speculatively reconstructing Al's earlier life events (which were likely to be formative in determining his premorbid personality, assets, and limitations), it appeared that his increasing social isolation, lack of a peer network, and parental criticism all contributed to his symptomatic impairments. Many who have studied schizophrenia believe that either *under*stimulating or *over*stimulating social environments can lead to symptoms and their worsening. Al was exposed to both types of stressors, alternating between total isolation and family criticism and overconcern.

It is also likely that his parents' cajolery may have served as a reinforcer of his growing negativism and isolation, i.e., their emotional responses to his attempts to reduce intolerable levels of arousal may have inadvertently increased his withdrawal. Al's lack of peer relationships deprived him of age-appropriate models from which he could have learned social skills to use in acquiring friends. In attempting to reduce external pressure on Al, his parents may have gone too far by "excusing" him from reasonable work responsibilities. Instead of receiving recognition and acknowledgment for chores and continuing in a remunerative job, Al received his parents' concern and solicitude for being increasingly helpless and dependent.

A functional analysis such as the above, despite its reliance on retrospective guesswork, can be helpful in the goal-setting process. In Al's case, it seemed important to alter the contingencies of reinforcement and communication patterns in the family, to find a reasonable work role for Al to develop, and to start Al on the pathway toward social relationships with peers.

Reinforcement survey

Reinforcers that could be utilized in Al's treatment program came from two general sources: social and symbolic rewards and more tangible rewards. Once neuroleptic medication had restored Al's responsiveness to reinforcers, nursing staff, psychiatrist, therapists, and family members were able to use social attention, recognition, and praise to reinforce Al's progress in attaining his treatment goals. For example, therapists liberally praised Al for giving correct answers and responding assertively in the social skills training scenes. Praise was paired with credits to reinforce Al's improvements in self-care and work. Tangible reinforcers, such as Al's favorite beverages and candy, were effective in backing up the value of the credits he received for grooming, showering, dressing, and interacting. As time went on, Al experienced reinforcement from higher level rewards such as the feeling of mastery at having successfully engaged a stranger in a ten-minute conversation on the hospital grounds. A high probability behavior of Al's, his preference for social isolation, was identified as a reinforcer and was used contingently to build up social involvement. Al was given access to his room for privacy *after* he first engaged in brief conversations with three different staff members or patients on the unit. This was part of a "contract" that Al negotiated with the unit treatment team as a prerequisite to being promoted to the highest level of autonomy and privileges in the credit system.

Monitoring progress in therapy

Al's progress was assessed in a continuing way through methods that were integral to his treatment program. His getting up, dressing, washing, grooming, and bed making were evaluated by the nursing staff who noted the number of prompts required for his completing these tasks. The assessment of prompts was the criterion for his receipt of credits. His credit earnings per se were another indication of his level of functioning—initially they were nil, as he required constant one-to-one prompting and assistance; later they increased as he moved up the hierarchical credit system to higher levels of self-initiation, self-evaluation, and individual responsibility.

In the social skills training sessions, the counts of errors made to questions assessing his perceptual and cognitive processing abilities reflected his progress. His ratings of verbal and nonverbal emotional expression also showed improvement. At one point, when he encountered interpersonal scenes involving assertion with his parents, his error rate went up and his nonverbal performance deteriorated.

This was an indication to his therapists that these situations needed to be broken down into smaller steps and that he required more modeling and positive feedback for his efforts. Perhaps the most important method of monitoring his progress through the social skills training was his completion of homework assignments. Al had little difficulty completing assignments related to talking with hospital staff and store clerks. When he was given assignments to converse with peers, however, he reported several times a failure to follow through on the assignment. Again, this was useful information for the therapists who increased their level of intervention, accompanying Al into the "field" to provide closer prompts and feedback for his peer contacts.

In the weekly family therapy sessions, Al and his parents were observed for signs of spontaneously using the communication skills that were taught in the group. The leaders looked for examples of giving positive feedback to each other for desired actions; making positive requests of each other; and expressing negative feelings directly and nonaccusatively. When no sign of spontaneous expression of negative feelings was noted, the leaders prompted the family to practice "feeling" statements in relation to a common problem.

The Social Interaction Schedule, with ratings of Al's socializing four times a day, provided a good indication of generalization or "transfer" of learning from skills training sessions to the more spontaneous give-and-take of the unit. When the data revealed an increase in social isolation, this became a signal to the staff to inquire of Al what might be stressing him. The BPRS enabled the psychiatrist to monitor Al's level of psychopathology and to modify his neuroleptic dose accordingly. The questions from the Present State Examination elicited core symptoms of schizophrenia and other types of psychopathology.[38] When the characteristic symptoms of schizophrenia had disappeared one month after admission, the psychiatrist used that information to make the decision to discharge Al from inpatient care.

Practitioners of behavioral analysis and therapy firmly adhere to specification and measurement in their clinical work. With observations and ratings conducted in an ongoing manner, the therapist and clinician can detect changes in behavior and make judgments about the effectiveness of the treatment and the appropriateness of the goals.

Discussion of Clinical Vignette

A behavioral analysis and treatment plan for the depressed patient in the case vignette developed by the editors in the introductory chapter provide the opportunity to demonstrate the kinds of clinical data and procedures for obtaining them used by behavior therapists in dealing with a nonpsychotic, depressed patient.

PROBLEM IDENTIFICATION

In assessing the 42-year-old businessman presenting with complaints of sadness, anorexia, insomnia, and loss of interest in his business, hobbies, and family over a period of six weeks, the behavioral clinician begins by pinpointing these problems in multimodal and operational terms. A multimodal behavioral assessment of the depressed businessman would include evaluating his:

1) *reduced rate of engaging in overt motoric, constructive, instrumental role-behaviors*—grooming and self-care deficits, diminution or cessation of work, household tasks, and recreational activities; and increased rate of nonproductive activities such as pacing, rubbing of hands and face, and lying down
2) *verbal and nonverbal expressions of lowered mood and dysphoria*—self-depreciation, somatic complaints, anhedonia, lowered rates of smiling, vocal monotones, slouched posture, frowning, and whining; and *failure to respond to events, people, and items* that were previously reinforcing and pleasurable
3) *social withdrawal* and qualitative changes in his relations with family, friends, and coworkers
4) *distorted attitudes* and views of himself, the future, and the world in consistently negative and critical terms
5) problems with *vegetative symptoms*—anorexia, constipation, insomnia (including changes in the sleep EEG), and loss of libido
6) *dream content and fantasy life* that contain masochistic and self-depreciative themes

For each of the problems, the frequency, intensity, duration, form, and quality need to be determined. A functional, behavioral analysis is conducted to determine the environmental antecedents and consequences that are contributing to the depressive behaviors.

Goal setting and a search for reinforcers available for motivating change precede the formal introduction of treatment techniques. A modular, sequential approach to treatment is recommended that enables the clinician to utilize the least expensive and time-consuming methods first before employing more ambitious and complex interventions.

Overt motoric and instrumental behavior

The clinical note states that the patient has lost interest in his business, hobbies, and family. Which aspects of his business? Are there some business tasks or certain times when he is interested in his work? Which hobbies has he lost interest in? Does he enjoy some hobbies with some people? In answering these questions, the clinician attempts to specify the actual scope of the patient's "loss of interest."

As depressed patients may exhibit overt motoric signs of depression—such as lack of smiling and reduced activity levels—it may be useful to measure "depressive behaviors" for charting the progress of treatment.[39] This has been done by using time sampling or frequency counts.

The patient has "excessive commitment to work." How does this translate into behavior? Does he work until late at night? Does he bring work home? Does he ruminate about his work, even while eating or watching television? Since "excessive commitment to work" may be associated with so-called Type A behavior, the clinician may want to look for other Type A behavior patterns. For instance, does he interrupt others' conversations, exhibit bursts of speech, and report feelings of being burdened by time pressure? The behavioral clinician does not attempt to develop criteria to classify the patient globally as a compulsive personality, but rather to identify specific behaviors that are interfering with his functioning and subjective well-being and that can become targets of intervention.

Similarly, to know what he means by "trying to be perfect" would be important. Does he complete all tasks? Are there tasks he can leave undone? How does he determine when a job is finished? Do certain people or situations increase his feelings of needing to be perfect? Can he admit weakness to his wife, colleagues, or children? Perfectionist behavior, like any other behavior, has been learned and maintained because it has been functional and can be rechanneled and mitigated by relearning. This patient's work history is a major asset, and it should be built upon in therapy as well as modulated.

For this patient we rely on self-reporting for much of the data, but securing information from his wife and observing him interact directly with his family in his home might be valuable.

Affective problems

The clinical note reports that the patient has periods of profound sadness. To rate this sadness, the clinician may use one of the many brief and convenient affect measures available (e.g., the Mood and Affect Checklist, Beck Depression Scale, Hamilton Depression Scale, Hopkins Symptom Checklist, Zung Self-Rating Scale, the Target Complaint Scale, Raskin Depression Scale, or the Profile of Mood States).[40,41,42,43,44,45] Maintaining repeated records of affective state on a weekly basis for continual evaluation of therapy progress is useful. Alternatively, a mood graph or mood record may be maintained by the patient on a daily basis. With this method the patient rates each hour or longer interval in terms of intensity of mood and/or other associated events. This type of record allows the patient and therapist to assess the reactivity of the patient's mood on ongoing daily events and to identify for treatment purposes events that are associated with increases or decreases in mood to supplement self-ratings of mood made by the patient.

Interpersonal relations

The clinical note states that the patient is "unable to express affection" and that his marriage has worsened for several years. To define what he means by being unable to express affection, the clinician would inquire about the time, place, and duration of this problem. For instance, are there some people to whom he can express affection? Since definitions of "affection" are culture bound, it would be important to interview the wife and patient together to clarify their values and formulations of their affectional needs.

To determine what he means by his marriage worsening, we would certainly conduct joint interviews with his wife; in fact, the entire assessment and therapy might take place in a couple context. In addition to interviews and observations, the use of one of many questionnaires and rating scales available for evaluating marital satisfaction and its ingredients might be considered.[46,47] These tools are best used in cooperation with the spouse. It is possible to directly rate marital interaction using audio or videotapes and one of several procedures that have been developed may be used.[48] If, when observing or rating the tape, it is apparent the patient interrupts his wife, then this specific behavior may become a target of therapy.

Cognitions

This patient has recurrent thoughts of death, is usually serious, tries to be perfect, and "needs to be in control of every social situation." Each of these cognitions can be better specified. The therapist wants to know the specifics of the patient's recurrent thoughts of death—when, where, and under what circumstances they occur. It is particularly vital to ask specific questions regarding the patient's suicidal ideation—the frequency, elaboration, and urgency of self-destructive thoughts.

Many depressed patients have a distorted thinking pattern, and measurement of these cognitive distortions may be obtained from the patient's self-report.[12] Also, specific rating scales have been developed to measure cognitive or thinking patterns. These scales include the Automatic Thought Questionnaire, the Cognitive Response Test-36, and the Dysfunctional Attitude Scale.[12,49]

The Automatic Thought Questionnaire presents the patient with 36 statements that the patient rates for frequency of occurrence over some specific time period. The statements themselves have been gathered from depressed patient self-reports and represent statements commonly found in the stream of consciousness of depressed patients.

The Cognitive Response Test-36 is a sentence completion format consisting of 36 situations in which the patient gives his or her first response to the stimulus event. For example, the patient is presented with the stimulus, "When I think of an upcoming family reunion, I think to myself. . ." The patient completes the sentence, and the response is scored for the presence or absence of irrationally negative and other thinking patterns.

The Dysfunctional Attitude Scale consists of 40 items in a Lykert-type format. The patient is asked to identify to what degree he or she endorses each of the attitudes or assumptions listed. These assumptions are derived from cognitive theory and are hypothesized to be associated with a vulnerability to depression.[49] Items include notions such as "in order to be happy I have to be successful."

Finally, cognitions or conceptualizations of situations may be measured through induced stimulus situations created through role playing, group interactions, or videotape stimuli. After specific interactions, patients are asked to express their first automatic thoughts or ideas relevant to the situation at hand. A distorted negative bias (i.e., one in which the patient sees himself as personally defective) might constitute an indication for behavioral or cognitive therapies. These tests of cognitive distortions are then used to pinpoint specific treatment targets, to indicate the utility of certain treatment modalities, and to monitor the ongoing success of treatment. In a similar way, the clinician would want to operationalize the patient's sensations, imagery, and fantasy.

Biological, somatic, and physiological

Just as with clinicians from other theoretical persuasions, the behavior therapist would want to know about the extent of the patient's weight loss, his eating patterns, type of insomnia, and severity of fatigue. These could be specified by using self-reporting, reports based on observations of family members, a weight scale, and physiological measures for insomnia. The severity and impairment produced by the vegetative-somatic symptoms might dictate the use of medication.

While multilevel assessment and monitoring of the depressed patient is vital to the therapeutic enterprise, reliable and valid specification of depressive phenomena are limited by our measurement tools and tactics, which are still in an early stage of development. Naturalistic observation, confederate tests, time-sampling behavioral codes, and standardized, role-played test situations are infusions from behavioral therapy that are adding new approaches to the still important, but older, methods of self-report inventories and structured interviews. Assessment of an individual's environment through recently developed instruments such as the Ward Atmosphere Scale, the Behavior Observation Instrument, the Reinforcement Survey Schedule, and the Pleasant Events Schedule, adds another important dimension to behavioral analysis of depression and to the development of an individualized treatment program.

As with other approaches, the behavior therapist would want to know about the patient's genetic or familial history of depression and the occurrence of other problems, which might integrate the symptoms and problems thus far defined. From this analysis it would be possible to develop a list of specific behavioral deficits and excesses that are the components of the patient's problems and can become the object of treatment interventions.

Behavioral deficits, excesses, and assets

With elaboration and further information gathering, the patient's behavioral deficits might include:

- Before the onset of current symptoms, the patient spent one or two hours per night reading, played bridge on Friday nights, and went to dinner on Saturday night with his wife. He no longer does any of these.
- The patient has periods of profound sadness when he is alone.
- The patient spends only twenty minutes talking with his wife on an average day.
- The patient does not reinforce wife for help or support.
- The patient makes no positive statements about himself.
- The patient has had no sexual activity in the past six weeks.

The patient's behavioral excesses include:

- The patient spends twelve hours per day, six days per week at work.
- The patient interrupts others before they finish a sentence.
- The patient drinks three ounces of whiskey at bedtime to help himself sleep.
- The patient frequently says to himself, "I am worthless," or "I am a failure."

The patient's assets are important for grafting on behavioral changes that will alleviate the depressive symptomatology. They include his long and successful work history, his commitment to work and sense of family responsibility, his former hobbies, and his concerned wife.

FUNCTIONAL BEHAVIORAL ANALYSIS

The previous analysis has helped to define the problems in terms of behavioral excesses, deficits, and assets. A more precise analysis of the environmental antecedents and consequences for each of these problems needs to be accomplished. For example, for the problem of "periods of profound sadness," the settings, situations, stimuli, or people who serve as occasions or precipitants for the occurrence of the problem need to be explored. Even people who report that they are "profoundly" sad have periods during most days when they are less sad than at other times. The events that may have precipitated the patient's depression also need to be explored and examined. Were changes at work and/or in his marriage contributory to the onset of depression?

It is noted that the patient's wife responds with sympathy to the patient's sadness. How does she do this? Does she always respond with sympathy? How the patient's life would be different if the problems were diminished needs to be known. For example, would he have to resume an even heavier work schedule than he currently has? Who persuaded or coerced the patient into treatment?

Starting with the onset or acquisition of depression, it is important to identify the environmental factors that can help to explain the businessman's depressive episode. These might include a lowered rate of positive reinforcement for adaptive behaviors; modeling of depressive behaviors; aversive or punishing experiences; and stimuli and symbolic events associated in the past with happiness, sadness, or a reduction in activity level.

One possible causative factor may be a lowered rate of positive reinforcement from the environment. This could impinge on the patient through fewer *potentially* reinforcing events (e.g., if the businessman had recently moved to a *new* locale or work situation where there were fewer potential interactions with friends, neighbors, coworkers, and supervisors) as well as a reduction in the *real* availability of reinforcement (e.g., if the patient experienced an actual loss of interpersonal contacts through the death of a friend). The most important type of reinforcer deficiency for the onset of depression is a decrease in social or interpersonal interaction. This is illustrated in the case of depression precipitated by job promotions where status, prestige, and financial rewards increase but where, at the same time, there are fewer opportunities to gain supportive and positive reactions from those higher in the organization and there are greater demands to give support and help to those below in the organization. The frequency of social reinforcement received to that given is a ratio that can decrease with job rises. Low rates of reinforcement result in low rates of constructive behavior and concomitant symptoms and negative feelings about oneself and one's environment.

Modeling of depressive behaviors by others may also contribute to the patient's depression. Here is where family history and the role of his wife's affective problems need clarification.

Aversive and traumatic events might contribute to the evocation of the patient's depression such as in the "learned helplessness" model.[50] It should be noted, however, that threats, bodily assaults, or physical illness must be persistent or prolonged, not isolated incidents, to produce depressive behaviors. Punishing experiences are also characteristically accompanied by a loss of lowered rate of positive social reinforcement.

A final possible antecedent of the businessman's depression might derive from "stimulus control," whereby an event or locale symbolizes and reminds the individual of a past period of grief, helplessness, sadness, or depression. The anniversary of the death of a loved one or a return to the site of unhappy experiences can evoke mood changes that, given other factors of susceptibility and reinforcement loss, can escalate into a full blown clinical episode of depression.

In the temporal sequence of events, it may be assumed that the above types of environmental antecedents can evoke or elicit depressive symptoms such as sadness, insomnia, anxiety, anorexia, and reduced activity levels.[51,52] These elicited behaviors then likely lead to cognitively-mediated self-statements such as, "I am weak, sick, depressed, unhappy, helpless, or bad"; "The world is bleak, threatening, and rejecting"; and, "The future is hopeless, grim, and not worth living for." Through self-attribution of distorted negative views of the evoked affective changes, the individual tends to exaggerate his faults and the obstacles in his path. This verbal labeling of affect magnifies the dysphoria and instigates further decrements in feelings and performance.[53]

Beck and his colleagues have amassed data bearing on the role of cognitions in depression and posit that the negative thinking patterns by which the depressed person views himself or herself, the future, and the world are developed throughout childhood and adolescence when the maturing individual is exposed to frequent critical evaluation by significant others. The individual adopts these highly critical standards as his or her own through the normal social learning process, with the result being a person who gets little reward in life because he or she is constantly debasing his or her performance.

Continuing our speculative odyssey from the acquisition to the *maintenance* of depression, the vicious cycle of dysphoria, negative self-statements, and greater dysphoria may be fueled by the attention, concern, sympathy, and nurturance provided to the depressed person by relatives, friends, physicians, and other "helpers." The positive social reinforcement of depressive affect, verbal and nonverbal expressiveness, can put the depression into a maintenance phase that can become a chronic, persistent problem. Iatrogenic factors may contribute to the chronicity of depression when medical personnel focus on the depressive symptoms or persistently investigate physical explanations for the symptoms. Another element in the maintenance of depression is the social withdrawal and isolation that occurs, principally as a result of anhedonia, social anxiety, and self-attribution of worthlessness, hopelessness, and negative world views. Isolation and alienation from others produce even greater obstacles to reconstituting interpersonal sources of reinforcement for adaptive behaviors and positive verbalizations. Social alienation also moves into a vicious cycle, because the depressed individual fails to provide reinforcement to friends and relatives and thus gradually tends to be avoided. Greater isolation from others leads to greater unpleasantness as a companion that, in turn, leads to mutual avoidance and further isolation.

Figure 4 is a diagram of the environmental processes that, given our current understanding of depressive disorders, might be considered as relevant to the evocation and maintenance of the businessman's depressive behaviors. This diagram, while seemingly complex, actually oversimplifies the dynamic flux among premorbid and current behavior, coping style, and environmental factors that account for the considerable inter- and intraindividual variation found in depression. Even the most elaborate behavioral and interactional observation codes are not likely to capture the subtle nuances in the behavioral-environmental interchanges that serve as modifiers of depressive phenomena. The content of a person's depressive feelings and behavior is also an outcome of the individual's idiosyncratic familial, cultural, and personal premorbid experiences. For example, individuals tend to fall back to anachronistic responses that successfully procured reinforcement during childhood or at times of real physical illnesses.

While behavior therapy approaches have sometimes been viewed as short term, it can be seen from the above description of multimodal behavioral assessment and functional analysis that behavior therapy can be as complicated as psychoanalytic investigation of psychiatric disorder. To avoid getting bogged down in long-term reconstructive therapy, however, the behavioral clinician would delineate and set priorities for the behavioral assessment and analysis of those environmental antecedents and consequences most immediately germane to the patient's decompensation from the previous level of functioning. Thus, in the case of the depressed businessman, investigation of recent life changes in both work and familial arenas would likely point to the critical environmental stressors that could be targeted for intervention.

Goal setting

The behavioral analysis of these problems can then be translated into goals for treatment. The goals for treatment should be derived logically from this analysis and should be specific and clear; chosen by the patient; short term, but linked to longer-term goals; salient; and attainable. Since little is known about this patient, and since behavior therapy decisions are made in an ongoing fashion depending upon the patient's changing clinical status, it is difficult to formulate a total behavior therapy plan at this juncture. However, to show how initial problems can be translated into treatment goals and interventions and how evaluative data are used to monitor progress of therapy and interact with ongoing treatment decisions, behavioral approaches to the treatment of depression will be described.

BROAD SPECTRUM BEHAVIOR THERAPY FOR DEPRESSION

The tremendous individual diversity among depressed persons has important implications for the design of treatment programs.

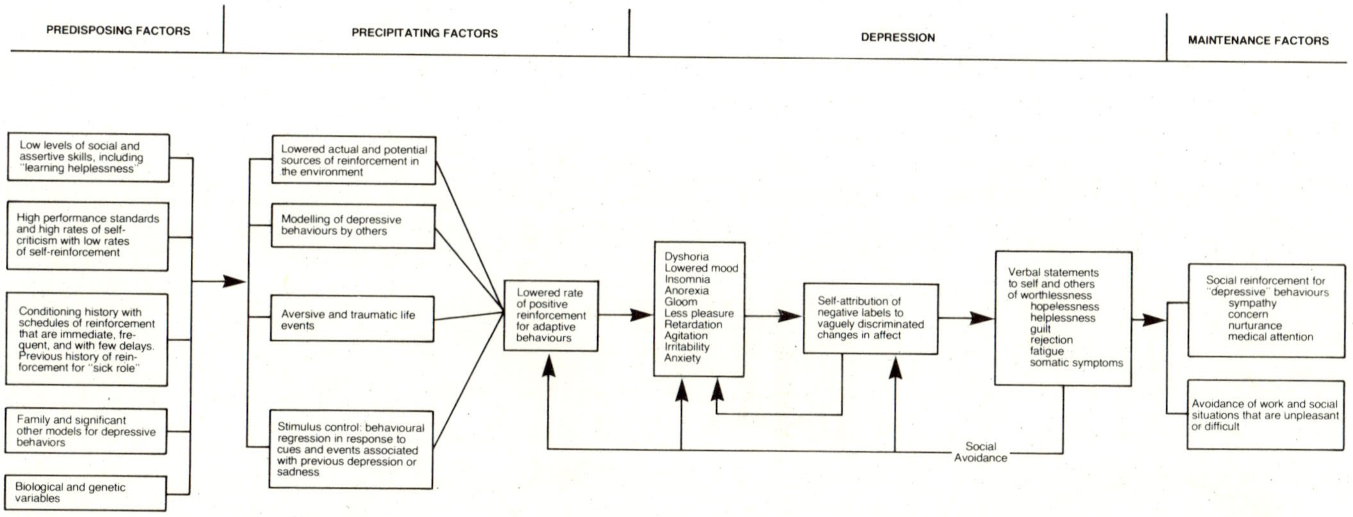

FIGURE 4

DIAGRAM OF THE ENVIRONMENTAL ANTECEDENTS AND CONSEQUENCES RESPONSIBLE FOR THE INDIVIDUAL VARIABILITY IN THE ONSET AND MAINTENANCE OF "DEPRESSIVE" BEHAVIOR

(adapted from Lewinsohn, 1975)

Diversity stems from variations in the multilevel phenomenology of depressive behaviors; from variations in the acquisition and maintenance of depressive behaviors; from differences in history, personal assets and resources that serve as sources of vulnerability to depression; and from variations in the depressed person's environmental dynamics and social support networks. These sources for diversity, together with their implications for treatment, are outlined in Table 6. Full appreciation of the diverse potentialities for the development, manifestation, and course of depressive phenomena—including interactions between the biological, behavioral, and environmental influences—suggests that therapeutic interventions must be responsive to the varied needs of each depressed person. For example, there may be many forms of depression with differential antecedents and consequences. Most experienced clinicians would agree that some combination of underlying organic disorder, life events, social skills deficits, lack of engagement in constructive and rewarding activities, and cognitive distortion may be implicated in many cases of depression. Yet the balance or the amount of variance in each clinical case accounted for by each of the implicated factors may be different for every case.

One option for designing treatment that takes into account individual differences is to construct a comprehensive therapeutic "package" that incorporates key interventions aimed at remediating most problem areas. For example, a broad-spectrum approach might be suitable for the needs of the depressed patient described in the case vignette. One component of broad-spectrum therapy for depression would re-engage the patient in previously enjoyable hobbies through the use of graded "homework" assignments and positive feedback from wife, children, and therapist. As a corollary, the therapist would work with the patient and his wife conjointly to alter the contingencies of reinforcement away from his wife's solicitousness for his being depressed and toward more constructive, albeit graded, task completion. Specific social skills training in areas where the patient appeared to have deficits would be another ingredient of the broad-spectrum strategy; examples are assertively expressing his feelings (especially affection), requesting assistance and contributions to family life from his wife, and saying "no" to excessive and unreasonable expectations of his work performance from colleagues. Marital and family therapy would be helpful in reconstituting his

TABLE 6
SOURCES OF DIVERSITY IN DEPRESSION THAT HAVE FUNCTIONAL TIES TO THE CHOICE OF TREATMENT INTERVENTION

Level or Dimension	Example	Treatment Implication
Biological/genetic	Bipolar manic-depressive phenomena	Use of lithium
Subjective affect	Presence of anxiety	Use of anxiety management or desensitization
Motor behavior	Anergic apathy and idleness	Graded assignments with positive feedback
Cognitive	Negative self-evaluation	Cognitive therapy
Social competence	Unable to ask others to help or assist self	Social skills or assertion training
Social network	Presence of concerned spouse	Involvement of spouse in couple therapy
Vocational	Job promotion precipitated depression	Target changes in work setting
Social system	Pension for disability due to depression	Changing social security regulations to provide incentives for rehabilitation

immediate support system. Emphasizing skills training in communication and problem solving, recreational-social restructuring, negotiating a contingency contract, and behavioral marital therapy have been described in a manual that enables clinicians of all persuasions to replicate the procedures.[46] Cognitive restructuring, a form of therapy developed first from a cognitive behavioral analysis of depressives, would be helpful in changing the patient's ways of derogating himself, his world, and his future and would aim to lower his scrupulously high standards of self-reward and perfectionism.[53]

The comprehensive, broad-spectrum approach to treating depressed patients has wide appeal. It satisfies the proponents of each of the major theoretical "schools" within the behavioral camp since it draws component techniques from each of them. In fact, most of the published reports of behavioral treatment of depression, both controlled and case studies, utilize a comprehensive, multicomponent approach, despite the highlighting of one or another of the techniques by the authors.[54]

While the broad-spectrum treatment approach is attractive because of its potentially wide applicability and likely efficacy, it is costly in terms of time, training of personnel, and its multidimensional evaluation of ongoing progress. The broad-spectrum approach is also intrusive and encumbers the patient with many interventions and assignments, some of which may not be necessary or applicable. An alternative to the broad-spectrum approach, but one that still meets the tremendous variability in the needs of depressed individuals, is a modular strategy in which the therapist uses flexible levels of intervention depending upon the response of the patient.

MODULAR STRATEGY FOR TREATMENT OF DEPRESSION

The modular approach starts with the assumption that "less is better than more treatment." Only those limited interventions and number of sessions required to bring about satisfactory improvement are employed. The full array of problem-specific treatment techniques is available to the clinician in the modular approach; however, techniques are selected and implemented only when the patient's specific problems or lack of response to previous interventions call for them. The training methods in the spheres of cognition, contingency, self-control, pleasurable activities, anxiety management, and social skills are tailored to the individual case. The preliminary assessment and the ongoing feedback provided by the patient's response to treatment guide the therapist in deciding which components of the broad-spectrum approach to utilize with the individual case and how much time and emphasis to place on each of the chosen components.

This modular approach to treatment is congruent with the process of most clinical endeavors in medicine, psychiatry, and psychology. It follows the Hippocratic imperative to do no harm to the patient. It gives maximum influence to the patient in the therapy process as each time a choice point is reached regarding the utilization of an additional module, the patient participates fully in the decision making. Thus, there are many more opportunities for active involvement by the patient in deciding the type, duration, and outcomes of therapy. With such a strategy, advantages also accrue to the therapist who self-consciously and regularly must evaluate and review clinical progress, consider treatment alternatives for goals and methods, and question whether or not he or she has something of value to offer the patient. This empirical approach to therapy derives from the flow chart depicted in Figure 1.

Initial modules

How might this approach be adapted and used with the depressed patient described in the common case vignette? The flow chart in Figure 5 outlines the first few decision points facing the therapist who begins to evaluate and treat such a depressed person. The initial visit or contact, whether it be in a clinic, mental health center, or private office, is filled with a variety of tasks. Regardless of one's theoretical and clinical orientation, the first session usually includes history taking, relationship building, ventilation of feelings and symptoms, and evaluation of the extent and severity of the problem.

Many times, especially in cases of mild disorders where depressive symptoms are precipitated by transient situational events, the first visit may suffice as an intervention in itself. Research on the process of psychotherapy suggests that significant symptomatic relief occurs between the time a patient enters a waiting room and is interviewed by a clinic secretary; thus, it should not be surprising that some patients with mild depressions can be sufficiently helped through the clarification, catharsis, and hopefulness of an evaluation interview. It appears from the case vignette, however, that the depressed businessman's disorder is not likely to respond to this superficial and brief initial intervention.

If the clinician deems the depression severe or life threatening at the time of the initial session, a choice point is reached for the utilization of antidepressant medication. If the decision to use anti-

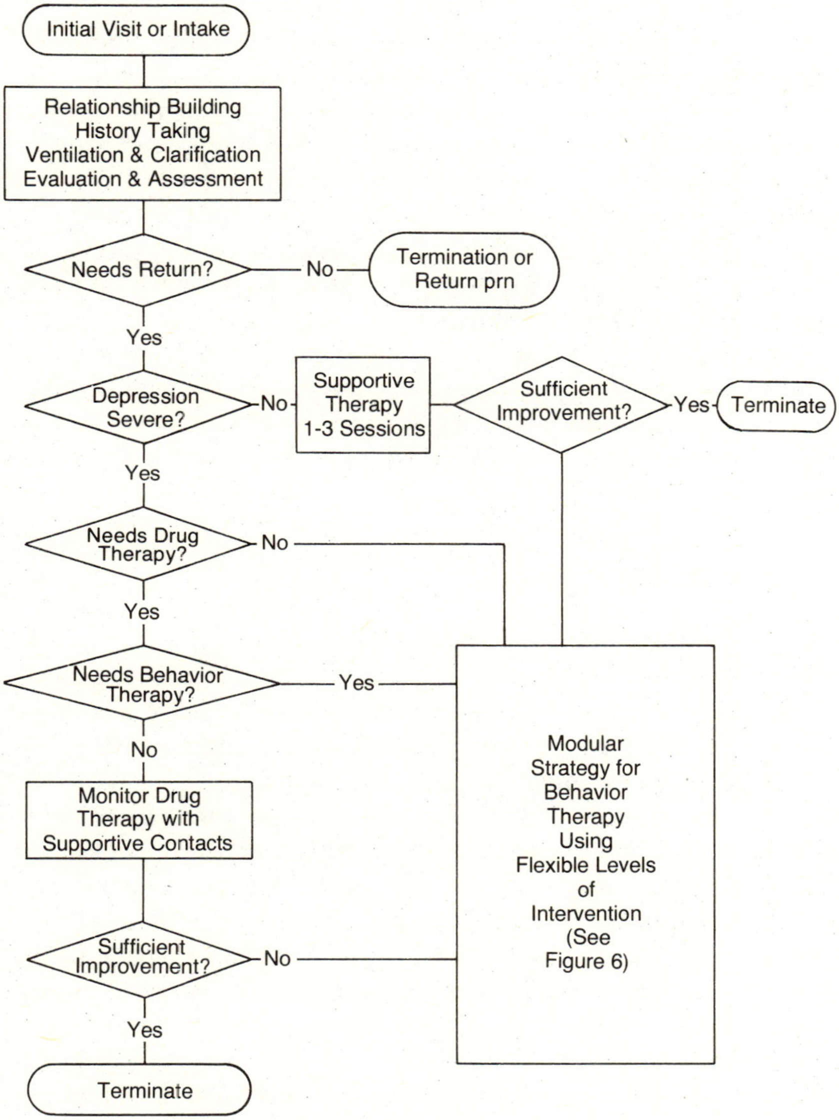

FIGURE 5

FLOW CHART DEPICTING INITIAL PHASES OF A MODULAR STRATEGY FOR THE TREATMENT OF DEPRESSION depressant drugs is made, another question arises at to whether the drug therapy should be given either alone with only supportive contacts, or whether drug therapy should be accompanied by systematic behavior therapy. The best criterion for making the decision comes from the work of Weissman and Paykell who found suggestive evidence that patients with social skill deficits prior to becoming depressed might require some form of psychosocial treatment beyond drug therapy for satisfactory clinical outcomes.[55] The prototype patient, with clear-cut and severe vegetative symptoms and social skills deficits, is likely to benefit from both drugs and systematic behavior therapy. If behavior therapy is chosen, with or without concomitant drug therapy, the clinician can draw treatment modules from the techniques developed in the past ten years and described as promising in a literature still marked more by clinical enthusiasm than by hard, controlled data.

Initial and ongoing assessment

Whether drug therapy, supportive therapy, or some combination behavior therapy is offered to the depressed businessman, a basic requirement for the empirically-based, modular strategy is a thorough initial assessment and ongoing evaluation of the patient's progress. An initial assessment can help the clinician in the step-wise decision-making process from minimum to maximum levels of intervention. For example, if the initial assessment of the businessman uncovered a marked paucity of recreational and leisure time activities, the clinician might set goals and give graded assignments to develop such outlets. If, as implied, the patient showed social withdrawal and scored low on assertiveness questionnaires, a decision might be made to offer social skills training.

The initial assessment, in addition to the conventional social and psychiatric history, should include measures of the extent and intensity of the depression—measures that can be used in a repeated way throughout therapy as a way of gauging progress. The clinician can use one or more of the many depression scales to monitor the patient's symptomatic changes as time passes, thereby obtaining information necessary for deciding, with the patient, when treatment should be continued, altered, tapered or terminated.

Besides an ongoing measure of symptomatic status, the clinician utilizing the modular treatment strategy will want to have other measures, at the time of initial evaluation and for repeated monitoring, that tap dimensions such as available reinforcers (e.g., a reinforcement survey); the patient's range and amount of activity (e.g., behavioral diaries or logs); social adjustment (e.g., ratings from the patient and significant others); and assertiveness (e.g., the Rathus Assertiveness Scale).

Behavior therapy modules

A flow chart depicting the choice points of a step-wise, minimum-to-maximum use of behavioral modules in the treatment of depression is shown in Figure 6. The discussion that follows would be equally applicable to patients who are being treated with behavior therapy alone or in combination with drugs. At each point in the progress of the patient through the behavior therapy modules, the therapist and patient should review the amount of improvement gained and decide whether additional therapy is needed. The informational resources from which the therapist can borrow in making treatment decisions include: 1) the changes occurring in the patient's symptoms and other behavioral and social measures; and 2) the available techniques that have been reported to be helpful to depressed patients.

A. PROBLEM FORMULATION AND GOAL SETTING. Before introducing more complex and time-consuming techniques, the therapist should begin with one to three sessions using a problem-solving focus. The patient is helped to view his problems, including symptoms, not as hopeless burdens but rather as challenges to cope with and solve. The first step in this process is to identify the problems—the symptoms, functional impairments, and their antecedents and consequences. It is important for the therapist to help the patient describe the problems in the patient's terms and then to translate feelings and concerns into behavioral terms. The focus is on pinpointing what the patient is *doing and saying* and in what environmental context. The patient and therapist together ask the following questions in a spirit of inquiry:

- Which problems are most interfering with the patient's functioning (e.g., if the patient's preoccupation with death converts into self-destructive fantasies, the immediate priority may be

FIGURE 6

FLOW CHART DEPICTING THE MODULAR USE OF BEHAVIORAL TECHNIQUES IN THE TREATMENT OF DEPRESSION.

Sufficient improvement can be determined by a multiple method, and sources of assessment. The sequence of modules in the large box does not necessarily reflect priorities or temporal ordering of treatment.

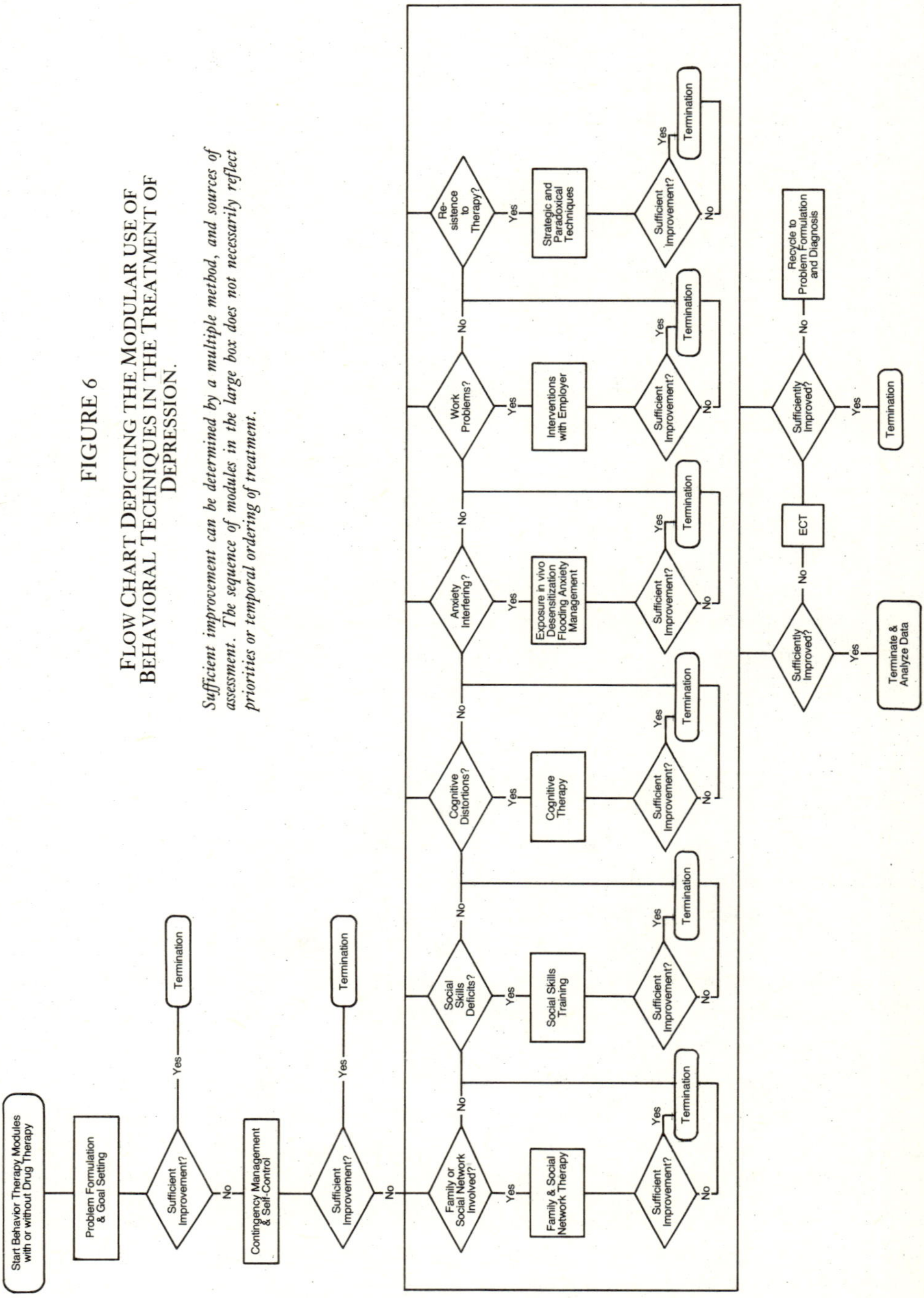

hospitalization and close supervision; if the patient is about to lose a cherished job, then the immediate intervention may be intercession with the employer or behavioral rehearsal of a scene with job supervisor aimed at obtaining sick leave)?

- Which problems are most responsible for the patient's being maintained in a state of depression (e.g., the patient's symptoms are being reinforced by a sympathetic wife, which suggests the need for intervention with the relative to change the reinforcement contingencies)?
- Which assets, if strengthened, can serve as a wedge to break the depressive cycle (e.g., if the patient has had good social relationships that have recently been dormant, the therapist may initially aim at social skills training to reconstitute these relationships)?
- Which specific behavior patterns require change in their frequency of occurrence, intensity, duration, or in the conditions under which they occur?
- What are the best practical means to produce the desired changes in this individual (e.g., manipulation of the environment or self-attitudes of the client)?

Once some problem definition has occurred, the therapist helps the patient set goals for the therapy. The therapist asks the patient for possible alternative behaviors to those currently producing an impasse. The therapist also offers suggested alternatives for the patient's evaluation. Questions are asked such as, "What would you like to do that you're not now doing?"; "How would you like your everyday life different from the way it is now?"; "What changes would you like to make in your routines and relationships?"; "How might you cope with the problems confronting you?" In the problem-solving approach, generating alternatives is accompanied by evaluating their probable consequences or outcomes. Once the various alternatives for dealing with the problem are evaluated, the therapist assists the patient in choosing one that seems reasonable.

Problem formulation and goal setting are enterprises that can provide the necessary impetus for the patient to cope better and get symptomatic improvement sufficient for termination. The problem-solving approach can be carried out in one to three sessions that, with the initial visits, may bring the patient to a total of three to seven sessions. A brief therapy course, such as the one just described, is obviously cost-effective and will often be sufficient with patients like the one in the case vignette who come to therapy with many assets and a good premorbid adjustment.

B. Contingency management and self-control. If the businessman-patient needs additional therapy beyond the problem-solving phase, the therapist can use attention and praise as contingent reinforcers for adaptive verbalizations during the therapy session and for reports of attempting homework assignments between therapy sessions. The therapist will be able to use the already established, positive therapeutic alliance in a contingent manner to strengthen assets and to help the patient to accomplish goals selected during the earlier problem-formulating module. Thus, the contingency management and problem-formulating modules interlock in a natural way. If the patient is hospitalized because of functional incapacity and/or suicidal risk, contingencies can be used that stem from hospital privileges and from social reinforcement from the entire interdisciplinary staff. In using graded assignments for adaptive behavior reinforced with positive feedback, the therapist ensures that instructions are given clearly, specifically, affirmatively, and with the structuring of positive expectations for success. At times, this must be accomplished in subtle ways, including the use of paradoxical instructions. Shaping is also kept in mind as this module progresses.

While the therapist is using his or her therapeutic relationship as a contingent reinforcer for the re-establishment of verbal and motor activities as alternatives to depressive behaviors, the patient can also be taught to use self-control methods to increase desired behaviors and interactions. These methods can include:

1) The patient's performing highly probable behavior (e.g., work tasks, withdrawal to bed, smoking, time to be alone) being made contingent upon the patient's first engaging in positive, desirable, but less likely positive self-statements or activities.
2) Self-monitoring, self-evaluation, and self-reinforcement with an emphasis on monitoring positive events and setting realistic attainable behavioral goals that would be expected to reduce depressive affect.

This module might continue as long as good progress is being made, with termination for satisfactory improvement occurring after perhaps two to ten sessions.

C. Behavioral family therapy. A family therapy side-branch on the modular flow chart would be appropriate for the businessman-patient if he has not made progress after a few sessions of contingency management and self-control, since family interactions might be maintaining the depressive behaviors. The family or marital therapy itself can proceed along several flexible levels of intervention, ranging from simple instructions to patient's wife and children to provide differential attention for adaptive behaviors, to that plus scheduling social and recreational activities, communication skills training, and contingency contracting. Hence, both across and within modules, minimum to maximum levels of intervention are used.

D. Other modules. Beyond the problem-formulating/goal-setting and contingency management modules, the employment of other behavior therapies can be considered if there has not been sufficient progress to terminate therapy. A variety of methods has been well described in the literature with varying amounts of evidence supporting their efficacy—cognitive therapy, self-control techniques, anxiety management techniques, social skills training, and paradoxical or strategic methods. The decision to utilize any one of these techniques would come from 1) insufficient progress from previous modules, and 2) information regarding specific deficits of the patient that could be remediated by the technique.

The decision points for these modules are shown in Figure 6 as having "equal significance"; however, only the accumulation of empirical experience with large numbers of depressed patients can indicate how often and how valuable any one of these techniques might be. For example, while it appears that a sizeable majority of depressed patients demonstrate cognitive distortions described by Beck, it doesn't necessarily follow that all such patients would require specific cognitive therapy for relieving their depression.[11,12] Some of these patients would improve sufficiently with five sessions of ventilation, catharsis, and problem-formulating/goal-setting. Others would improve sufficiently with the addition of a few sessions of contingency management. Those who continue to show cognitive distortions, remain depressed, and are thus in need of further therapy, would be much better candidates for the cognitive therapy approach. The same is true for the other behavioral techniques currently in vogue for depression.

E. STRATEGIC THERAPY. Strategic or paradoxical therapy techniques deserve a special note because they can be employed with other more straightforward behavior therapies to enhance cooperation and commitment and increase compliance with instructions and assignments. As a wider body of techniques for depression is developed, it is apparent that the discovery of what people need *to do* to overcome their problems is not the most difficult clinical task. *Getting people to do* what they need to do is the most difficult task. A group of prescriptive methods is now available that, if followed properly by the patient, can yield meaningful improvement. But, as any experienced behavior therapist will admit, it is getting patients to do what is prescribed that usually provides the challenges to therapeutic acumen. These techniques have been described in a number of publications.[46,56]

In the horizontal sequence, the depiction of the various behavior therapy modules in Figure 6 does not denote a preferential ordering of each module's utility or priority of presentation. Figure 6 is presented as a hypothetical starting point for clinical and empirical testing. Even the depiction of a contingency management/self-control module prior to the use of other modules is offered as a speculative leap into the proposed modular approach. It is conceivable that a different module—e.g., cognitive therapy—may be more useful than the contingency management/self-control module. The provision of a module to a patient and its temporal priority in the therapeutic sequence would be determined by:

1) the specific needs of each patient as elucidated by the initial behavioral assessment and ongoing monitoring of progress
2) the empirically documented efficacy of any one module in the hands of the clinician and in the literature
3) the cost and intrusiveness of any one module

Thus, for the depressed patient described in the clinical vignette, it is likely that his presenting problems and premorbid deficits and excesses would point to the need for the following behavioral modules: problem solving, contingency management and self-control, marital therapy, social skills training, and cognitive therapy.

As clinical and research experience with the use of a modular approach to the behavioral treatment of depression accumulates, the utility of each module for remediating the specific deficits of the individual patient, as well as for improving symptoms and mood, will become more evident. For example, it may be found that social skills training is effective in helping depressed persons establish social relationships, but is less effective for improving symptomatic state. The number of patients exposed to each module should clarify the types of deficits that depressed persons have; furthermore, the modular approach should make clearer the need for additional treatment modules addressing deficits and problems that our current behavioral technology does not cover. By weeding out the less seriously depressed patients and those who would respond favorably to "nonspecific" factors in therapy, the modular strategy provides a more stringent test of the efficacy of each of the constituent treatment interventions. As time passes and experience with a modular strategy accumulates, both individual clinicians and the research community can "shake down" the various modules and adapt and evolve new techniques having greater impact on depressive behaviors.

Summary

The hallmark of behavior therapy is its reliance on specific measurement to characterize all dimensions of behavior, including affect, sensation, imagery, verbal and nonverbal elements of social interaction, thoughts, and biological phenomena. Thus, behavioral assessment must encompass all the levels of behavior that contribute to the clinical symptoms, role impairment, treatment outcome, and DSM-III operational criteria. Beginning with an operational description of the target behavior(s), the therapist proceeds with a determination of excess of maladaptive behavior and/or deficits of adaptive behavior to be modified. Problem behaviors are then categorized in terms of frequency, intensity, duration, latency, and situation. These determinations are made on the basis of self-report, including checklists, surveys, and diaries, or on direct observations. The result is a functional analysis of the antecedents and consequences of the target problems. We provide a model of the environmental process that, given our current understanding of depressive disorders, for example, might be relevant to evaluating and maintaining depressive behavior. Once a behavioral assessment and functional analysis are completed, it becomes possible to develop treatment goals. Such goals should be logically derived, specific, clear, and accomplished through short-term therapy though leading to longer-term goals.

Behavior therapy employs a broad range of treatment procedures and techniques in treating all levels of behavior, including affect, sensation, imagery, verbal and nonverbal elements of social interactions, cognition, and biological phenomena, as well as instrumental, observable actions. The particular treatment strategies a therapist plans to use must be logically chosen from this behavioral analysis and be appropriate to achieve the treatment goals. In behavior therapy, the patient's progress is carefully monitored; new goals are selected as previous ones are achieved; and there is an ongoing interaction among treatment, progress, and evaluation. DSM-III diagnoses are a first step in labeling problems that behavioral assessment can then more precisely define and quantify.

TABLE 2
OUTLINE OF BEHAVIORAL APPROACH TO HISTORY TAKING, ASSESSMENT & THERAPY

I. PROBLEMS AND GOALS

A. Define and translate problems and goals into *behavioral terms* using as dimensions the frequency, intensity, duration, form or quality, and the appropriateness of the context of the behaviorist(s).

B. Develop a *multimodal* inventory of the problems and goals, in which all levels of human behavioral expression and experience are covered:

overt, motoric and instrumental behavior
affects
sensations
interpersonal relations
cognitions
imagery and fantasy
biological, somatic, and physiological

C. Determine *behavioral deficits*: which behaviors need to be initiated, increased in frequency, or strengthened in form?

TABLE 2 (CONTINUED)

D. Determine *behavioral excesses*: which behaviors need to be terminated, decreased in frequency, or altered in form?

E. Determine *behavioral assets*: consider strengths in multimodal terms.

F. Determine if the patient's self-description of the problem is congruent with that of other observers.

II. ANALYSIS OF CONDITIONS MAINTAINING THE PROBLEMS

A. *Antecedents* of the behavioral problems: what are the settings, situations, stimuli, or people which serve as occasions or precipitants for the occurrence of the problems? Ask patient of the problem: where, when, and with whom? What "life events" have recently occurred that might be stressors?

B. *Consequences* of the behavioral problems: sometimes called "secondary gains," these are actually the primary and important ways the environment responds to maintain the problem behaviors or make less likely movement toward the desirable, alternative goals. Ask questions such as:
Who responds to the problems with sympathy, help, attention, or emotional reactions?
Who persuaded or coerced the patient into treatment?
What would happen if the problems were ignored or if the problems went away?
How would the patient's life be different if the problems were diminished?
What reinforcers or benefits would the patient gain if the problems were removed?

C. *Self-motivation:* how is the patient affected by the problems — comfortable, ambivalent, or troubled? Does the patient acknowledge the problems and desire change?

III. ASSESSMENT INSTRUMENTS

Ascertain the correspondence between *verbal self-report* by patient and *actions* observed by assessor and others.

A. *Fear Survey*: determines degree of fear associated with a wide range of items, places, stimuli, situations, and interpersonal events that patient may avoid.

B. *Reinforcement Survey* and *Pleasant Events Schedule:* determine activities, places, people, foods, and things that can be used to motivate progress.

TABLE 2 (CONTINUED)

C. *Behavioral diaries or logs*: counting frequencies or intervals promotes self-observation, self-monitoring, and more accurate depiction of scope and timing of problem behaviors.

D. *Symptom ratings and interviews*: Target Complaint Scale, anxiety inventories, Symptom Checklist, Marital Adjustment Test, Self-Rating Depression Scale, Beck Depression Inventory, Hamilton Depression Interview, Present State Examination, etc.

E. *Physiological measures*: heart rate, blood pressure, fingertip skin temperature, skin resistance, biofeedback devices.

IV. BIOLOGICAL ASSESSMENT

Relevant medical and surgical problems

Physical limitations and handicaps

Psychotropic drugs — they interact with behavioral interventions as well as affecting behavior directly

V. SOCIOCULTURAL ASSESSMENT

Recent changes in milieu — migration, intergenerational family conflicts, changes in residence or work

Recent changes in relationships — divorce, death

Language and values

VI. GOAL SETTING

Move focus from problems to goals as soon as possible

Behaviors selected as goals when possible should be:
- specific and clear
- chosen by patient
- short term as links to longer-term goals
- frequently occurring
- salient and functional
- attainable

VII. MONITORING PROGRESS

Using behavioral measurement means keeping track of changes in the behavior targeted as problems and/or goals. Measurement should be practical, convenient, and relevant to the clinical problems. Data can come from the treatment session and from the natural environment. Observing and recording can be done by the therapist, the patient, and by significant others. Some types of recording progress are:
- Frequency counts of the behavior
- Intervals noted when the target behavior has occurred

TABLE 2 (CONTINUED)

Duration or latency of the behavior
Intensity estimations (e.g., "How much did the anxiety bother you during the last week?")
Permanent products are tangible outcomes that indicate that the behavior occurred (e.g., ticket stubs to a movie; no dirt on face indicates face was washed)

VIII. BEHAVIOR THERAPY TACTICS

A. Develop trusting, caring, warm, and mutually respectful therapeutic alliance that serves as the foundation and lever for many of the behavioral techniques.
B. Develop time-limited treatment program.
C. Use behavioral rehearsal or role-playing to simulate "real world" problem situations.
D. Prompt, cue, signal, and coach patient to make improvements.
E. Give "homework assignments."
F. Reinforce small, discrete steps in adaptive directions.
G. Use therapeutic instructions and promote favorable expectations of outcome.
H. Have patient repeatedly practice the desired behavior.
I. Feedback information on behavioral changes to patient and periodically re-evaluate progress and reset goals.
J. Reinforce progress, underplay reversals.
K. Generalize gains to natural environment by involving family members and other aspects of the "real world."

REFERENCES

1. Agras, W. S., Kazdin, A. E., and Wilson, G. T.: *Behavior Therapy: Toward an Applied Clinical Science*, San Francisco: Freeman, 1979.
2. Kazdin, A. E.: *History of Behavior Modification*, Baltimore: University Park Press, 1978.
3. Skinner, B. F.: *Science and Human Behavior*, New York: Macmillan, 1953.
4. Eysenck, H. J.: Learning Theory and Behaviour Therapy, *Journal of Mental Science*, 195:61–75, 1959.
5. Pavlov, I. P.: *Conditioned Reflexes*, Oxford University, 1927.
6. Hull, C. L.: *Principles of Behavior*, New York: Appleton-Century-Crofts, 1943.
7. Mowrer, O. W.: *Learning Theory and Behavior*, New York: Wiley, 1960.
8. Wolpe, J.: *Psychotherapy by Reciprocal Inhibition*, Stanford, CA.: Stanford University Press, 1958.

9. Bandura, A.: *Social Learning Theory*, Englewood Cliffs, N.J.: Prentice-Hall, 1977.
10. Ellis, A.: *The Essence of Rational Psychotherapy: A Comprehensive Approach to Treatment*, New York: Institute for Rational Living, 1970.
11. Lazarus, A. A.: *Behavior Therapy and Beyond*, New York: McGraw-Hill, 1971.
12. Meichenbaum, D.: *Cognitive Behavior Modification*, New York: Plenum Press, 1977.
13. Beck, A. T., Rush, A. J., Shaw, B. F., and Emery, G.: *Cognitive Therapy of Depression*, New York: Guilford Press, 1979.
14. Ferguson, J. M., and Taylor, C. B.: *Comprehensive Handbook of Behavioral Medicine*, Vols. 1–3, Jamaica, N.Y.: Spectrum, 1980.
15. Liberman, R. P., and Davis, J.: Drugs and Behavioral Analysis, in M. Hersen, R. Eisler, and P. Miller (eds.): *Progress in Behavior Modification*, Vol. 1, New York: Academic Press, 1975, 307–330.
16. Liberman, R. P.: A Model for Individualizing Treatment, in L. Rehm (ed.): *Behavior Therapy for Depression*, New York: Academic Press, 1981, 231–254.
17. Jacob, R. G., Kraemer, H. C., and Agras, W. S.: Relaxation Training in the Treatment of Hypertension: A Review, *Archives of General Psychiatry*, 34:1417–1427, 1977.
18. Drury, R., DeRisi, W. J., and Liberman, R. P.: Temperature Biofeedback Treatment for Migraine Headaches, *Headache*, 19:278–284, 1979.
19. Cautela, J. R., and Upper, D.: The Behavioral Inventory Battery: The Use of Self-Report Measures in Behavioral Analysis and Therapy, in M. Hersen, and A. S. Bellack (eds.): *Behavioral Assessment: A Practical Handbook*, New York: Pergamon Press, 1976, 77–109.
20. Kanfer, I. H., and Saslow, G.: Behavioral Diagnosis, in C. M. Franks (ed.): *Behavioral Therapy: Appraisal and Status*, New York: McGraw-Hill, 1969.
21. Mash, E. J., and Terdal, L. G. (eds.): *Behavioral Assessment of Childhood Disorders*, New York: Guilford Press, 1981.
22. Ciminero, A. R., Calhoun, K. S., and Adams, H. E. (eds.): *Handbook of Behavioral Assessment*, New York: Wiley, 1977.
23. Caugela, J. R.: *Behavior Analysis Forms for Clinical Intervention*, Champaign, IL: Research Press, 1977.
24. Stuart, R. B.: *Action-Oriented Clinical Aids and Inventories*, Champaign, IL: Research Press, 1975.
25. Battle, C. C., Imber, S. D., Hoehn-Saric, R., Stone, A. R., Nash, E. R., and Frank, J. D.: Target Complaints as Criteria of Improvement, *American Journal of Psychotherapy*, 20:184–192, 1966.
26. Liberman, R. P., and Smith, V.: Multiple Baseline Study of Desensitization, *Behavior Therapy*, 3:446, 1972.
27. Liberman, R. P., Teigen, J., Patterson, R., and Baker, V.: Reducing Delusional Speech in Chronic, Paranoid Schizophrenics, *Journal of Applied Behavior Analysis*, 6:57–64, 1973.
28. Hersen, M., and Barlow, D. (eds.): *Behavioral Assessment: A Practical Handbook*, Elmsford, N.Y.: Pergamon Press, 1976.

29. Mash, E. J., and Terdal, L. G. (eds.): *Behavior Therapy Assessment*, New York: Springer, 1976.
30. Keefe, F. J., Kopel, S. A., and Gordon, S. B.: *A Practical Guide to Behavioral Assessment*, New York: Springer, 1978.
31. Wolpe, J.: *The Practice of Behavior Therapy*, New York: Pergamon Press, 1969.
32. Gambrill, E. D.: *Behavior Modification: Handbook of Assessment, Intervention, and Evaluation*, San Francisco: Jossey-Bass, 1977.
33. Clement, P. W., and Richard, R. C.: Identifying Reinforcers for Children: A Children's Reinforcement Survey, in E. J. Mash, and L. G. Terdal, (eds.): *Behavior Therapy Assessment*, New York: Springer, 1976, 207–216.
34. MacPhillamy, D. J., and Lewinsohn, P. M.: Depression as a Function of Levels of Desired and Obtained Pleasure, *Journal of Abnormal Psychology*, 83:651–657, 1974.
35. Guy W.: *ECDEU: Assessment Manual for Psychopharmacology*, Rockville, MD: U.S. Dept. of Health, Education, and Welfare, revised 1976.
36. Van Putten, T., and May, P. R. A.: Subjective Response as a Predictor of Outcome in Pharmacotherapy, *Archives of General Psychiatry*, 35:477–480, 1978.
37. Rathus, S. A.: A Thirty Item Schedule for Assessing Assertive Behavior, *Behavior Therapy*, 4:298–306, 1973.
38. Wing, J. K., Cooper, J. E., and Sartorius, N.: *The Management and Classification of Psychiatric Symptoms*, London: Cambridge University Press, 1974.
39. Jacobson, N.: The Assessment of Overt Behavior, in L. Rehm (ed.): *Behavior Therapy for Depression*, New York: Academic Press, 1981, 279–300.
40. Zung, W. W. K.: A Self-Rating Depression Scale, *Archives of General Psychiatry*, 12:63–70, 1965.
41. Raskin, A., Schuterbrandt, J., Reatig, N., Cook, T., and Odle, D.: Depression Subtypes and Response to Phenelzine, Diazepam, and a Placebo, *Archives of General Psychiatry*, 30:66–75, 1974.
42. Hamilton, M.: A Rating Scale for Depression, *Journal of Neurology, Neurosurgery, and Psychiatry*, 23:56–62, 1960.
43. Derogatis, L. R., Lipman, R. S., and Rickels, K.: The Hopkins Symptom Checklist, in P. Pichot (ed.): *Modern Problems in Pharmacopsychiatry*, Basel, Switzerland: Karger, 1973.
44. Beck, A. T.: *Depression Inventory*, Philadelphia: Center for Cognitive Therapy, 1978.
45. McNair, D. M., Lorr, M., and Droppleman, L.: *Profile of Mood States Manual*, San Diego: Educational and Testing Service, 1971.
46. Liberman, R. P., Wheeler, E., DeVisser, A. J. M., Kuehnel, J., and Kuehnel, T.: *Handbook of Marital Therapy*, New York: Plenum, 1980.
47. Weiss, R. L., and Margolin, G.: Marital Conflict and Accord, in A. R. Ciminero, K. S. Calhoun, and H. E. Adams (eds.): *Handbook for Behavioral Assessment*, New York: John Wiley, 1975.
48. Patterson, G. R., Weiss, R. L., and Hops, H.: Training of Marital Skills: Some Problems and Concepts, in H. Leitenberg (ed.): *Handbook of Behavior Therapy and Modification*, Englewood Cliffs, N.J.: Prentice-Hall, 1976.

49. Hollon, S. D., and Beck, A. T.: Cognitive Therapy of Depression, in P. C. Kendall, and S. D. Hollon (eds.): *Cognitive-Behavioral Intervention Theory, Research, and Procedures*, New York: Academic Press, 1979.
50. Seligman, M. E. P.: *Helplessness: On Depression, Development, and Death*, San Francisco: W. H. Freeman, 1975.
51. Liberman, R. P., and Raskin, D. E.: Depression: A Behavioral Formulation, *Archives of General Psychiatry*, 24:515–523, 1971.
52. Lewinsohn, P. M.: The Behavioral Study of Treatment of Depression, in M. Hersen, R. Eisler, and P. Miller (eds.): *Progress in Behavior Modification*, Vol. 1, New York: Academic Press, 1975.
53. Beck, A. T.: *Cognitive Therapy and the Emotional Disorders*, New York: International University Press, 1976.
54. Rehm, L. P., and Kornblith, S. J.: Behavior Therapy for Depression: A Review of Recent Developments, in M. Hersen, R. M. Eisler, and P. M. Miller (eds.): *Progress in Behavior Modification*, Vol. 7, New York: Academic Press, 1979.
55. Weissman, M. W., and Paykel, E. S.: *The Depressed Woman: A Study of Social Relationships*, Chicago: University of Chicago Press, 1974.
56. Haley, J.: *Uncommon Therapy*, New York: Norton, 1973.

Chapter Five

The Family and Marital Therapies

Lyman C. Wynne, M.D., Ph.D.
with the collaboration of
Alan Gurman, Ph.D.
Robert Ravich, M.D.
and
Ivan Boszormenyi-Nagy, M.D.

Drs. Lee Combrinck-Graham, Norman Paul, and James Lieberman also assisted with early drafts.

Introduction

The field of family therapy is undergoing rapid growth and change both clinically and conceptually. Fortunately, a recent and comprehensive overview of major diverse points of view in the field has been published.[1] Even with those published guidelines, most clinicians will have difficulty clarifying the level of consensus that exists today about the theoretical premises and clinical techniques of family therapy. Despite the risks of oversimplification, this overview will identify certain principles that are commonly accepted by many, but by no means all, family therapists. For those readers who may be challenged to explore more fully the rich complexity of the concepts and techniques that are discussed here, a sample of the pertinent literature is provided in the references.

Theoretical Premises

THE FAMILY AND SYSTEMS THEORY

Family therapists have sought a theoretical framework that clarifies the relevance of the family context to the understanding and treatment of a variety of clinical problems. Such a theory should be helpful in organizing clinical data obtained directly from family members, including observations during face-to-face (conjoint) family interviews. More broadly, the theory should link family processes to the functioning of individual family members (including their symptoms and disorders) and to the social networks within which families are embedded. Finally, the theory should address the ethical issues of the effects of treatment not only on the identified patient, but also on the other persons whom the therapy significantly affects.

A major premise of family therapy is that both health and dysfunction can be formulated in terms that are continuously contextual. In family oriented assessment, any kind of presenting problem, psychological or physical, is evaluated contextually. In principle, attention is given to the health and patterns of living of all persons who are likely to be affected by the treatment process and who can contribute to the resolution of the presenting problem.

More formally, family therapists think of contexts going beyond an individual patient, often formulating these contexts in terms of a systems theory. Not all family therapists *explicitly* use a systemic viewpoint to guide their specific treatment interventions, but they all do regard the family unit as a distinctive, complex, integrated organization of persons with a history together and the prospect of a future together.

The most commonly accepted version of a systems concept is that derived from the general systems theory of Weiss and von Bertalanffy and as applied to general medicine by Engel.[2,3,4,5] Engel has pointed out that a biopsychosocial medical model derived from systems theory has important implications for improved study and assessment of both medical and psychiatric patients. He has described how the assessment of data and the resulting treatment of a patient, for example, with acute myocardial infarction, differ if one is aware of factors beyond those of cardiac functioning alone.

Briefly, general systems theory begins with the observation that nature can be viewed in a hierarchically arranged continuum, with more complex, larger units superordinate to less complex and smaller units. What is distinctive about this view is that each level in the hierarchy is regarded as an organized whole, with distinctive properties and characteristics not reducible to, but intertwining with simpler levels. The cell, the organ, the person, the family, and the community are each a level in this hierarchy of organization, and each has distinctive and unique qualities. The methods and rules of study of the person as a person are not reducible to study of the cell as cell, or organ as organ, and the family as family cannot be reduced to the study of person as person.

Marriage and the family are the smallest, relatively enduring social units in these concentric contexts of general systems theory. Beyond the nuclear family, larger systemic organizations can be identified:

networks of extended families; social and occupational networks; and organizations and networks linked to diverse religious, ethnic, and other value systems.[6,7,8] Within the nuclear family, individual persons are subsystems that, in turn, have functional subsystems—biochemical, neurophysiologic, behavioral, psychodynamic, and so forth. In short, the "family *is* context and *has* context."[9]

Components of a system co-vary more fully with one another than with the components of other systems. This distinction is a matter of degree, for all living systems are "open" and linked to other systems, i.e., they are subject to influences from other system levels. Clinically, this means that the presenting problem of an individual identified patient may be the starting point for family therapy. Conversely, relief of family dysfunction can begin with individual treatment. Most family therapists believe that *both* family relationships and the well-being of individual family members can be enhanced through family therapy.

Beyond these general premises of systems theory, many family therapists apply systems principles in their daily clinical observations. For example, most family therapists observe closely the repetitious sequences of communication and behavior, the patterns of reciprocal "give-and-take" transactions in face-to-face conjoint family meetings. These repeated patterns are usefully conceptualized as systemic and not described adequately in terms of the individuals.[10]

General systems theory has been both criticized and praised because it is, formally, content-free; any specific content, including emotional functioning, can be encompassed within its framework. But this fluidity of the theory leaves so much latitude that critics believe the concepts in practice are not easily enough applied to pragmatic clinical problems. For example, Bowen believes that *general* systems theory is not specific enough to conceptualize the intense emotional processes that occur in families.[11]

MARRIAGE AS A SUBSYSTEM OF THE FAMILY

A number of family therapists, such as Framo and Bowen, are conceptually oriented to the family as a unit, but clinically focus on the subsystem of the marital couple.[17,18] Such family therapists usually regard the marital couple as the responsible leaders of the family who need to build a coalition before they can cope appropriately with children. In accord with the systems concept that the marital dyad is a subsystem of the family, marital therapy has more and more become integrated with the broader field of family therapy during the last 15 years.

Earlier, family therapy and marital therapy had rather different historical origins, and marital therapy still can be described and evaluated in a distinctive fashion.[14,15,16,17,18] For example, the "contractual" basis of marital relationships does not have a counterpart in two-generation nuclear families.[19]. Also, the comparative "simplicity" of marital interaction patterns has made the application of behavioral methods easier in marital therapy than in family therapy.[18,20] Clinical classifications for marriages appear to be more successful than for families.[12,15,19,21,22] The principles and methods of assisting couples troubled by impending divorce or by the consequences of divorce have recently evolved into a subspecialty called "divorce therapy."[23] On the other hand, the complicated family relationships created after remarriage, often blending children from two or more prior marriages, frequently make the distinction between marital therapy and family therapy arbitrary; marital and two-generational issues usually interweave or alternate in such situations.

ETHICAL PREMISES

Boszormenyi-Nagy builds upon systems concepts but takes a theoretical position also based upon premises of contractual obligations and accountability between persons.[24,25] He contends that "relational ethics" going beyond systems theory "allows no valid substitution" of one person for another, and that working out the accountability of family members directly with one another about past events and actions should be a treatment objective. Thus, "a debt incurred vis-à-vis mother through her merit can be repaid only to the mother."[25] A contrary view derived from systems theory is that persons can substitute for one another. For example, if one family member has been scapegoated but is relieved from the role, another family member may be thrust into the scapegoat role. A treatment goal based on this hypothesis is to achieve role flexibility within the family system so that no one person becomes enduringly scapegoated.

Boszormenyi-Nagy points out that the multilateral components of the family treatment system have significant theoretical and ethical implications that are not usually discussed in individual treatment. Regardless of who is initially identified as a patient, family therapists consider each of the other persons who, through deep-rooted relatedness, will be affected by the treatment process and can contribute constructively to successful therapy. Thus, family therapy is an approach that leads to concerns about persons beyond the identified patient and beyond those who are present in the consultation room at the time of the initial assessment or later interviews. This theoretical and ethical orientation has technical implications for who should be involved in therapy and how they can be most appropriately included.

These considerations actually apply to *all* therapy, not simply family therapy, with a chief difference being that the therapist treating only an individual can more easily remain unaware of the impact of individual interventions upon others who are significantly involved with the identified patient. The multilateral emphasis of family therapy is quite different from that of present-day Western society with its predominant orientation to an individual-based ethic. Family therapists recognize and assess the presenting problems of individual family members, but they do not *require* that an individual patient be identified. Many families and couples now present themselves initially as having *relationship* problems, without an identified patient. The problem for which such families and couples seek treatment is not a psychiatric diagnosis as such. Even when DSM-III diagnoses can be legitimately assigned to one or more family members, the symptoms justifying these diagnoses are often not the most keenly distressing difficulties from which the family seeks relief.

In addition to the here-and-now issue of mutual consideration versus mutual exploitation in current family relationships, loyalties and indebtedness transcend generations and need to be balanced between families of marriage and families of origin.[24] This is an approach to fairness and trustworthiness which extends from one system level to another. It is a theory of family therapy theories and has, therefore, been characterized as a "metatheory."[1] Despite its highly abstract premises, this approach does have consequences for clinical issues, e.g., in the formulation that symptoms develop when there has been a "breakdown of trustworthiness of relationship through disengagement of multilateral caring and accountability."[25]

THERAPIST-FAMILY RELATIONSHIPS

A premise derived from the general systems concept of multiple linked levels is that the physician or other health-care person relates reciprocally, not only with the identified patient, but also with the family unit. Furthermore, because each individual family member is a component of the family system as a whole, a family therapist necessarily has multilateral relationships affecting each of the family members, as well as involving the family as a whole. Most family therapists make a further concept explicit: that through the transactions of the therapist with the family, a new configuration of relationships develops, the treatment system.

Family therapists differ greatly in their views of whether it is possible or desirable for the therapist to minimize becoming emotionally and cognitively involved in the *family* system; the therapist obviously cannot avoid being part of the *treatment* system. At least five ways of formulating and approaching this problem have been advocated. In the first, exemplified by Bowen, the therapist tries to remain disengaged from the family because "as soon as a vulnerable outside person comes into viable emotional contact with the family, he becomes part of it, no matter how much he protests the opposite."[13] Therefore, Bowen advocates that the therapist make every possible effort to be "outside the family emotional system," or at least to remain "workably objective" within this intense emotional field. Behaviorally oriented family and marital therapists have many concepts not shared with Bowen, but they tend to take a similar viewpoint that it is both possible and desirable for the therapist to work "objectively" with the family unit.

A second point of view has been represented by Boszormenyi-Nagy who has developed a concept of "multidirectional partiality."[24] Boszormenyi-Nagy suggests that the therapist actively consider each family member's claim for fairness and empathic understanding. This is consistent with Boszormenyi-Nagy's therapeutic "intention to be concerned with every family member's emotional well-being and growth," but otherwise to abstain from controlling the therapeutic process.

A third approach involves more active multipersonal engagement of family members. For example, Zuk has stated: "Side-taking by the therapist is unavoidable in family therapy and must be considered a normal part of a group process."[26] Another version of this general point of view has been proposed by Selvini *et al.*, and by Stierlin *et al.*, who move in a "circular" interviewing process from one family member to another, asking each to comment upon the relation of two other members.[27,28] The therapist appears at any point in time to be allied to the person being addressed, but "the end result of the successive alliances is that the therapist is allied with every one and no one at the same time."[27]

A fourth approach to therapist-family relationships recognizes and facilitates the *active* involvement of the therapist in the treatment system, without an attempt to be neutral. When this involvement is on the experiential level, as exemplified by Napier and Whitaker, the hazards are reduced if the therapist first wins a "battle for structure" in the therapeutic relationship, and if he works with a co-therapist who can remain relatively "objective" about the family while the other therapist is letting himself become experientially a "member" of the family.[29]

A fifth view of the therapist-family relationship is expressed in the active interventions of structural family therapy and of strategic family therapy.[30,31,32] These therapists conclude that all therapy is inevitably manipulative because "one cannot do therapy without manipulating people in the sense of influencing them to change, since the change is the purpose of therapy."[31] If the goal of being objective and nonmanipulative is unobtainable, then, Haley argues, continuing efforts to obtain this goal are an expression of ignorance about the countless ways in which information is concealed and revealed across the therapist-family boundary. This formulation has direct consequences for a highly active, explicitly interventionist technique of therapy, including the view that the "primary feature" of strategic family therapy is that the therapist should take responsibility for planning strategies to solve the family problems.[32] After quickly engaging the family, structural and strategic family therapists generally disengage quickly, as soon as new family transactional patterns have emerged.

Thus, there are many variations about the details of how the family therapist and the family system can and should relate to one another. Overall, it may be necessary to characterize the family therapy field at present merely as acknowledging the potency and significance of the therapist-family relationship.

FAMILY HOMEOSTASIS

Following several 19th century physiologists who had described the self-regulatory maintenance of relatively steady states in biologic systems, Cannon applied the term homeostasis more generally to any condition of equilibrium "which may vary but which is relatively constant."[33] He suggested that complex social organizations also "must have more or less effective self-righting adjustments" to cope with "distressing perturbations."[33] Later, Jackson focused on family homeostasis as illustrative of the general principle.[34]

A common hypothesis in family theory has been that if a family becomes stuck in homeostatic equilibrium, growth and change are blocked. Acute conflictual symptoms may result and, later, deficit function may be the consequence of a dysfunctionally unchanging family system. The concept of family homeostasis was especially valuable in elucidating the high degree of apparent stability in some families with a severely disturbed member. For example, many clinical observers noted that when schizophrenic patients were starting to change and were ready to move out of a hospital, the anxiety level of the rest of the family increased. Thereupon they took action to transfer the patient to another hospital (change-reducing, "negative" feedback). In the prototypical case, the patient's symptoms then returned while the anxiety level of the rest of the family diminished. The family, patient, and hospital could be interpreted as being in repetitious, cyclic, homeostatic equilibrium.

An important premise based upon family homeostasis is that change of the individual is not possible without change in the rest of the family.[30] This premise, almost regarded as axiomatic by many family therapists, is linked to the proposition that individuals and their symptoms are adaptive to, or functional within, a dysfunctional family homeostasis. Clinically, this means that if an individual can be helped to change *other* family members, the individual will be able to change more easily. Also, this formulation suggests that by first focusing on change in family transactions, individual change will follow more easily or even inevitably.

Despite widespread acceptance of this formulation of family homeostasis, it has not been empirically established across a broad range of problems and clinical situations. The homeostasis concept, with its emphasis upon negative feedback loops that counteract deviance and change, has been most useful in the clinical study of chronically and severely disturbed families. More generally, homeostasis probably has been overemphasized as a *generalized* issue in family functioning and therapy. Clinically, many disturbed and normal families can be observed who do not counteract growth of a family member. Perhaps family therapists have been unduly impressed with the difficulties of changing those families in which everyone is stuck or at an impasse, and where individual change seems to be undone by counteractive changes in the family.

The primacy given by some family therapists to first changing the *family* system is actually contrary to a broader systems view that *each* systems level may be regarded as providing the starting point in a sequence of transactions, depending upon how the sequence is "punctuated." As Gurman has pointed out: "Individual dysfunctioning does not necessarily reflect relationship conflict; in fact, individual functioning at times may precipitate relationship conflict. Moreover, while individual symptomatology undoubtedly is often equilibrating for a relationship, the fact, well known to clinicians, should not be overlooked that such symptomatology also serves organismic functions, that is, has intraindividual, autoregulating consequences and purposes."[22] Wahlroos has similarly cautioned: "We just do not know under what conditions the theoretical postulates of family homeostasis apply, and under which conditions they do not apply."[35]

Another difficulty with using homeostasis too exclusively as an explanatory concept is that it fails to explain how change takes place during normal development or during therapy, especially discontinuous change and the phenomenon of runaway escalation of positive- or deviance-amplifying feedback. The application of both positive and negative cybernetic loops to concepts of stability and change has been described in systems theory as morphogenesis and morphostasis.[36,37] Morphostasis, or homeostasis, represents the tendencies within a system to use negative feedback loops to maintain a steady state or equilibrium, whereas morphogenesis represents the tendencies to disequilibrate, with positive feedback loops escalating or amplifying deviance.

The concept of discontinuous change in the structure of an entire system needs to be distinguished from ordinary day-to-day fluctuations, called "first-order changes."[38] Watzlawick and colleagues have exemplified this distinction. A person having a nightmare can do many things within a dream—run, fight, scream, jump off a cliff, and so forth, but changing from one behavior to another would not terminate the nightmare.[39] This kind of change has been called first-order: the details differ, but the state remains the same. One way out of the dream would be a change from sleep to a waking state. Waking is no longer a part of the dream but a second-order change to an altogether different state.

Ordinarily, when a second-order change occurs in family systems, there is a transitional period of crisis or instability, when deviance-amplification has pushed the system's "tolerance" to near the breaking point.[37] At that point, three outcomes appear to be possible:

1) Homeostatic, counteractive processes may reassert themselves and reestablish the prior conditions.
2) Deviance-amplifying feedback loops may escalate change in a runaway fashion, leading to breakdown of the family system and/or the individual's functioning, i.e., the family may be dissolved or broken up and the patient may become suicidal or psychotic, or at least more disorganized. This negative outcome is obviously feared and is a hazard in the course of ordinary developmental change as well as during therapy.
3) More positively, discontinuous and evolutionary change may transform functioning at both the family and the individual levels. For example, a family with enmeshed authoritarian/dependent relationships of parents and adolescents sometimes makes surprisingly abrupt shifts to greater autonomy of the generations, or new resources of trustworthiness may be tapped for a fresh start. The possibility of such transformations clearly depends upon the latent assets and resources of individuals and families that they can draw upon either from within themselves or from external sources, including the therapist and health-care systems.

Recognition of the balance between opposing processes—to

amplify deviance and to counteract it—underlies a relatively new approach to therapy of the family system. In this approach, the dangers and fears that can be aroused by change are explicitly acknowledged, and the family and patient are advised "to go slow" with change. At the same time, small controlled changes are prescribed and often ritualized.[40,41,42,43] Under these conditions, the therapist expects that the family will oppose these tasks and, instead, will actively initiate change.

Although the subsequent changes (but not their content) are predictable, these transformations of the family are initiated from within, appear to be "spontaneous," and often are abrupt. Interventions intended by the therapist to produce such changes have been somewhat inappropriately termed "paradoxical."[32,37,39,41,42,43,44] This approach to therapy currently is arousing considerable interest, but the actual practice of family therapy still rests more on the premise that families are resistant to change because of overly rigid family homeostasis and that considerable activity on the part of the therapist is necessary to cope with this resistance. Further work linking these theoretical premises and the techniques of family therapy is clearly needed.

Another important premise is based upon deviance-amplification and states that change can begin anywhere and will lead to change in the rest of the system. A number of family therapists have argued, using a systems point of view, that treatment can begin at *any* level, including that of the individual, and yet remain conceptually part of a "family therapy" orientation. This premise has led to the assertion that individual therapy conducted with this orientation is actually a form of family therapy and that it is not very important who is in the consulting room so long as the therapist is thinking in family systems terms.[13,25]

At a theoretical level, it seems unreasonable to expect that individual change would reverberate *automatically* into the rest of the family system. Families, like other living systems, are never fully integrated, and the resonance of change beginning in an individual may or may not be transmitted and experienced in other members of the family. It also can be noted that individual persons participate not only in family systems but also in occupational systems, school systems, peer group relationships, and so forth. Although spillover from one of these systems to another certainly occurs, it is clinically apparent that some people compartmentalize their lives quite successfully. Thus, successful occupational performance may be associated with abysmal family life, or conversely. Also, treatment "success" within a hospital setting or within the family context may or may not be associated with much change in community or work settings.

Thus, it is hazardous to make facile hypotheses about the consequences of change and to contend as a generalization that it does not matter where the starting point may be. Empirically, studies of treatment outcome appear to suggest that improvement in relationship difficulties occurs most effectively and readily when the persons in the relationship actually meet in face-to-face, conjoint therapy. Thus, when the treatment problem is marital conflict, conjoint marital therapy appears to be more effective and leads less often to deterioration than does therapy with an individual partner.[45]

At this point, it seems wise to reserve the concept of family therapy for therapy that is at least predominantly involved with the face-to-face or conjoint meetings of the family members and, similarly, with marital therapy. Until there is empirical evidence to support the hypothesis that family or marital change can effectively and regularly occur through therapy with individual family members, this idea should be recognized as a working hypothesis that is not yet established.

CIRCULAR, NOT LINEAL, CAUSALITY

Family therapists generally regard traditional medical concepts of "etiology" as resting upon the inadequate Aristotelian premises of a lineal view of causality. Instead, they emphasize reciprocal transactions unfolding through time recursively in circular (or, more accurately, spiral) sequential patterns.[46] This view of causality is systemic and moves away from concepts of individual blame. The concept of circular causality makes it impossible to specify unidirectional or external causes after a problem has involved multiple persons, each of whom contributes to its maintenance. The issue then becomes more one of sustaining and perpetuating factors, rather than specific and ultimate etiologies with historically defined starting points.

Family therapists differ in how completely they adopt a systemic paradigm. As yet, there is no convincing, empirical evidence to support an *exclusive* emphasis upon circular causality. It is quite easy to identify multiple factors that plausibly are contributing to any specific clinical situation, but more difficult to weigh their relative salience. Here, longitudinal studies appear helpful in revealing and comparing directional trends that began under definable antecedent conditions which in that sense can loosely be regarded as "causal." Unfortunately, only a few studies using family variables are presently available for drawing such conclusions. An example is found in the risk research of Goldstein.[47]

THE FAMILY'S PERSPECTIVE TOWARD TREATMENT

An implicit premise in any therapy is that the participants bring with them a set of expectations or beliefs, a "theory" of what is going wrong and how it should be corrected. In family therapy these ideas can be formulated in terms of myths.[48,49,50] Such myths draw upon the value systems and expectations of ethnic and religious groups as well as more specifically from the families of origin of both parents and the nuclear family's own past history. These myths and expectations may be subtle and complicated in detail or they may be commonplace as, for example, the belief that psychiatric symptoms result from individual willful disobedience of family rules and that more forceful orders will correct the problem. Another common family myth is that everyone in the family is harmonious and that conflict or deviance from this family norm must have resulted from the intrusion of someone or something from the outside, such as an illness.[50]

This formulation of family expectations about treatment can be added to a tripartite model of mental health treatment presented by Strupp and Hadley.[51] They proposed that the perspectives of at least three major interested parties need to be considered in treatment:

1) society—including significant persons in the patient's life
2) the individual patient
3) the mental health professional

Family therapists would add a fourth perspective, that of the family. The family's perspective is often at variance with that of the general society or of the neighborhood or community and, hence, it should be specified separately. This point of view is consistent with the systems level concept described above.

Different mental health professionals tend to emphasize one perspective more than others. Thus, a psychoanalyst emphasizes the individual's sense of well-being; some forensic psychiatrists emphasize society's expectations; family therapists give special attention to the perspective of the family. A thoroughgoing systems viewpoint does not set up these perspectives as competitive but, rather, as complementary.

TOWARD A DEFINITION OF FAMILY THERAPY

Many family therapists have strongly insisted that family therapy rests on premises that involve a radical shift of paradigm from that used in somatic, individual, or group therapy. The difference, it has been claimed, is not merely of modality but, more fundamentally, of orientation. For example, Haley expressed this view as follows: "By the end of the 1950s it was becoming clearer that family therapy was a different concept of change, rather than merely an additional method of treatment to be added to individual and group therapy. The focus of family treatment was no longer on changing an individual's perception, his affect, or his behavior, but on changing the structure of a family and the sequences of behavior among a group of intimates. With this shift, it became clearer that neither traditional individual therapy nor group therapy with artificial groups was relevant to the goals and techniques of family therapists. The problem was to change the living situation of a person, not to pluck him out of that situation and try to change *him*."[52]

Haley thus defines family therapy in terms of the therapist's orientation and goal (e.g., to change family structure and behavioral sequences) rather than as a modality in which the therapist meets face-to-face with two or more family members. Other therapists have proposed other goals such as the building of trustworthiness and empathy in family relationships.

For day-to-day clinical work and for comparative studies of treatment efficacy, criteria are needed to determine when such therapy is taking place. First, does the therapist actually behave in ways that are consistent with the avowed goal? Second, does the family actually participate with the therapist in a manner that could possibly achieve the goal? A full definition of a treatment approach probably should incorporate criteria for answering such questions about whether a given treatment has actually taken place. If a pharmacotherapist does not follow through with the prescription of a specified medication, or if the patient does not take it when prescribed, the noncompliance itself is important information, but the treatment cannot be said to have occurred. Similarly, with family therapy, if the therapist merely *intends* to change the family system but conducts interviews in a manner inconsistent with this goal, or if the family does not participate on the therapist's terms in the treatment plan, then "family therapy" was attempted but not provided.

Most family therapists have believed that family system changes will be manifest in *observable* changes in the reciprocal transactions of the family members during the family meetings. For example, changes in family coalitions (marital versus cross-generational) and in empathic understanding of one another may be quite readily inferred from direct observations. The widespread use of face-to-face, conjoint family meetings reflects the theoretical premise that observable, direct, here-and-now transactions are a significant setting for therapy.

Because family therapy has been almost routinely observed by consultants and supervisors and/or tape-recorded for later review, this treatment approach has the potential for unusually excellent access to data on what actually takes place, compared to what is retrospectively reported. Nevertheless, it seems both premature and contrary to the free spirit of family therapists to insist that *only* the events of conjoint family meetings provide the relevant data for defining and evaluating family therapy. For example, interposed meetings with individual family members and with relevant non-family members may be consistent with the general assumptions of family therapy. Also, inquiries and explorations outside of the face-to-face sessions with family members about their transgenerational relationships are regarded as useful by some therapists, although evidence of subsequent change *within* conjoint meetings still could be expected in order to help assess treatment efficacy.

Nevertheless, even if some treatment activities that do not take place within conjoint meetings are regarded as part of family therapy, it still seems useful on both theoretical and pragmatic grounds to give special attention to the directly observable transactions of family members with one another. After all, this is the most distinctive modality, though not the only one used by family therapists. In short, it seems parsimonious at least to *begin* with a definition in terms of modality: the participation in face-to-face conjoint meetings of the members of a marriage or family. As indicated above, the available research evidence indicates that the composition of those persons meeting together does make a difference in treatment outcome.[45]

The concept that the family and the therapist begin with distinctive perspectives toward treatment suggests that the *sharing* of perspectives could even be a defining aspect of family therapy that has succeeded in getting under way. In contrast, for those meetings prior to the point of reaching a collaborative perspective, perhaps a term such as "family consultations" or just "family interviews" would be more accurate than "family therapy." The latter term clearly implies that the family as a unit is engaged in therapy. It appears dubious on both ethical and conceptual grounds to believe that family therapy can or should take place without a family.[53] At least an informal "contract" or understanding with a family unit would appear to define the beginning of family or marital therapy in this sense.

In summary, both for practical, clinical purposes and for research on treatment process and outcome, an operational distinction is needed between:

1) family *therapy* in which the therapist joins with the family in reaching or at least striving toward a shared perspective or goal, and

2) a family *orientation* in which the impact on nonparticipant family members is considered and sought. The second approach requires different intervention techniques and different methods of initial assessment and later outcome.

When family therapy focuses on reciprocal, sequential transactions unfolding over time, a further, quite widely accepted premise is implied: family assessment and family therapy are interwoven. Before a therapeutic plan has been reached, assessment typically builds upon data obtained during preliminary interventions; the family's responses help assess the potential usefulness and directions of therapy. Hence, the discussion in the remainder of this chapter about *assessment* procedures and assessment data for treatment planning will merge with description of *treatment* procedures.

Clinical Data Necessary for Family Treatment Planning

The clinical data used to plan family treatment can be grouped under seven headings:

1) the presenting problem and its context
2) the composition of the nuclear and extended family
3) the family's expectations of treatment
4) the treatment-relevant history
5) the strengths and resources within the family and available to the family, and the nonsymptomatic deficits and liabilities
6) the therapist's observations of family transactions
7) the therapist's subjective use of self as a source of data

THE PRESENTING PROBLEM AND ITS CONTEXT

Central in family treatment planning is an orientation to the presenting problem and its context. Later, in evaluating outcome, resolution of the presenting problem is a *minimal* (though incomplete) criterion of "successful" family therapy. Contextual data about the presenting problem include much more than the traditional phrase in individual psychiatric records: "overdosed with sleeping pills"; "the voices won't stop"; "she won't eat"; and so forth. In a family approach, the presenting problem is multifaceted and is conceptualized around the issues of "who," "what," and "where."

Who believes a problem exists? This includes the persons or agencies making the referral as well as all the family members who are involved and knowledgeable.

What does each person believe is the problem? Clarifying discrepant views of what each person believes should be changed in treatment is not only crucial initially but also may continue to unfold as a central issue throughout therapy. Indeed, when this "starting point" for treatment planning is successfully evaluated, the need for treatment may be over! The family then may be in sufficient accord to go ahead without professional help.

Where is the problem located? The diverse initial views of family members, as well as later revisions, will need to be considered. In hospitals and medical offices, families usually begin by locating the problem as in an "identified patient." In other settings, such as family and marriage clinics, the problem is more apt to be presented as a complaint about a relationship such as: "There is no discipline in our family," or "Our marriage is on the rocks." In such instances, later inquiry usually can reveal symptoms justifying a DSM-III diagnosis, and family treatment may relieve these symptoms. But family therapists usually do not formulate therapeutic problems as beginning, and never as ending, with an individual DSM-III diagnosis.

Symptoms, syndromes, and disorders may be the "problem" from the perspective of many mental health professionals, but the problem as presented from the family's perspective is nearly always quite different. This distinction has been documented by McPartland and Richart who showed that psychiatrists tend to inquire about and to treat symptoms and disorders and to ignore and leave untreated the problem for which the patient and/or family sought help, a problem that was little changed at follow-up.[54]

With the advent of the Problem-Oriented Record (POR) in psychiatry, the distinction between "disorders" and "problems" has become more generally recognized. A problem has been defined as "anything important enough to . . . try to do something about," and one that suggests "possible interventions."[55] The POR is concerned with physiological, psychological, or social dysfunctioning of *individual* patients. A further shift in thinking is required to consider problems as relational and as located in the family unit rather than in an individual family member. From this perspective about the location of the "problem," a distinctive difference is the explicit concern with all family members, including the expectation that therapeutic interventions (pharmacologic, behavioral, psychotherapeutic) affecting any individual family member will have consequences for the other persons who have major relationships with this individual.

Historically, the family doctor with personal knowledge of the family unit, its individual members, and their relationships with one another and with the surrounding social network and community, provided general health care from the perspective of family therapy. In a sense, this traditional family medicine point of view has been applied and developed further in the field of mental health by family therapists.[56] However, simply filing individual records of family members together, without concern for or knowledge about the impact of the family members upon one another, is "family practice" from a bookkeeping, not from a therapeutic standpoint. Family medicine that gives genuine attention to family-wide relationships illustrates an approach to health care in which somatic, psychological, and social points of view are integrated in the planning of both treatment and prevention.

Child abuse provides a good example of a presenting problem that needs to be assessed contextually, and it is one in which treatment planning does not begin with an individual DSM-III diagnosis. DSM-III makes this point explicit: "A category for child abuse is not included in DSM-III as a mental disorder (of the abusing parent) since child abuse as an act can be a symptom of many different disorders or not be associated with any mental disorder."[57] Yet, everyone would agree that this problem is serious and requires attention and treatment. Child abuse is a relational and contextual problem, not an illness that can be located neatly in one person. Family-oriented treatment planning of such a problem first requires clinical data relevant to contextual questions: How has the problem been brought to professional attention? Who perceives that a problem exists and wants changes? Do the family members and the referral sources agree about what the problem is? How does the nonabusing parent fit into the picture? Does he or she provoke or collude passively in the problem? What are the detailed sequences through which the problem escalates? What are the contributions to the escalation from each family member, including the abused child? What supports are available or lacking for individual family members and for the family as a whole?

Answers to such questions provide clinical data with which family treatment can be planned. Clearly, data from and about individual members are an integral part of family assessment, but prolonged diagnostic inquiry about individual symptoms in a noncontextual, check-list fashion is apt to distract from the more comprehensive approach recommended here.

NUCLEAR AND EXTENDED FAMILY CONSTELLATIONS

Although a family-based approach to the presenting problem will provide much information about the composition of the household and the family, additional and more systematic information on family membership may be useful in family treatment planning. Family therapists differ considerably on this point. Intergenerational data about the families of origin of each parent are used by some family therapists as background information for planning and by others as a framework for active inclusion of a large family network in the treatment itself. Bowen, Boszormenyi-Nagy and Spark, Framo, Guerin and Pendergast, Paul, Speck and Attneave, and Whitaker, are among those who have emphasized the connectedness of the presenting family with extended family and social networks [1,23,17,58,59,60,61,29,53]

The most comprehensive, formal schema for assembling data about family composition was prepared by the Group for the Advancement of Psychiatry (GAP) Committee on the Family.[62] This outline is too detailed for ordinary clinical use but provides a format for potential information that may be pursued when the clinical problem leads beyond those present in the initial family assessment interviews. The GAP method of representing the family field is unique in its "double entry" system for each individual, recognizing that any person who has married is a member of at least two families (the family of origin and the family of marriage or procreation).

The sheer facts of the family constellation can suggest important preliminary hypotheses about the expectable location and quality of distress in the family life. The treatment needs and plans clearly will be enormously different for family constellations which vary as follows:

1) a divorced mother with five adolescent and preadolescent children and no supportive relatives
2) a middle-aged couple living with an aging parent who refuses to go into a nursing home
3) a "blended" family with both parents bringing into the household children from prior marriages and with one parent actively enmeshed with the family of origin

THE FAMILY'S EXPECTATIONS OF TREATMENT*

A crucial, but all too often neglected, aspect of data for effective treatment planning involves the family's (and individual members') theories of what is going wrong and their plan to correct it. The salient issue here is the degree of congruence between the perspectives or expectancies for treatment of the family and therapist. An openly collaborative treatment approach will require that the therapist and family understand one another's expectations. Even in strategic family therapy in which the therapist does not explain to the family the rationale for the treatment intervention, he or she needs to have a detailed grasp of how the family expects change to take place and already has attempted to bring about change.[32,63,64]

Thus, whatever the therapist's assessment of the family situation is, the family's assessment (i.e., its own "diagnosis" and "treatment plan") must be given enormous weight in treatment planning, whether their plan or multiple plans are identical to or orthogonal to that of the therapist. More commonly, they are somewhere in the middle. For example, if the family's own "diagnosis" unanimously and rigidly attributes their collective suffering to the immutable "character" of the identified patient (and especially if he or she concurs with this view), certain styles of intervention are likely to fail, at least early in therapy. For example, discussion of each family member's *interactional* contribution to a family problem and overt attempts to shift the focus to the family as a whole, or to the marital relationship, are likely to meet with significant resistance. Conversely, with those couples who already have adopted a "theory" of relational incompatibility to explain their dilemma, an individual diagnostic study of one spouse may seem irrelevant. The issue here, it should be clear, is how to assess and establish a shared framework with a family, not to decide about all the subsequent investigations that may be indicated later on.

Family members do not ordinarily perceive their own theories and attempts to resolve the problem as part of the problem. From the family therapist's standpoint, the family's self-diagnosis and attempts to change may seem to have converted a minor difficulty into a serious, escalating clinical problem, e.g., a controversy about an

*Dr. Alan Gurman particularly contributed to this section.

adolescent's bedtime may turn into a battle about incipient delinquency. Individuals and families come for help stating that they do not have any ideas about the nature of the problem or what should be done about it, e.g., they may regard a family member's hallucinations as coming completely out of the blue. However, their view that the professional is the possessor of a diagnosis and plan for treatment that will be given to them is, in itself, an expression of a rudimentary theory, i.e., that a problem exists in which they are not participant and have no resources or contributions to make to its resolution. Thus, no matter how a problem is presented, explicit or implicit treatment expectations exist, and these expectations need to be assessed in terms of *where* the family members, individually and collectively, locate the need for change, *whether* they believe change is possible, and *who* is believed to have the capability and responsibility for bringing about change.

The theories that families bring to treatment about their problems can be roughly arranged along a continuum:

1) The difficulty may be viewed by all family members as arising from a *fixed* characteristic of an identified patient. Examples include a physical disability, heredity or temperament, or a psychiatric diagnosis such as chronic schizophrenia which the family may understand to be an untreatable handicap. Depending upon the severity and quality of the patient's incapacity, the rest of the family may or may not ask the identified patient about his or her views before requesting a family consultation. Whether or not the consultant agrees with the family's viewpoint, a family systems approach may be introduced quite easily (with more difficulty if excessive blame and responsibility have complicated the problem). For example, if the identified patient has a chronic physical or psychiatric illness, such as a cerebrovascular accident or chronic schizophrenia, the collective suffering and reverberations in the family are apt to be profound. The impact on the rest of the family and on their resources to help one another *currently* may be taken as the starting point for family therapy, deliberately and explicitly setting aside issues of remote causes, blame, and responsibility.

2) The situation is more complicated when the family members have differing views of the problem and its treatment. A common situation is that the identified patient rejects the family's theory of his or her fixed character or biologic illness and insists that the

difficulty lies either elsewhere in the family or external to the family. The patient's objections may intensify the insistence by the rest of the family that he or she must be forced or induced into somatic treatment, individual psychotherapy, or psychoanalysis. Here the elements of blame and responsibility, combined with the family's view of the cause and treatment of the problem, must be carefully assessed and modified before family-wide participation in therapy can take place.

3) The mirror image of this situation occurs when the patient claims that he or she is hopelessly "stuck" (e.g., with an eating problem, a phobia, or depressive feelings) and wants to be left alone, but the rest of the family is enmeshed in "helping" and taking responsibility.

4) The "trading of dissociations" is an especially important and common situation for family assessment.[65] Each family member insists on individual treatment of another person's disorder. Reciprocal but lineal attributions of pathology are exchanged. Each person sees the other as "causing" the problem and each regards himself or herself as *only* reacting to provocations from the other. In effect, a *quid pro quo* of pathological attributions is allowed to continue as a trade-off for relief from self-blame. In marital relationships, this frequently takes the form of collusive blame in which, e.g., the wife blames an unhappy marriage on her husband because he is so uncommunicative that she is "forced" to nag, or the husband places the blame on his wife's nagging which "forces" him to withdraw.[66] Similarly, in family relationships, the parents may view "the problem" as their adolescent's irresponsibility and secretiveness, whereas the adolescent sees the problem as parental overcontrol and intrusiveness. In terms of individual psychology, each person is denying or dissociating his or her own contribution in order to obtain relief from both self-blame and responsibility for change. Typically, each person seeks the therapist as an ally in locating the blame and responsibility in the other. The reverse may also occur with some depressed patients who insist on locating *all* blame and responsibility in themselves.

The family or marital therapist will need to assess these treatment expectancies systematically, hearing all perceptions and eschewing the lineal, unilateral epistemologies of the family members. Family therapists have observed that the very act of hearing from only one family member tends to confirm that person's hopes and perceptions. Even though the therapist can try to elicit from the individual, seen alone, what he or she believes to be the viewpoints of other family members, such assessment is vulnerable to speculative misunderstandings if the other persons are not present and do not have an opportunity to contribute their own observations.

The therapist may see clear evidence that intrusive pushing by the family is stimulating passive withdrawal of the identified patient, and the patient's passivity is stimulating the family's pushing. Either perception by the patient or by the rest of the family implies a lineal, unidirectional theory of causality. But if the family therapist starts to push the idea of circular causality against the family's lineal view, the difficulty within the family system may be recreated within the therapeutic system: a therapeutic impasse will replace the intrafamilial impasse. Thus, the skillful therapist will assess not only the expectations of treatment within the family, but also how these expectations mesh with his or her own expectations.

5) Probably, most couples or families will work on their problems themselves without seeking therapy if they truly see the need for change in both or all persons in the relationship. More often, such perceptions emerge after therapy is underway and expectancies have shifted. Nevertheless, even initially there are some couples and some families who do see themselves as caught up in a vicious circle where they both provoke and are provoked, but they feel unable to break out of this pattern. In short, their insight is not enough.

In summary, the assessment of treatment perspectives and expectations requires special care, because it often is not obvious whether the therapist and family have really reached an agreement about what kinds of changes are needed and are desirable. For example, if one family member has pushed the idea of treatment in order to obtain change in the other while staying individually unchanged, this covert goal will not only be at odds with other family members' goals, but also may be at odds with the therapist's goal of achieving reciprocal and multilateral support for all family members. This broader, multilateral perspective of the family therapist may lead him or her to conclude that there are serious drawbacks or hazards of change for one or more family members. The assessment process, therefore, may require a working, multilateral relationship with the family in which assessment and treatment processes are interwoven.

THE TREATMENT-RELEVANT HISTORY

Most family therapists emphasize here-and-now interaction much more than retrospective reports of family history. Some family therapists belittle the meaningfulness of history; most selectively incorporate data about the past as it appears relevant to the current family patterns. Paul has used shared mourning experiences as a means of increasing empathic relatedness of family members.[60] Boszormenyi-Nagy and Spark examine the "invisible loyalties" that carry over from the past and contribute to alienation and distrust in current and future family relationships.[24] Bowen and Framo relate current marital difficulties to ties with the families of origin of both spouses.[12,13,58] Whitaker, Ackerman, and Skynner are among the large group of family therapists who view current family relationships as deriving from what various family members learned in their families of origin.[29,53,67,68] Additionally, the content of family myths serves to "blot out or selectively distort certain aspects and implications of the members' real task and prevent involvement with each other."[49]

Another issue relevant to history concerns the developmental stage of the family as a unit. Family sociologists in earlier years and, more recently, family therapists have given recognition to the expectable sequences of family formation and the tasks associated with "normal" stresses of changing family structure.[69,41,70] Family developmental stages include establishing the marital pair, establishing boundaries from the families of origin, developing a new type of unit with the birth of a child, a child's entry into school and departure from home, deaths of a family member, and so forth. Just as in the developmental psychology of individuals, certain family tasks need to be solved at each stage of life before the family is prepared to go on with the next developmental stage. Failure to establish a workable marital coalition will make more difficult the parental functions that follow developmentally. A frequently important issue in family assessment involves the continuation of ties to the families of origin of adults, often with serious adjustment disorders and many symptomatic manifestations within the context of these conflicting or ambiguous loyalties. One hypothesis has been that individual symptoms may develop during periods of family developmental crises, not only as a response but also as a solution to the stress of transition. Hadley and colleagues conducted one of the few empirical studies of this hypothesis and found a positive statistical correlation between individual symptoms and a family developmental crisis.[71] On the other hand, for a substantial number (39%) of families, individual symptom onset did not occur within nine months after either the loss or the addition of a family member. Other kinds of developmental crises were not studied.

When a child is the identified patient, assessment should consider whether the family may have a "developmental misfit" pattern. For example, the family can be too differentiated to integrate young children, too variable and complex to facilitate internalization of family patterns by young children or, on the other hand, the family may be too enmeshed to allow for adolescent differentiation and departure.

Numerous formats for organizing the current and historical data from a family vantage point have been developed. Examples are presented by Epstein, Duhl, Guerin, and Carter and McGoldrick.[59,72,73,70] The family case history format prepared by the GAP committee provides a useful though elaborate framework for obtaining family history material systematically.[62]

THE FAMILY'S STRENGTHS AND RESOURCES, DEFICITS AND LIABILITIES

A major thrust of most family therapists is attention to the assets and healthy functioning of families (cf. Axis V of DSM-III). Regardless of the severity and specificity of an individual family member's disorder, the resources of the family as a whole can be marshalled in most family treatment approaches. A valuable schema for assessing these features has been provided by Lewis and colleagues in their study of psychological health in families.[74] They have compared families producing mentally healthy and dysfunctioning children in terms of a number of dimensions of the family, including power structure, differentiation of individual identities, presence of clear communication, presence of a firm parental coalition, ability to interact spontaneously with humor and wit, and the ability of various family members to take initiative flexibly. Other approaches to assessing the nonsymptomatic functioning of families along a variety of dimensions of these kinds have been proposed by Epstein and the Duhls.[72,73]

The assets and resources within families clearly provide means by which problems can be ameliorated or counteracted. An exclusive orientation toward pathology during assessment of either individuals or families will fail to evaluate strengths that are clearly important for effective treatment planning. Indeed, many families with assets such as high energy level are prone to turmoil and conflict, but also creative, lively interaction. Whitaker, in particular, has labelled such creativity as "craziness" that needs to be tapped as a resource for family growth.[53]

Other aspects of family assessment that have been given increasing attention in recent years are the evaluation of the nonsymptomatic skill deficits of the various family members, their difficulties in correcting and compensating for one another's deficiencies, and their ability to draw upon extrafamilial sources of assistance. Particularly in educational and behavioral approaches to family therapy, special attention is given to deficient skills that can be taught both within and outside the family context. If a family member has been protected from expectable life experience for a long period of time within the family context or has been hospitalized and has not had opportunities to develop skills at an ordinary developmental stage, recognition of these deficits may be important to consider, not only with the identified patient but also with the family as a whole. The potential contribution of family members to "catching up" in deficit areas, particularly in social skills, is a practical matter requiring explicit attention during treatment planning. If the family is in a current, overwhelming crisis, obviously these considerations must come later.

Some families show very little overt symptomatology, but have an amorphous, plodding, pervasive dullness; lack of initiative; and lack of social skills. In many ways, such families are much less interesting and, hence, more difficult to treat than are the overtly disturbed but more energetic and lively families. Where there are areas of skill deficits, without much explicit ambivalence or conflict, behavioral and skill training programs may be an important aspect of family treatment.[75] Some therapists prefer not to call such approaches "therapy," but rather label them somewhat pejoratively as counselling or education. Nevertheless, these methods are increasingly recognized as making major, integral contributions to a comprehensive treatment program, both with individuals and with families.

Family boundaries which are either dysfunctionally rigid or permeable need to be assessed in relation to both the family as a whole and each individual member.[30,50] Some families are socially isolated with poor interchange with others and with little to draw upon in times of crises; other families have such vague or unstable boundaries that the members, especially the children, have great difficulty in identifying a stable framework within which their personal growth can proceed.

In summary, a treatment plan that is family-oriented will include efforts not only to alleviate the presenting symptoms of an index patient, but also will consider the nonsymptomatic functioning in the family system as part of treatment planning. More supportive relationships are likely to forestall relapse of the presenting symptoms and may help the family to mobilize its resources so that gains in adaptive functioning in one area will extend to other areas. The likelihood of subsequent symptoms in other family members thus may be reduced. A family orientation does not primarily focus on pathology, but on resources, especially the potential for building trustworthy relationships with concern for fairness, caring, and giving.

THE THERAPIST'S OBSERVATIONS OF FAMILY TRANSACTIONS

The details of internal family organization, described in terms of the sequences and patterns in which family members relate to one another, cannot be reported by the family members themselves. Family beliefs about their own alliances and conflicts do not include information about sequences in which symptomatic behavior is embedded, such as, e.g., the incoherent talk of the identified patient that regularly intrudes into tension between two other family members. Such information can be obtained by direct observation of verbal and nonverbal transactions of family members with one another. Nevertheless, it should be noted that even though direct observation of family interaction is clinically economical, the multidirectional concern and caring by the therapist about all family members, and the family as a social unit, is not confined to the conjoint family meetings.

Quite apart from biologically and legally defined roles that can be diagrammed, the therapist needs to assess the ongoing transactional patterns within the family system: who communicates with whom; who makes alliances and emotional ties; and what sequences of change take place in these alliances, coalitions, splits, and subsystems in response to changing circumstances. This level of assessment is distinctive and central to family therapy and will be discussed further in a later section. As shall be noted, the family's capacity to make use of therapy can be assessed through observation of preliminary efforts to bring about change. Some therapists may, for example, ask two family members to sit next to each other and talk about a problem that they have had with one another in the here-and-now of the session itself. Their clarity in doing so, their emotional involvement, and the response or intrusions of the rest of the family all consititue data for family assessment.

THE THERAPIST'S USE OF SELF AS A SOURCE OF DATA

As part of the assessment process, family therapists usually regard their own presence as a type of intervention. Especially crucial to the assessment is the response of the family to the presence and interventions of the therapist. The boundaries of some families are so tightly drawn that the therapist is regarded as alien, a threat, or incapable of understanding the special dilemmas of the family. Other families try to incorporate the therapist, to have the therapist take over one or more of the family roles and, at the same time, often depriving him or her of professional skills. Therefore, the interviewer should consider which treatment strategies are likely to be effective in the light of the family's responses to comments, inquiries, and preliminary recommendations. The family's ability to communicate clearly and to respond within a generationally appropriate authority hierarchy is another important aspect of their initial response that needs to be assessed. Also, preliminary indications of the family's flexibility in restructuring itself in response to the therapist's comments or directives is important prognostic information.

As particularly exemplified by Whitaker and Skynner, the therapist's use of his or her own fantasies and the expression of them not only can facilitate treatment, but also will help assess from the beginning what access the family already has to subjective experiences.[53,76] In turn, such access may help the family become open to new options and greater flexibility.

A quite different approach to the use of self is found in structural family therapy and in strategic family therapy which include a vast array of treatment procedures with an emphasis on giving the family specific directives and tasks to be accomplished both within the interview and as "homework."[30,31,32,64,77] The active participation of the therapist as a member of the therapeutic system is a key feature of these approaches that inextricably meld assessment and therapy.

FAMILY DIAGNOSIS

In addition to the above seven categories of data attended to by the family therapist in assessment and treatment planning, consideration needs to be given to the issue of "diagnosis" at the family systems level. Family therapists generally use the term "family diagnosis" in the broad sense of assessment or evaluation rather than the narrow typologic classification of individual disorders in Axes I to III in DSM-III. The question has been raised whether an analogous or parallel set of diagnoses specific to the family system level is possible or desirable. In DSM-III, a start is made with three rudimentary V Codes listed "Conditions Not Attributable to a Mental Disorder That Are a Focus of Attention or Treatment." These are Marital Problem (including marital conflict), Parent-Child Problem (including child abuse), and Other Specified Family Circumstances (including "interpersonal difficulties with an aged in-law, or sibling rivalry").[57] Going beyond these V Codes, can, or should, a classification of "Family and Marital Disorders" comparable to "Mental Disorders" be constructed? If so, they might be accorded a more distinctive place in future classifications than they were in DSM-III.

Certainly the failure to give classificatory attention to family and marital dysfunctions is not because they are uncommon. For example, Sager and colleagues found that 50% of patients requesting psychotherapy did so largely because of marital difficulties, and another 25% had problems related to marriage.[78] In a nationwide survey, Gurin found that among the reasons why people seek help for emotional problems, marital concerns rank first, followed by other family problems.[79] If relevance to treatment were the primary rationale for classification, then psychiatry should be classifying "problems," not disorders, a point discussed earlier concerning Problem-Oriented Records. An orientation to problems implies attention to multiple system levels, which assuredly should include the family but also wherever else the difficulties and distress occur and may be ameliorated. Hence, while family therapists object to prevailing excessive preoccupation with the individual and with somatic levels of functioning, an interest in family diagnosis does not imply a one-sided preoccupation *only* with family systems.

Nevertheless, at present, no clinically useful family classification has yet been agreed upon, although a number of suggestions have been made that go beyond the DSM-III V Codes. Most family classifications have been constructed for theoretical or research purposes and have not been regarded generally as useful for family treatment planning, but further work on this problem is warranted.[80]

The first step, already taken, toward constructing a classification useful in family therapy was to drop the earlier custom of classifying families in terms of individual diagnoses: families of schizophrenics, families of drug addicts, and so forth. Clearly, the concept of distinctive, irreducible system levels was inconsistent with this basis for identifying families, despite interesting research correlations between patient diagnosis and various family features.

The second step, still in progress, was to sort out certain dimensions of functioning along which families can be described and classified. Olson, Russell, and Sprenkle have developed a model for marital and family systems that attempts to locate families in a matrix created by the two dimensions of family cohesion and family adaptability.[81] This method has been tested with families participating in a structured family interaction game and with a questionnaire.[82] These authors recommend that dimensionalized diagnosis of families precede family treatment.

One of the most elaborate dimensionalized approaches to family assessment is the McMaster Model of Family Functioning.[83] Six dimensions are assessed, involving both areas of strength and problem areas, in order "to understand the family structure, organization, and transactional pattern dysfunctions associated with family difficulties." These include problem-solving, communicating roles, affective responsiveness, affective involvement, and behavioral control.

As previously noted, Lewis and colleagues developed a family classification that can be condensed into three levels of functioning: severely disturbed, mid-range, and healthy. These summary assessments are composites from multiple family system scales rated in five areas:

1) family structure (overt power, parental coalitions, closeness, and "pecking order")
2) family mythology
3) goal-directed negotiation
4) autonomy (communication of self-concept, responsibility, invasiveness, and receptiveness)
5) family affect (expressiveness, mood and tone, conflict, and empathy)[74]

Several other family classifications have emphasized issues that are specifically relevant to the proponent's treatment method. Thus, Minuchin, who is especially concerned with structural changes in family therapy, conceptualizes a continuum of dysfunctional family boundaries, classifying the extremes as enmeshment and disengagement.[84,85] Treatment can be oriented to modifying these family dysfunctions.

Ford and Herrick advocate a treatment approach in which certain overriding family transactional patterns of "rules" that have not been commented upon within the family are made explicit by the therapist. Therefore, they have classified families in terms of these family rules, giving pithy labels such as "Children Come First," to families where there are no leaders and all members are children behaviorally or psychologically.[86] Andolfi has proposed a classification of flexible and rigid family systems based on the balance between tendencies toward homeostasis and toward transformation.[87] This approach appears especially, but not exclusively, relevant to interaction in families with a schizophrenic member.

Many of the classifications mentioned in this brief sampling apply to marriages as well as to families. In addition, there have been several noteworthy attempts to classify marriages alone. Lederer and Jackson classified couples in terms of their rules for defining power in the relationship.[88] Cuber and Harroff proposed a classification by level of intimacy.[89] Ravich and Wyden have identified types of couples on the basis of their decision-making manifested in a Train Game.[90] Martin described four pathological marriage patterns that are directly relevant to marital therapy and can be used in comparative outcome studies.[15] Sager has presented a comprehensive "typology of relationships" derived from seven behavioral profiles that are descriptive of how a mate can react to his or her partner, leading to 28 possible combinations of two partners.[21]

None of these approaches, nor numerous others not mentioned, has been generally adopted by a large number of therapists or, for that matter, thoroughly evaluated as to their helpfulness in treatment planning. There appears to be a dilemma between the complexity of a multiple dimensional diagnosis that is necessary for comprehensive appraisal and the need for a less cumbersome approach for ordinary clinical use, especially with the current emphasis on brief family therapy. Additionally, there is a belief in several schools of family therapy that the best diagnosis *for therapy* emerges by allowing the family to respond to attempts to bring about change.[31] Also, some object to *any* classification that locates the treatment problem in the individual or the family and does not give explicit attention to the family therapist and the other professionals who are part of the therapeutic system, nor to the therapeutic method used. This viewpoint implies that a classification would need to take into account the "fit" of patients/families, therapists, and therapies. Despite these difficulties of assessment and "diagnosis," further work in this area continues and may provide useful treatment guidelines in the future.

Specific Treatment Procedures

Although family assessment and treatment procedures usually overlap, it may be helpful to provide an overview of the broad classes of treatment procedures currently used with families. Each of the various schools of family therapy tend to favor one group of procedures over another.[1] Additionally, in actual practice these procedures vary with the family constellation available to participate in the treatment, the setting in which the therapy is carried out, the type of clinical situation or problem presented, and the family's expectations about change and treatment.

Three very broad classes of treatment techniques can be identified in terms of goals:

1) communicational and problem-oriented approaches
2) techniques for building empathy, trust, and differentiation/belongingness
3) family restructuring and skill building approaches

COMMUNICATIONAL AND PROBLEM-ORIENTED APPROACHES

Continuing with the initial effort to clarify the presenting problem as seen by the multiple viewpoints of family members, one set of procedures involves assisting family members to clarify their communication with each other so that they can agree upon goals, resolve problems and conflicts, and open channels for new ways of relating. Ordinarily, communicational and problem-solving approaches call for conjoint meetings of the family as a whole or the most relevant family subsystems, especially the marital couple. Here-and-now communications, rather than reports about the past, are the data preferred by most family therapists. Although the family's awareness of the origins of their current ways of relating may grow, few family therapists attempt to impart insight interpretively in a way comparable to the use of transference in psychoanalysis. A great variety of techniques for facilitating communication are used by different therapists. Haley, Epstein, Sager, and others exemplify the great diversity of approaches which have a major goal of solving problems as presented.[17,52,72]

TECHNIQUES FOR BUILDING TRUSTWORTHINESS, EMPATHY, AND DIFFERENTIATION/ BELONGINGNESS

Another group of procedures tend to defocus the presenting problem quite soon after the initial difficulties are assessed and to work toward a different kind of subjective experience for the family members. The ways in which different therapists achieve this goal vary, particularly in the extent to which the therapist joins the family. Napier and Whitaker, Skynner, Kramer and, in the earlier days, Ackerman have given strong emphasis to the therapist's use of himself/herself in opening up an immediacy of new experience which the therapist models for the family.[29,67,76,91,92] The playful use of fantasy, an emphasis on humor and irony, and vivid, direct confrontation are all used to jar the family into opening up new levels of experience and, hopefully, improved ways of relating to one another. The same goals of improved belongingness of the family members, together with improved differentiation of each generation and of each person as an individual, are also sought by Boszormenyi-Nagy, Stierlin, and Bowen, but with methods quite different from Whitaker.[13,25,28] Boszormenyi-Nagy's contextual approach emphasizes the goal of trustworthy relating that follows from responsible caring. He aims to elicit creative options for family members so that they may gain entitlement to autonomy and growth through appropriate consideration of each other's needs and life interests.[25] Bowen attempts to stay out of the emotional field of the family, but also attempts to enhance the way in which the family members relate to one another, both with their families of origin and within the nuclear family. These approaches usually bring experiences from the past into the here-and-now experiences of the family.[60,93] Paul has already shown how an unresolved grief reaction of one of the parents may be opened up both for sharing with the other family members and for helping the grieving parent become more understandable to the others.

Additionally, a whole set of techniques for eliciting a deepened family experience has been adapted from psychodrama and has been called family sculpting and family choreography.[94] These approaches are intended to help clarify the nonverbal manifestations of family relationships. Kwiatkowska's use of family art therapy had a similar goal.[95]

FAMILY RESTRUCTURING AND SKILL BUILDING APPROACHES

A third broad group of approaches directs and re-arranges family behavior in ways that are distinctive for family therapy. Frequently, tasks are assigned, both within the conjoint family meetings and as homework between sessions. These procedures include "enactment" of a problematic situation, such as eating a meal together in a family where an offspring is anorectic.[96] Other restructuring techniques involve having family members move their seating arrangement so that they can each more directly see one another, to help strengthen a marital coalition, or some other objective of the therapist.[30]

Other interventions in this broad group include both straightforward directive and paradoxical interventions.[32] Straightforward directive approaches also may draw upon behavioral therapy for building skills in problem-solving, which differs from solving a presenting problem. Although behavioral approaches have been particularly applied to marital therapy, they also have been introduced into two-generational family therapy.[18,20,97] Many of these procedures, particularly paradoxical intervention, are used when the family is stuck in an impasse and has considerable perplexity and ambivalence about change.[43,87] When a family's intentions to change have become clear, direct skill training and education may be introduced usefully, although most family therapists have not regarded such procedures as part of "therapy."[75] Social skills that are approched in this way have a great diversity and overlap with the treatment of sexual dysfunctions and the educational opening up of more diversified personal and family experience.

The above outline of three major classes of interventions in family therapy can be subdivided into many more roles and functions of the therapist. A longer list of therapist functions for marital therapy has been presented by Gurman, and this same list can be regarded as applicable to family therapy more generally.[98] Gurman compares importance of these therapist functions from the standpoint of family therapists with a psychodynamic orientation, a behavioral orientation, and a "systems" orientation; the latter is subdivided into those following Bowen's theory and those following communicational theory. It should be noted that, in one form or other, systems theory now is so much a part of the orientation of nearly all family therapists that even such designations as "psychodynamic" and "behavioral" can be encompassed within this broad framework.

Family Assessment Processes and Procedures

REFERRAL PROCESS

Systems-oriented family therapists give detailed attention to how the referral itself has taken place. Examples of the data that emerge from the referral process are given in the clinical vignette at the end of this chapter. Contextually, those persons who participate in the referral to the family therapist have inevitably helped shape the presenting problem, highlighting certain aspects and dismissing other features that may emerge later. If a school counselor or a probation officer, for example, has made the referral of the identified patient and the family, the identity of this referral source will continue to need to be taken into account. Not only *what* the referral source conveys to the therapist, but *how* it is conveyed, and *who* does the transmitting of the information, are items of crucial, clinical information for family treatment planning. In some instances, the referral source may be included usefully in the actual intake interview, particularly if the presenting problem involves a conflict between the family and the referral source. The interviewer then has the initial role of a consultant prior to reaching a treatment plan.

The identity of the family member who calls to make the appointment is a crucial item of assessment information. If this person is someone other than the identified patient, the family therapist assumes that the relationship between the person who called and the identified patient should be explored during treatment planning. Sometimes the person who calls is actually in more distress than the identified patient, but the fact of making the call is a manifestation of that person's involvement and concern in the presenting problem. At the very least, this person will be important as a resource, not only for information, but also as a likely participant in the process of problem resolution.

During the intake process, the family interviewer should obtain an initial statement of the presenting problem and the names and relationships of all the persons who are knowledgeable about and concerned with the presenting problem. This aspect of treatment planning involves bringing together what Skynner has called a "minimum sufficient network."[68] Other family therapists, such as Whitaker, invite participation of "the largest system possible."[53] Still other family and marital therapists are willing to begin with an individual family member, with the understanding and expectation that others will contribute as soon as feasible.[99] Some therapists regard the ability of the family to mobilize themselves to come for the family interviews as an essential piece of assessment data, highly relevant to the prognosis of treatment. Bowen regards the central subsystem of the family, usually the marital couple, as sufficient.[13] A more common view is that valuable contributions can be made by all the members of the current household, plus those who continue to be actively involved with the family and with the presenting problem. It needs to be stressed that the composition of the family meeting with the family interviewer constitutes a datum of assessment, not merely a source of data.

OBSERVATIONS OF INITIAL TRANSACTIONS

During the initial meeting, behavioral and nonverbal assessment data for family treatment planning are often richly available prior to verbal description of the presenting problem. Who takes the leadership in reaching out to the interviewer to shake hands, how the family members arrange themselves in subgroups in the interview room, and how willing various family members are to engage in social amenities and to "join" are essential items helping to shape the treatment plan.[30,85] It may quickly become apparent that one of the family members, or a pair, or even the whole family, is taking a hostile or suspicious attitude toward the interviewer or, conversely, rushes in with effusive familiarity. Although such information is given some attention in other approaches to therapy, the predominant focus in family treatment on the transactional patterns among the family members, and with the therapist and others in their immediate social network, make these observations about the initial relationships not merely helpful and interesting, but crucial for effective treatment planning. Data obtained include not only initial moves made by the family members toward the therapist, but also the responses of the family members to the therapist's actions.

Especially when a father has not participated in the referral calls, many family therapists believe that efforts are needed to "join" with the father, both to stay in tune with cultural expectations and to recognize that fathers tend to be somewhat more alienated from the rest of the family than mothers and, yet, can readily sabotage treatment planning. Thus, the accessibility of each of the family members to the interviewer helps determine the next steps in treatment planning.

THE CONTEXT OF THE PRESENTING PROBLEM

The therapist commonly will inquire why the family is present or what problem has brought them to the session. The assessment data that result are not only the content of what is said but also how and by whom the response is made. Because the family has its own established hierarchy, the family interviewer must not only obtain data about the hierarchy within the family but also must recognize that procedures used in obtaining information shape the information that will be obtained. Thus, if the interviewer directs the opening inquiry to no one in particular, or explicitly invites "anyone" to respond, then information is obtained by noting who volunteers to take the leadership role, or who assigns or designates the task of responding to another person. Some interviewers prefer to speak first to the adult who seems least involved with the problem.[31] For example, if a mother has made an appointment call expressing concern about a child, and the father has appeared the more peripheral both during the referral call and during the initial social stage of the interview, it may be well first to ask the father about the problem in order to define him as a participant in the meeting and to begin to assess whether he is willing to take responsibility for action when requested. Because the interviewer already has obtained some picture of the involvement of the person who made the referral phone call, and after the interviewer has repeated the information given, most interviewers will address someone other than the person who made the call and also other than the person designated as the index patient. As suggested above, some interviewers address the family as a whole, letting them select who will first respond. In certain families, the members instantly become engaged in controversies with one another which begin to give a picture of the hierarchies, alignments, and splits within the family, at the same time providing visible data about the nature of the presenting problem in transactional terms.[100]

In any event, the viewpoint of *each* of the participants about the nature of the presenting problem, and *how* it is a problem for each individual and for the family as a whole, are crucial items for assessment. Family therapists assume that each problem is idiosyncratic to its context, that different facets of the problem will be perceived by the various family members, and that they bring different resources to modify the problem. The context of the presenting problem also includes data about what makes this a problem *now*, compared to the past. Finally, a vital piece of information relevant to treatment planning is a picture of who most wants the presenting problem to change, who is content with or resigned to its continuation, and who may be defiantly opposed to any change. Usually the person most actively interested in change is not the person with the presenting symptoms, but may well be the key one for family therapy. The presenting problem, including the symptoms as only one component, involves both the person with the symptoms and those both wanting and opposed to change.

Another part of the context of the presenting problem is the family's ideas about what kind of change would be desirable and what should be avoided. Very often it is useful to inquire what changes the family members believe should *not* take place.

Another aspect of the context is the account of attempts to find a solution, what attempts are continuing, and what the family's expectancies are about the quality and prospects of change. The data about attempted solutions will be valuable in treatment planning, not only as a warning about what actions not to propose initially, but also what to try to block. Some family therapists believe that misguided attempts at the solution of "normal" problems of living generate more serious problems requiring professional intervention.[64]

An additional aspect of the presenting problem and of possible goals for treatment may be elucidated by inquiring about the *smallest*, specific change that they would find helpful. This information is likely to be extremely valuable in planning treatment which is oriented to helping the family experience noticeable and useful changes as soon as possible.

While listening to the presentation of the problem as viewed by the various family members, the interviewer will assess their expectancies in terms of their definitions of the problem. For example, do they see the problem as a defined, labeled, mental disorder of the identified patient? Do they see the problem in terms of blaming someone within the family or someone outside of the family for "bad" behavior, attitudes, or character? Is the problem viewed as within the willful control of the identified patient or someone else? Or is the problem viewed as a misfortune with immutable characteristics to which everyone must compensate or adjust?

BACKGROUND ASSESSMENT

Some family therapists collect background information during the course of exploring the presenting problem and its context. Others obtain background information systematically after the initial presentation of the problem. Still others ask some background questions prior to inquiring about the presenting problem. A commonly used device for organizing such information is the genogram which diagrams the structure of the family in terms of membership and major boundaries.[59,62] Often, the genogram is written on a blackboard or a piece of paper for view by the family during the interview; sometimes it is constructed afterwards by the interviewer. When fully constructed, a genogram provides a wealth of information about the family structure and leads into initial data about current and past illnesses, family similarities and differences, and so forth. This approach to the family history can be useful also for understanding the familial distribution of mental disorders and personality characteristics.

As in all clinical situations, a balance needs to be achieved between obtaining data directly relevant to treatment and more comprehensive information which may turn out to be useful only later during therapy.

ASSESSMENT THROUGH INTERVENTION

As noted earlier, family therapists observe the quality of involvement of the family in response to treatment as an essential mode of continuing assessment. Three kinds of interventions used in this manner are enactment, directives, and opening or recreating communication channels.

Enactment

Minuchin has stressed the assessment treatment procedure of asking family members to enact problematic relationships in the interview session itself.[30] For example, he asks the family of an offspring with an eating disorder to have lunch together so that he can observe directly their difficulty in coping with this problem. Enactment often is combined with active manipulation of spatial relationships of family members. During a session, family members are asked to change seating arrangements in order to address one another more directly, thus suggesting the possibility of new alignments and points of connectedness that may have been difficult within the family. Similarly, many family therapists give special attention to delineating the generation boundaries between parents and offspring. This is related to the common clinical observation that an intense cross-generation tie between one parent and one offspring may be part of the dysfunctional family pattern at odds with an effective parental coalition.

Directives

More than in other forms of therapy, family therapists use the response to directives to assess the family's capacity to make use of therapy. This often begins by defining the conditions under which the therapy might best take place and specifying certain rules for communication such as not talking simultaneously or not answering for someone else. Some of these directives take place within the sessions; other directives involve homework to be conducted between meetings. The elaborateness of these homework tasks varies greatly. Sometimes these involve behavioral techniques to improve parenting skills or, for couples, to deal with sexual dysfunctions.

Still other tasks are intended to set in motion patterns that will have a "paradoxical" effect.[43] For example, prescribing a ritual such as having certain days of the week for one person in the family to do something for another, with a reciprocal arrangement for the other family member on other days of the week. Such rituals set in motion new transactional sequences that may arouse the family to take the initiative in redefining relationships in more compatible terms, at the same time providing them with an opportunity to get out of the "stuck" relationship patterns which led them into treatment.

Whereas paradoxical interventions generally are oriented to slowing down change and minimizing stressful conditions, other therapists attempt to modify homeostatic impasses by deliberately escalating stress through blocking certain patterns of interaction, by emphasizing differences between family members, and by temporarily joining in alliances with certain family members against others.[30]

Family therapists now commonly supplement directives with explicit educational and supportive guidance procedures that traditionally were not regarded as part of therapy. Within the family context they are more and more viewed as useful interventions. Behaviorally oriented therapists include such techniques as having family members help one another to build social skills. This approach may be facilitated by group therapy and group educational procedures.

Opening or Recreating Communication Channels

One of the more universally agreed upon procedures of family therapists is to facilitate more direct communication among family members, although Bowen prefers to emphasize the communication of the family members with the therapist rather than with each other.[13] Some therapists give special emphasis to assessing how family members are able to imagine what the other persons in the family are experiencing. This information is valuable both in evaluating the quality of their relatedness and in increasing their empathy with one another. Boszormenyi-Nagy has particularly emphasized the therapist's consideration of relational integrity as a part of building trustworthy relationships between family members.[25] Other therapists emphasize the more cognitive aspects of improved clarity of communication. Others stress attention to the kinesic and nonverbal aspects of communication.[101] Still others give special attention to particular content areas, such as grieving and unresolved relationships with deceased parents or relatives that continue to alter the current family relationships.[60,102]

Clinical Vignette to Illustrate Family Treatment Planning

The description of this clinical vignette will include a diversity of procedures for assessment, some, or most of which, would be used by many family therapists. Options will be indicated because not all of the possibilities mentioned here would be regarded as necessary or personally congenial to different therapists. One of the more important variations would be that some family therapists would explicitly identify one or more sessions as "assessment," while others would blend assessment and therapeutic moves from the very beginning. Often the early meetings are designated as consultations, interviews, or "meetings" before an explicit decision and "contract" is made about proceeding with treatment. Further treatment planning then proceeds hand-in-hand with the expansion and deepening of the assessment process. Obviously, treatment planning of this sort does not begin or end with a DSM-III diagnosis.

The clinical vignette, described in the Introduction of this volume, begins: "A 42-year-old businessman presented with complaints of loss of interest in his business, hobbies, and family over a period of 6 weeks." We later learn that his wife has been "solicitous and obviously concerned" since the onset of his symptomatology. This suggests that the wife may have made the phone call to the psychiatrist in order to request the initial appointment, especially if the husband was so deeply depressed that he had difficulty taking the initiative on his own behalf. His wife's making this call would be regarded as important assessment information, suggesting a current marital relationship in which the husband may take a passive, dependent role in relation to a more assertive and dominant wife. Family therapists ordinarily would use the initial phone call to invite both husband and wife to come to the initial meeting and to make a supportive inquiry to the wife that her husband's depression must be a strain for her. Most family therapists would comment that her picture of the problem would be helpful, and that she would be a valuable resource in coping with the problem. The family therapist would go on to inquire who else is knowledgeable about the problem and who is currently living in the house.

Let us assume that the wife explains that the family consists of a

12-year-old daughter and an 18-year-old son who has been away at college for two months, but who will be coming home for Thanksgiving holiday the next week. Some family therapists would invite the son and daughter to come to the session, while others would begin with the marital couple and perhaps have the children attend in the next session, especially if they were in any way caught up in the problem. Let us imagine that the wife also mentions that her husband is greatly worried about his aging mother who has been ailing for as long as the wife has known her. Recently the husband's main activity outside work has been to drive 200 miles to visit his mother since she is not well enough to travel. The therapist might say, "Hopefully we can get to know her later."

Although the wife probably has given some of the presenting symptoms in her initial request for an appointment, the family therapist usually does not ask for an elaboration at this time but instead explicitly suggests that further details should be brought up when they get together for the first meeting. In this hypothetical scenario, before hanging up, the wife might inquire if it is actually necessary that the children come to the meeting. The therapist might respond that it must be difficult for them, too, to see their father so depressed and they may well have some useful observations and contributions to make.

Either during the initial referral contact or the first interview, the psychiatrist should inquire about the physical health of the family members and especially ask if the symptomatic father has had a recent physical examination; if not, he would request that the father obtain one. The family therapist would, optimally, express an interest and willingness to establish a collaborative relationship with the general practitioner or internist or others involved in the care of family members. Particularly if there has been a family doctor who has seen more than one member of the family, the therapist would request permission to share information about all family members with this physician. In this way, the therapist would receive assessment information and also could provide information to the colleague that might be relevant to medical care. Careful attention to the biologic or somatic functioning is part of a systems-oriented approach to treatment planning.

Another referral scenario could involve the referral coming from the family's general practitioner who had been consulted by the husband because of his insomnia, fatigue, anorexia, and weight loss. The general physician did a physical examination and there were no positive findings. He prescribed a course of tricyclic antidepressants (or, more likely, but less usefully, might have prescribed diazepam). Because this treatment had not been successful, the general practitioner called the psychiatrist, reporting that the identified patient recently had had business and family difficulties and had been troubled by recurrent thoughts of death. After this call, the identified patient or the wife might call for an appointment, and the arrangements for the initial interview would be as described above.

At the beginning of the initial interview, a family-oriented therapist would give more attention to the "social" or "joining" phase than is customary in individual interviews. This phase is important both as a source of further data for the therapist and as an introduction for the family to the type of therapy that will follow. Although styles of family interviews vary considerably, most interviewers find that it is useful to be more informal and to participate in social amenities that might be considered unnecessary or inappropriate in individual meetings.

Certain features of the family structure will emerge immediately, even in the waiting area. Let us imagine that the interviewer notices that the mother and daughter are having a noisy conversation in one area of the waiting room while the father and son are quietly speaking on the opposite side of the room. When the interviewer comes out to greet them, the father abruptly interrupts his conversation with the solemn son. The daughter, however, continues to talk with the mother who tries ineffectually to interrupt and tell her it is time to go into the office. The wife gets up to shake hands with the therapist, but the husband stands stiffly and waits until the interviewer extends his hand first. The son follows the father's example, but the daughter asks to go to the bathroom and she and her mother leave. The interviewer turns to the son and expresses pleasure that he has been able to come. The son is unresponsive. The father comments that the son has two mid-term papers to write over the weekend. The son immediately corrects his father: one of the papers is not due until next Wednesday. The father says, "But you won't get it done unless you write it over the weekend." The therapist comments to the son: "It must be complicated for you to come today when you have other things on your mind." The son sourly comments: "All those courses are dumb." The mother and daughter return and, although the father and son are nearer the office door, the father waits for his wife to precede him. The daughter insists that she wants to wear her coat into the office; the mother insists she leave it in the waiting room. The daughter walks into the room with her coat on and neither parent comments about this.

In the interview room, the parents hesitate to take a seat, the mother asking where she should sit. The daughter has already taken a seat on the sofa. After the interviewer says, "It's up to you," the mother seats herself next to the daughter on the sofa. The son and father take separate chairs. The two children are now positioned between the parents.

Even before the session begins, the interviewer has gained an initial picture of the family relationship structure: the daughter and mother are aligned; the father and son are aligned; there appears to be no marital coalition. The interaction in the waiting room also has shown qualitative and affective differences in each family member's style of interaction. Although there may have been some mention in the telephone contact that the couple had been having marital difficulties, links between the marital problem and the context of the larger family system are emerging. The interviewer also will have noted (to himself/herself) that the family, with the recent departure of the son from the household, is moving into a new phase of its developmental life cycle.

Exploration of Presenting Problem

Most family therapists give considerable attention to a detailed exploration of the presenting problem as perceived by the various family members. Many family interviewers will begin this phase of the assessment by asking each individual in turn what he or she regards to be the problem. This approach usually brings out the multiple facets of a presenting problem. Such differences provide the family interviewer with both assessment and therapeutic leverage for working toward the common ground of a shared perspective. The presence of less involved, even peripheral members of the family or the social network may be valuable because such persons, including children and adolescents, often see the family more objectively and sometimes in relationship terms rather than as simply the fault of one person. The discovery that they have something constructive to offer may help bring them in as an integrative and otherwise underutilized resource.

How the family describes the presenting problem is often fully as informative as its content. Many family interviewers begin by asking a deliberately open-ended and undirected question in order to see who takes the responsibility for directing the process. In this scenario, the wife speaks first: "Why don't you tell him what's been bothering you, Bill?" Although the wife *seems* to give the stage to her husband, she has, in fact, assumed leadership by initiating the sequence of interaction and choosing the "spokesman."

Some interviewers deliberately address the opening question to a family member who was *not* involved in the referral call. If the wife had called for the appointment, the interviewer might briefly describe the content of the call and then ask the other family members for their understanding of the reason for the appointment. Other interviewers, at this point, explicitly inquire of the identified patient how his understanding of the problem compares with that reported. The technique of going systematically from one family member to another is oriented to having some participation early on from all family members. In any event, the family interviewer takes the position that the presenting problem will need to be understood from the point of view of all of those concerned with and affected by the problem.

In this vignette, the husband is asked what he sees as the problem. He responds, "Nothing specific. I don't understand it. I just can't get going anymore. I'm too tired to get out of bed in the morning." His wife adds, "He tosses and turns all night," and he says, "I wake up at 3:30 and can't get to sleep again." The wife interrupts this last comment to say to the daughter, "Quit wiggling! Can't you sit still?" The daughter impudently responds, "No!" The husband turns to his wife and in a plaintive but critical tone says, "Can't you keep her under control?" She responds, "I certainly don't get much help from you!"

At this point, the interviewer could use a considerable variety of comments and interventions. Some would continue the process of joining with the family by commenting on the difficulties of reaching parental agreement, perhaps asking the daughter: "Are you able to keep them on their toes as parents? They might start to get lazy in their old age." Another interviewer might inquire whether there also is a problem about control at home, e.g., at dinner time, and elicit from the wife: "She won't clean her plate, and he makes a big fuss about it." The husband says, "We have a rule that everybody should eat what is prepared for the family. When she won't eat, I send her away from the table and tell her she can't have anything more until breakfast. Then you (to wife) let her have peanut butter and jelly sandwiches a half-hour later." (The daughter looks overweight.) Daughter (to father), "I'd eat if you weren't so grouchy about it." Mother (to father), "We get along perfectly fine until you come in the door." The father responds, "I guess I should just stay away." The interviewer may interject, "When did this start to be a problem?" The wife answers, "It's been a fight every night this fall." The interviewer asks: "What else was going on this fall?"

Another approach might omit inquiring about further history for the time being and ask the parents to talk together about what they can do now about this problem with the daughter. This would provide further assessment data at the same time that the family might gain the positive experience of coping with a specific, focused issue. Their ability to have such experiences is part of the assessment process but, if they fail to do so, this information also provides prognostic data.

A contextual approach would explore the positive behaviors of the scapegoated daughter by asking the parents: "When has your daughter been helpful to you?" This would involve obtaining a broader picture of assets and resources. This approach to healthy aspects of the family functioning usually opens up surprising material that is overlooked when the focus is only on the symptoms and other difficulties.

Let us assume then that one of the problems that has emerged as a context for the presenting symptoms of the husband is a triangular relationship in which cross-generational ties between mother and daughter are strong, leaving the husband relatively isolated and alienated. Further, it emerges that this pattern has intensified during the period in which the husband's symptoms have grown to their present severity.

A second area may then emerge:

Interviewer: "What else has been going on this fall?"

Wife: "He's very worried about his business and thinks we'll all starve the way it's going. I want to go to work, but he objects!"

Husband: "You can't manage the house now and you can't control Josie (daughter). What would happen if you worked all day? (turning to interviewer) The business lost its two biggest contracts this fall. Maybe I'm in the wrong line of work. Sometimes I feel like giving up and doing something else, or maybe just giving up." (This could lead into exploration of concerns about suicide.)

Interviewer: "Has your family known about these worries?"

Daughter: "He's always gloomy, talking about life not being worth living."

Wife: "His chief assistant whom he counted on for the last ten years got another job a month ago. He's hired three replacements since then and isn't satisfied with any of them. So he ends up working all the time, brings work home at night and weekends, and complains if anybody wants to have any fun."

Husband: "There's just a lot of work and it has to be done. I don't appreciate the house being in turmoil all the time. The meals aren't even ready on time."

Wife: "You don't eat enough to feed a fly lately."

The above dialogue illustrates how considerable data relevant both to the family relationships and to the symptoms of the identified patient can emerge within the context of a family interview. In order to assess the seriousness of the clinical picture, including possible suicidal risk, individual meetings with the identified patient or the spouse would be held by many family therapists.

In the above scenario, let us assume that up to this point the son has been quiet. The interviewer might bring him in with a comment:

Interviewer: "You've been gone from home about two months now. What's your picture of how things have changed?"

Son: "It was good to get out."

Wife: "You're not doing anything at college."

Father: "He wants to quit college and he's just barely started."

Son: "It's dumb."

Father:	"Well, I can't *make* you go! I'm ready to give up on you too."
Wife:	(to interviewer) "They used to do everything together. Going camping and canoeing until last summer when Fred (son) said he just didn't want to go. Then he just sat around. They used to go hiking or camping almost every weekend, and this fall Bill hasn't done anything except work."
Interviewer:	(to wife) "Did you and Josie go along too?"
Wife:	"My back has bothered me for years, and Josie had to have her piano lessons on Saturday."

The immediate context for the presenting problem that has emerged thus far includes the cross-generational tie of mother-daughter, the developmental disruption of the tie of father-son, and the husband's impaired or dissolved work relationships leading him to experience still greater pressure to support his family. The wife's willingness to be helpful by working is rejected by the husband, perhaps because this would involve unacceptable changes in "old-fashioned" roles and values and because of the implicit depreciation of his capabilities in supporting the family. At the same time, this gives him the impression that she is erratic and flighty and not attending properly to her role as a mother.

Either in a subsequent interview or perhaps within or before the initial family interview, many family therapists would request that there be a session with the marital subsystem in which additional assessment data might emerge. The marital context of the presenting problem very likely involves long-standing problems that have come into focus more recently. The couple had married 20 years ago when they both were leaving unhappy families of origin. Family interviewers differ considerably in the degree to which they explore this historical background, though nearly all will agree that primary attention to historical patterns should involve those features that are reverberating in the here-and-now.

Both husband and wife have gradually become aware that their life experiences outside of the marriage were constricted, with neither having close relationships with anyone else prior to their marriage. They now differ in their view of the early sexual relationship, with the husband recalling it as quite satisfactory, but the wife describing herself as compliant, without affection or orgastic satisfaction. She describes having been helped during the last several years by individual psychotherapy which began when she was upset and depressed over the death of both of her parents in rapid succession. At that time she discovered that she had been chronically and diffusely discontent about her marital relationship. She had begun to think about getting a job when her daughter began school; however, she had not worked before marriage and had no career to which she could return. Recently she had taken a few courses and was encouraged by her individual therapist to get a job outside the home. At the same time, the individual therapy had alerted her to her dissatisfaction with the marital sexual relationship and, indeed, she recently had refused to have sex with her husband unless he was gentler and more loving. She long had been angry with him for being too precipitous in his sexual demands. She further complained that he always had premature ejaculations and that this was the reason that she could never build to an orgasm. Above all, she said, there was his lack of lovingness. He complained, on the other hand, that her unwillingness to take part in sex made his sexual needs so intense that this caused the premature ejaculations. During the past eight months, she had been in a women's group where issues of work and sex had been discussed, and she had been reinforced in her angry view of the role in which she had found herself over the years, a role she was no longer willing to continue.

More recently, there was a partial reversal of the pattern. The husband was overtly depressed and this led her to feel solicitous and concerned but, at the same time, she felt that he should get help from someone else, just as she had done. In turn, this led him to be reluctant to take part in therapy, both because he felt pushed and because he felt that her therapy had not helped their marriage. Her individual therapist was supportive of marital therapy for the couple, although he was not prepared to add marital therapy to the individual relationship. A crucial aspect of the assessment process would involve exploring the nature of the wife's continuing treatment relationship and, often, making contact with the other therapist.

Still another aspect of the context of the presenting problem emerged during the marital interviews when the husband complained that his wife wanted to control everything, whether it was a vacation or the timing of their sex lives. She angrily retorted, "Don't confuse me with your mother." In her individual therapy she had become aware of her tremendous resentment against his mother, because he seemed willing to give time and attention to his mother even though he complained that his mother was so highly controlling and disagreeable. On the other hand, the husband excused his mother as having had many hardships in her early life. He didn't think that his wife appreciated what his mother had gone through and how much she needed support. The wife replied, "You knock yourself out doing things for your mother, and your younger brother doesn't do anything for her, but he's the apple of her eye." The husband explained, "My mother became so upset when my youngest brother was killed in an automobile accident that she blamed me because I was the only one around at the time. My other brother lives across the country. So when he comes to visit her, it's easier for them to be friendly and nice to each other." At the same time, when describing his mother's angry rejection of him, he seemed to be closer to showing open distress and grief than at any other time in the assessment interviews.

In terms of treatment planning, the preceding material might enable a family therapist to take an orientation toward the marital subsystem as the primary unit for intervention, with perhaps some of the meetings involving the parents and offspring. At a future point, meetings involving the husband's mother might be helpful. Most family therapists would add pharmacotherapy to the treatment plan if the husband showed persistent major manifestations of depression. Most family therapists, given the above scenario, would doubt that pharmacotherapy *alone* would be sufficient to deal with the problems that have emerged in the described context. They also would expect that a symptom-oriented, diagnostic individual interview would be unlikely to uncover many of the important contextual features that have been noted above.

Still other features of the history, including early responsibilities of the husband for younger siblings and an alcoholic and depressive family history could be interpreted in both genetic and experiential frameworks. Some family therapists, particularly those following the leads of Bowen and Framo, would ask the father to explore the relationships with his family-of-origin in greater depth and ask the wife to do the same. Other family therapists would explore aspects of the historical past only insofar as they emerged as relevant to the current presenting problems. It could be anticipated that the initial presenting problem of the depressive symptomatology of the husband would be replaced in a matter of weeks or a few months by more concern about the long-standing issues in the marital relationship. At such a point, other approaches, possibly including behavioral and sex therapy techniques, might be incorporated into the family and marital treatment program.

An expansion of this vignette might indicate how a family therapist would continue the evaluation or assessment process beyond the presenting DSM-III symptoms into other aspects of the psychosocial context. Most importantly, this beginning phase of assessment with the family has already illuminated a series of pressing problems that differ in scope and quality from those identified with a DSM-III diagnosis.

REFERENCES

1. Gurman, A. S., and Kniskern, D. P.:*Handbook of Family Therapy*, New York: Brunner/Mazel, Inc., 1981.
2. Weiss, P.: Tierisches Verhalten als "Systemsreaktion": Die Orientiering der Ruhestellunger von Schmetterdingen (Vanessa) gegen Licht und Schwertkraft, *Biologia Gen.*, 14:168-248, 1925.
3. von Bertalanffny, L.: *Problems of Life*, New York: John Wiley & Sons, 1952.
4. von Bertalanffny, L.: *General Systems Theory*, New York: Braziller, 1968.
5. Engel, G. L.: The Clinical Application of the Biopsychosocial Model, *American Journal of Psychiatry*, 137:535-544, 1980.
6. Speck, R. V., and Rueveni, U.: Network Therapy, a Developing Concept, *Family Process*, 8:182-190, 1969.
7. Beels, C.: Social Networks, the Family, and the Schizophrenic Patient, *Schizophrenia Bulletin*, 4:512-521, 1978.
8. Beels, C.: Social Support and Schizophrenia, *Schizophrenia Bulletin*, 7:58-72, 1981.
9. Bloch, D. A.: The Future of Family Therapy, in M. Andolfi, and I. Zwerling (eds.): *Dimensions of Family Therapy*, New York: The Guilford Press, 1980, pp. 273-280.
10. Spiegel, J. P.: *Transactions*, New York: Science House, 1971.
11. Bowen, M.: Theory in the Practice of Psychotherapy, in P. J. Guerin (ed), *Family Therapy: Theory and Practice*, New York: Gardner Press, Inc., 1976, pp. 42-90.

12. Framo, J. L.: The Integration of Marital Therapy with Sessions with Family of Origin, in A. S. Gurman, and D. P. Kniskern (eds.): *Handbook of Family Therapy*, New York: Brunner/Mazel, Inc., 1981, pp. 133-158.
13. Bowen, M.: *Family Therapy in Clinical Practice*, New York: Jason Aronson, 1978.
14. Broderick, C. B., and Schrader, S. S.: The History of Professional Marriage and Family Therapy, in A. S. Gurman, and D. P. Kniskern (eds.): *Handbook of Family Therapy*, New York: Brunner/Mazel, Inc., 1981, pp. 5-35.
15. Martin, P. A.: *A Marital Therapy Manual*, New York: Brunner/Mazel, Inc., 1976.
16. Paolino, T. J., and McCrady, B. S. (eds.): *Marriage and Marital Therapy: Psychoanalytic, Behavioral and Systems Theory Perspectives*, New York: Brunner/Mazel, Inc., 1978.
17. Sager, C. J.: *Marriage Contracts and Couple Therapy*, New York: Brunner/Mazel, Inc. 1976.
18. Stuart, R. B.: *Helping Couples Change: A Social Learning Approach to Marital Therapy*, New York: The Guilford Press, 1980.
19. Sager, C. J.: Couples Therapy and Marriage Contracts, in A. S. Gurman, and D. P. Kniskern (eds.): *Handbook of Family Therapy*, New York: Brunner/Mazel, Inc., 1981, pp. 85-130.
20. Jacobson, N. S.: Behavioral Marital Therapy, in A. S. Gurman, and D. P. Kniskern (eds.): *Handbook of Family Therapy*, New York: Brunner/Mazel, Inc., 1981, pp. 556-591.
21. Sager, C. J.: A Typology of Intimate Relationships, *Journal of Sex and Marital Therapy*, 3:83-112, 1977.
22. Gurman, A. S.: Contemporary Marital Therapies: A Critique and Comparative Analysis of Psychoanalytic, Behavioral and Systems Theory Approaches, in T. J. Paolino, and B. S. McCrady (eds.): *Marriage and Marital Therapy: Psychoanalytic, Behavioral and Systems Theory Perspectives*, New York: Brunner/Mazel, Inc., 1978, pp. 445-566.
23. Kaslow, F. W.: Divorce and Divorce Therapy, in A. S. Gurman, and D. P. Kniskern (eds.): *Handbook of Family Therapy*, New York: Brunner/Mazel, Inc., 1981, pp. 662-696.
24. Boszormenyi-Nagy, I., and Spark, G. M.: *Invisible Loyalties: Reciprocity in Intergenerational Family Therapy*, Hagerstown, Md.: Harper & Row, Publishers, Inc., 1973.
25. Boszormenyi-Nagy, I., and Ulrich, D. N.: Contextual Family Therapy, in A. S. Gurman, and D. P. Kniskern (eds.): *Handbook of Family Therapy*, New York: Brunner/Mazel, Inc., 1981, pp. 159-186.
26. Zuk, G. H.: *Family Therapy: A Triadic-Based Approach*, New York: Behavioral Publications, Inc., 1971.
27. Selvini, M. P., Boscolo, L., Cecchin, G., and Prata, G.: Hypothesizing—Circularity—Neutrality: Three Guidelines for the Conductor of the Session, *Family Process*, 19:3-12, 1980.
28. Stierlin, H., Rücker-Embden, I., Wetzel, N., and Wirsching, M.: *The First Interview with the Family*, New York: Brunner/Mazel, Inc., 1980.

29. Napier, A. Y., and Whitaker, C. A.: *The Family Crucible*, New York: Harper & Row, Publishers, Inc., 1978.
30. Minuchin, S., and Fishman, H. C.: *Family Therapy Techniques*, Cambridge, Mass.: Harvard University Press, 1981.
31. Haley, J.: *Problem-Solving Therapy: New Strategies for Effective Family Therapy*. San Francisco: Jossey-Bass, Publishers, 1976.
32. Madanes, C.: *Strategic Family Therapy*, San Francisco: Jossey-Bass, Publishers, 1981.
33. Cannon, W. B.: Self-Regulation of the Body, in W. Buckley (ed.): *Modern Systems Research for the Behavioral Scientist*, Chicago: Aldine Publishing Co., 1968, pp. 256-258.
34. Jackson, D. D.: The Question of Family Homeostasis, *Psychiatric Quarterly Supplement*, 31:79-90, 1957.
35. Wahlroos, S.: Some Limitations of Family Therapy, *Journal of Family Counseling*, 4:8-11, 1976.
36. Maruyama, M.: The Second Cybernetics: Deviation-Amplifying Mutual Causal Processes, *American Scientist*, 51:164-179, 1963.
37. Hoffman, L.: *Foundations of Family Therapy: A Conceptual Framework for Systems Change*, New York: Basic Books, Inc., 1981.
38. Ashby, W. R.: *Design for a Brain*, New York: John Wiley, 1954.
39. Watzlawick, P., Weakland, J. H., and Fisch, R.: *Change: Principles of Problem Formation and Problem Resolution*, New York: W. W. Norton & Co., Inc., 1974.
40. Selvini, M. P., Boscolo, L., Cecchin, G., and Prata, G.: Family Rituals a Powerful Tool in Family Therapy, *Family Process*, 16:445-453, 1977.
41. Haley, J.: *Uncommon Therapy: The Psychiatric Techniques of Milton H. Erickson, M.D.*, New York: Ballantine Books, 1974.
42. Hoffman, L.: Deviation-Amplifying Processes in Natural Groups, in J. Haley (ed.): *Changing Families: A Family Therapy Reader*, New York: Grune & Stratton, 1971, pp. 285-311.
43. Selvini, M. P., Boscolo, L., Cecchin, G., and Prata, G.: *Paradox and Counterparadox: A New Model in the Therapy of the Family in Schizophrenic Transaction*, New York: Jason Aronson, 1978.
44. Watzlawick, P., Beavin, J. H., and Jackson, D. D.: *Pragmatics of Human Communications: A Study of Interactional Patterns, Pathologies, and Paradoxes*, New York: W. W. Norton & Co., Inc., 1967.
45. Gurman, A. S., and Kniskern, D. P.: Deterioration in Marital and Family Therapy: Empirical, Clinical, and Conceptual Issues, *Family Process*, 17:3-20, 1978.
46. Keeney, B. P.: Ecosystemic Epistemology: An Alternative Paradigm for Diagnosis, *Family Process*, 18:117-129, 1979.
47. Goldstein, M. J., Rodnick, E. H., Jones, J. E., McPherson, S. R., and West, K. L.: Familial Precursors of Schizophrenia Spectrum Disorders, in L. C. Wynne, R. L. Cromwell, and S. Matthysse (eds.): *The Nature of Schizophrenia: New Approaches to Research and Treatment*, New York: John Wiley & Sons, 1978, pp. 487-498.

48. Ferreira, A. J.: Family Myths and Homeostasis, *Archives of General Psychiatry*, 9:457-463, 1963.
49. Stierlin, H.: Group Fantasies and Family Myths—Some Theoretical and Practical Aspects, *Family Process*, 12:111-125, 1973.
50. Wynne, L. C., Ryckoff, I., Day, J., and Hirsch, S.: Pseudo-mutuality in the Family Relations of Schizophrenics, *Psychiatry* 21:205-220, 1958.
51. Strupp, H. H., and Hadley, S. W.: A Tripartite Model of Mental Health and Therapeutic Outcomes: With Special Reference to Negative Effects in Psychotherapy, *American Psychologist*, 33:187-196, 1977.
52. Haley, J. (ed.): *Changing Families: A Family Therapy Reader*, New York: Grune & Stratton, 1971.
53. Whitaker, C. A., and Keith, D. V.: Symbolic-Experiential Family Therapy, in A. S. Gurman, and D. P. Kniskern (eds.): *Handbook of Family Therapy*, New York: Brunner/Mazel, Inc., 1981, pp. 187-225.
54. McPartland, T. S., and Richart, R. H.: Social and Clinical Outcomes of Psychiatric Treatment, *Archives of General Psychiatry*, 14:179-184, 1966.
55. Ryback, R. S., Longabaugh, R., and Fowler, D. R.: *The Problem Oriented Record in Psychiatry and Mental Health Care*, Rev. Ed., New York: Grune & Stratton, Inc., 1981.
56. Richardson, H. S.: *Patients Have Families*, New York: Commonwealth Fund, 1945.
57. *Diagnostic and Statistical Manual of Mental Disorders (Third Edition)*, Washington, D.C.: American Psychiatric Association, 1980.
58. Framo, J. L.: Family of Origin as a Therapeutic Resource for Adults in Marital and Family Therapy: You Can and Should Go Home Again, *Family Process*, 15:193-210, 1976.
59. Guerin, P. J., and Pendagast, E. G.: Evaluation of Family System and Genogram, in Philip J. Guerin (ed.): *Family Therapy: Theory and Practice*, New York: Gardner Press, Inc., 1976, pp. 450-464.
60. Paul, N.: The Use of Empathy in the Resolution of Grief, in *Perspectives in Biology and Medicine 11*, no. 1, Chicago: University of Chicago, 1967.
61. Speck, R. V., and Attneave, C. L.: *Family Networks*, New York: Pantheon Books, 1973.
62. Group for the Advancement of Psychiatry, (GAP), *The Case History Method in the Study of Family Process*, Vol. VI, Report No. 76, New York: Group for the Advancement of Psychiatry, 1970, pp. 323-331.
63. Haley, J.: *Strategies of Psychotherapy*, New York: Grune & Stratton, 1963.
64. Stanton, M. D.: Strategic Approaches to Family Therapy, in A. S. Gurman, and D. P. Kniskern (eds.): *Handbook of Family Therapy*, New York: Brunner/Mazel, Inc., 1981, pp. 361-402.
65. Wynne, L. C.: Some Indications and Contra-indications for Exploratory Family Therapy, in I. Boszormenyi-Nagy, and J. L. Framo (eds.): *Intensive Family Therapy: Theoretical and Practical Aspects with Special Reference to Schizophrenia*, New York: Harper & Row, Inc., 1965, pp. 289-322.

66 Wynne, L. C.: Collusive Blaming: A Commentary, in R. Lang and the Editorial Board (eds.), *International Journal of Psychoanalysis and Psychotherapy, Vol. 8, 1980-81*, New York: Jason Aronson, 1980, pp. 457-460.
67. Ackerman, N. W.: *Treating the Troubled Family*, New York: Basic Books, Inc., 1966.
68. Skynner, A. C. R.: *Systems of Family and Marital Psychotherapy*, New York: Brunner/Mazel, Inc., 1976.
69. Hill, R., and Rodgers, R. H.: The Developmental Approach, in H. T. Christensen (ed.): *Handbook of Marriage and the Family*, Chicago: Rand McNally & Co., 1964, pp. 171-211.
70. Carter, E. A., and McGoldrick, M.: *The Family Life Cycle: A Framework for Family Therapy*, New York: Gardner Press, Inc., 1980.
71. Hadley, T. R., Jacob, T., Milliones, J., Caplan, J., and Spitz, D.: The Relationship between Family Developmental Crisis and the Appearance of Symptoms in a Family Member, *Family Process*, 13:207-214, 1974.
72. Epstein, N. B., and Bishop, D. S.: Problem-Centered Systems Therapy of the Family, in A. S. Gurman, and D. P. Kniskern (eds.): *Handbook of Family Therapy*, New York: Brunner/Mazel, Inc., 1981, pp. 444-482.
73. Duhl, B. S., and Duhl, F. J.: Integrative Family Therapy, in A. S. Gurman, and D. P. Kniskern (eds.): *Handbook of Family Therapy*, New York: Brunner/Mazel, Inc., 1981, pp. 483-513.
74. Lewis, J. M., Beavers, W. R., Gossett, J. T., and Phillips, V. A.: *No Single Thread: Psychological Health in Family Systems*, New York: Brunner/Mazel, Inc., 1976.
75. L'Abate, L.: Skill Training Programs for Couples and Families, in A. S. Gurman, and D. P. Kniskern (eds.): *Handbook of Family Therapy*, New York: Brunner/Mazel, Inc., 1981, pp. 631-661.
76. Skynner, A. C. R.: An Open-Systems, Group-Analytic Approach to Family Therapy, in A. S. Gurman, and D. P. Kniskern (eds.): *Handbook of Family Therapy*, New York: Brunner/Mazel, Inc., 1981, pp. 39-84.
77. Andolfi, M.: *Family Therapy: An Interactional Approach*, New York: Plenum Press, 1979.
78. Sager, C. J., Gundlach, R. H., Kremer, M., *et al.*: The Married in Treatment, *Archives of General Psychiatry*, 19:205-217, 1968.
79. Gurin, G., Veroff, J., and Feld, S.: Americans View Their Mental Health: A Nationwide Interview Survey, *Joint Commission on Mental Illness and Health Monograph Series 4*, New York: Basic Books, 1960.
80. Fisher, L.: On the Classification of Families: A Progress Report, *Archives of General Psychiatry*, 34:424-433, 1977.
81. Olson, D. H., Russell, C. S., and Sprenkle, D. H.: Circumplex Model of Marital and Family Systems II: Empirical Studies and Clinical Intervention, in J. P. Vincent (ed.): *Advances in Family Intervention, Assessment and Theory*, Greenwich, Conn.: JAI Press, 1979, pp. 129-176.
82. Russell, C. S.: Circumplex Model of Marital and Family Systems: III. Empirical Evaluation with Families, *Family Process*, 18:29-45, 1979.

83. Epstein, N., Bishop, D. S., and Levin, S.: The McMaster Model of Family Functioning, *Journal of Marriage and Family Counseling*, 40:19-31, 1978.
84. Minuchin, S., Montalvo, B., Guerney, B. G., Rosman, B. L., and Schumer, F.: *Families of the Slums: An Exploration of Their Structure and Treatment*, New York: Basic Books, Inc., 1967.
85. Minuchin, S.: *Families & Family Therapy*, Cambridge, Mass.: Harvard Univ. Press, 1974.
86. Ford, F. R., and Herrick, J.: Family Rules: Family Life Styles, *American Journal of Orthopsychiatry*, 44:61-69, 1974.
87. Andolfi, M., Nicolo, A. M., Menghi, P., and Saccu, C.: Interaction in Rigid Systems: A Model of Intervention in Families with a Schizophrenic Member, in M. Andolfi, and I. Zwerling (eds.): *Dimensions of Family Therapy*, New York: Guilford Press, 1980, pp. 171-204.
88. Lederer, W. J., and Jackson, D. D.: *The Mirages of Marriage*, New York: W. W. Norton & Co., Inc., 1968.
89. Cubor, J. F., and Haroff, P. B.: *Sex and the Significant Americans*, New York: Penguin Books, 1960, pp. 43-65.
90. Ravich, R. A., and Wyden, B.: *Predictable Pairing*, New York: Wyden, 1974.
91. Kramer, C. H.: *Becoming a Family Therapist: Developing an Integrated Approach to Working with Families*, New York: Human Sciences Press, 1980.
92. Ackerman, N. W.: *The Psychodynamics of Family Life: Diagnosis and Treatment of Family Relationships*, New York: Basic Books, Inc., 1958.
93. Paul, N. L., and Paul, B. B.: *A Marital Puzzle: Transgenerational Analysis in Marriage Counseling*, New York: W. W. Norton & Co., Inc., 1975.
94. Papp, P.: Family Choreography, in P. J. Guerin (ed.): *Family Therapy: Theory and Practice*, New York: Gardner Press, Inc., 1976, pp. 465-479.
95. Kwiatkowska, H. Y.: *Family Therapy and Evaluation through Art*, Springfield, Ill.: Charles C. Thomas, 1978.
96. Minuchin, S., Rosman, B. L., and Baker, L.: *Psychosomatic Families: Anorexia Nervosa in Context*, Cambridge, Mass.: Harvard Univ. Press, 1978.
97. Barton, C., and Alexander, J. F.: Functional Family Therapy, in A. S. Gurman, and D. P. Kniskern (eds.): *Handbook of Family Therapy*, New York: Brunner/Mazel, Inc., 1981, pp. 403-443.
98. Gurman, A. S.: Dimensions of Marital Therapy: A Comparative Analysis, *Journal of Marital and Family Therapy*, 5:5-16, 1979.
99. Fogarty, T. F.: Marital Crisis, in P. J. Guerin (ed.): *Family Therapy: Theory and Practice*, New York: Gardner Press, Inc., 1976, pp. 325-334.
100. Wynne, L. C.: The Study of Intrafamilial Alignments and Splits in Exploratory Family Therapy, in N. Ackerman, F. L. Beatman, and S. N. Sherman (eds.): *Exploring the Base for Family Therapy*, New York: Family Service Association of America, 1961, pp. 95-115.
101. Scheflen, A. E.: Susan Smiled: On Explanation in Family Therapy, *Family Process*, 17:59-68, 1978.
102. Williamson, D. S.: New Life at the Graveyard: A Method of Therapy for Individuation from a Dead Former Parent, *Journal of Marriage and Family Counseling*, 4:93-101, 1978.

Chapter Six

Special Perspectives on Treatment Planning for Children

John G. Looney, M.D.
and
Mark J. Blotcky, M.D.

Introduction and Overview

The process of designing treatment for a child is different enough from that used for an adult to warrant special focus. Therefore, there is a need to include in this volume a chapter devoted to treatment planning for children. Treatment modalities for adults, and indications for their use, have been described well in previous chapters; however, the types of treatment previously described may have to be used with major modifications when used with children.

That treatment planning is an exercise more difficult than simply giving a disorder a name is particularly true with children, because of the impact upon their psychological balance of such things as rapid growth, constitutional differences, cognitive changes, the effect of the family and other support systems, the changing balance between

---

*The authors have written this chapter at the request of the American Academy of Child Psychiatry for inclusion in this volume.

Dr. Looney is Director, Department of Child and Adolescent Psychiatry, Timberlawn Psychiatric Center, Dallas, Texas. He serves as Research Psychiatrist at the Timberlawn Psychiatric Research Foundation.

Dr. Blotcky is Director, Children's Inpatient Unit, Timberlawn Psychiatric Center, Dallas, Texas.

The authors wish to express appreciation to the following representatives of the American Academy of Child Psychiatry who served on a Corresponding Committee that assisted in formulating the concepts of this chapter:

Robert L. Stubblefield, M.D.,
President
Dennis P. Cantwell, M.D.
Joseph Fischhoff, M.D.
Saul I. Harrison, M.D.
Virginia Q. Bausch, M.D.,
Executive Director
Jack Martin, M.D.
Lillian H. Robinson, M.D.
John Schowalter, M.D.

ego strengths and pressure of drives, the changing nature of defense mechanisms, the changing quality of object relationships, fluidity of personality organization, age-related developmental tasks, and other such factors affecting childhood psychological balance.

The authors will attempt to achieve several goals in this chapter. The first is to present a brief overview of the process of child development. Biologic and psychodynamic changes, as well as the child's changing relationship to the social milieu, will be emphasized particularly. This review is presented to stress that children change constantly, and that these changes have to be taken into account in assessing normality or pathology and in planning effective interventions for troubled children. Second, a review of types of data needed for careful treatment plan formulation is offered. Third, a brief review of the types of procedures used to gather information about children is presented. Finally, the authors will review the process of synthesizing the collected information to formulate a treatment plan. An illustration will be offered of synthesis of data gathered from the following multiple levels:

1) Psychological or intellectual problems within the child
2) Problems of the child within the family
3) Problems of the child with peers
4) Problems of the child with social institutions such as school
5) The effect on the child of sociocultural and religious forces
6) The level of the child's physical health and development

To achieve this last goal of synthesizing the data and planning a treatment program, the problem of matching available treatment modalities to the needs of a youngster will be described. The issue of determining the points of intervention that offer maximum benefit will be addressed.

For purposes of achieving the stated goals, the needs of two children will be considered throughout the chapter.

> *Amy and Bill are different in age, family situation, socioeconomic status and ethnic background. Yet for similar reasons they are referred to clinicians for evaluation. Both children manifest symptoms of depression. Both break rules in school, at home, and in other places in a serious, and sometimes illegal, manner. Both lose control of angry feelings and hurt people. Both have had enough trouble with reading to impede their school performance. Both children have*

> *asthma. These similar problems have interfered with their normal activities to approximately the same degree. Each child has experienced similar degrees of stress over the past year.*

Clinicians planning treatment approaches for the two children would need to assess a kaleidoscopic array of developmental variables in order to synthesize approaches offering maximum opportunities for beneficial change. Toward the end of the chapter, a detailed description of these children's problems is offered and treatment plans are developed to meet their needs.

Before pursuing the major goals of the chapter, some significant preliminary points, as they affect the process of treatment planning, need to be made about the development of children. Although these points are self-evident, they warrant emphasis to illustrate how different children's needs may be from those of adults. First, it should be noted that tremendous growth and change occur during the childhood years, e.g., body weight may increase fifteen- to twenty-fold between birth and puberty. Changes in function are similarly dramatic. Although helpless at birth, by puberty the child has made such progress that he or she seems almost a different organism. Vast changes take place in physical, mental, and social relationship capabilities. Therefore, one cannot state that a person is a child and convey much information other than the person is not an adult. Differences between infants, pre-school children, and school age children are as great as between any other three life stages.

Further, development does not take place at an even, steadily accelerating pace. There are spurts and regressions. There are modal tasks that must be accomplished at reasonably predictable ages. Children take time to accomplish these tasks. In order to move to a new task, the previous ones must be mastered and the new task must appear intriguing or, at least, not excessively frightening.

Lastly, it should be stressed that a child's biological, psychological, and social development are intimately related. For example, early attachment and bonding between a mother and an infant is a process that has biologic determinants, that initiates important psychodynamic process, and that is the anlage of all later social relationships. The child comes into the world with a genetically determined program for human development. Imposed upon the child's "biologic" substrate is the impact of the environment. Sameroff offers a conceptually helpful "transactional model" of child development that postulates a progressive interplay between the biologic attributes of the child and the forces within the environment.[1] Deviant outcome, therefore, results from an insult to the biological adaptive capacity of the child, or to the influence of destructive environmental forces, either or both of which over time prevent the child from an effective organization of his or her experience. Thus, the following descriptions of development along different dimensions is artificially separated for clearer illustration in a brief space.

Biological Aspects of Childhood Development

Psychiatric treatment planning for children must take into consideration biologic developmental processes because:

1) the rate and amount of change are greater during childhood than during any other phase of life
2) these predetermined biological changes are functionally associated with psychological changes

Physical maturation is necessary for psychological progression, e.g., children with chronic illnesses, severe trauma, or constitutional handicaps usually do not progress normally through the predicted stages of psychological development. The reverse is also true, psychological nurturing may significantly affect physical development. Spitz demonstrated convincingly that infants who do not receive the normal amount of handling and cuddling fail to grow at the same rate as other children.[2]

To be maximally helpful to children in diagnostic assessment and treatment planning, the clinician pays attention to the child's achieved point along the line of physical development, as well as noting whether the child appears to be moving or fixated on that line. It would, therefore, be helpful to review thoroughly important contributions to knowledge about biological development, and yet a thorough review would be encyclopedic in scope. The authors' purpose is only to remind the clinician of selected important issues. The reader desiring more comprehensive reviews of normal changes is referred to several sources.[2–6]

Although biological issues important to child development can be defined and catalogued in a variety of ways, the following categorization offers some utility in organizing information for treatment planning:

1) Genetics
2) Pregnancy, labor, and delivery
3) Neurological maturation
4) Biological bases for "physiological processes of development"
5) The effect of general health status on development

GENETICS

Although selected aberrations of development (e.g., amino acid disorders) are clearly genetically determined, the relationship between genes and most developmental problems is not absolutely clear. The problem is to separate genetic programming from environmental molding, e.g., behavioral differences between sexes may be determined by either genetic or environmental influences. "Maleness" is thought to be determined by androgenic influences on the fetus. Without the genetically determined presence of a Y chromosome, and the resulting production of androgen, the fetus is thought to progress naturally to phenotypic "femaleness."[7] Behavioral differences are thought to be observed between boys and girls.[8,9,10] Are these differences due to genetically determined androgenic influence throughout development, or due to different responses to boys and girls by parents, or both? Another important, but currently unclear, issue is whether constitutional differences in temperament and behavioral traits are due to genetic, intrauterine, or other influences. Somewhat better established by research data is the presumption that certain major psychiatric syndromes (e.g., the schizophrenias and a spectrum of related disorders, as well as some types of affective disorders) have genetic predisposition.[11,12]

PREGNANCY, LABOR, AND DELIVERY

The fetus is both responsive and vulnerable, e.g., it is known that the fetus is responsive to auditory stimulation fairly early in gestation.[13] Of course, it is well established that the fetus is vulnerable to the effects of multiple infectious agents, toxins, drugs, and malnutrition. More controversial is whether the fetus is vulnerable to emotional turmoil of the mother. Stott and Latchford's comprehensive epidemiologic study demonstrated correlations between a pregnant woman's interpersonal stress and behavioral problems in the child several years after birth.[14] Pasaminick and Knobloch and others demonstrated a spectrum of developmental difficulties related to prematurity and accidents of labor, which, in turn, are related often to socioeconomic factors.[15,16]

NEUROLOGICAL MATURATION

An aspect of physical development of particular interest to the psychiatrist is neurologic maturation. The brain increases in mass from about 350 grams at birth to about 1500 grams by the end of puberty. The degree of anatomic complexity, the amount of myelination, and the degree of localization of specific functions also increase enormously. Although the rate of change is greatest during the first several years of life, changes take place throughout childhood. Maturation of the nervous system is neither linear in rate nor independent of environmental stimulation. Nonlinearity is demonstrated by such things as spurts and slowing in the development of new capabilities and by longitudinal electroencephalogic studies demonstrating changing patterns at ages that psychological developmental theory, or naturalistic observation, predict major behavioral changes to occur.[17] It also appears that the brain does not develop its functional capabilities without stimulation. For example, Spitz, in the study already mentioned, learned that foundling home children were slower in the development of mental capabilities as well as physical stature and health.[2] The massive amount of neurologic maturation that must take place during childhood means that special problems are posed for children whose maturation is arrested or slowed by congenital or acquired central nervous system (CNS) disease.

BIOLOGICAL BASES FOR "PSYCHOLOGICAL PROCESSES OF DEVELOPMENT"

Special comment must be made about the biologic bases for the psychological processes of development. One example is changes in object relatedness being dependent upon physical growth and increasing function. The early formation of the mother/infant dyadic bond can be viewed from a biologic or psychological perspective depending on training, interest, and theoretic perspective of the viewer. Biologically programmed tendencies lead to a fulfillment of relatedness imbued with a high order of "human emotion." Maturation of the ocular system and visual cortex facilitates the child's recognition of the mother's face. The smile that is a reflexic response to the visual perception is a powerful stimulus to unlock the mother's potential for caring. Biologic changes are also necessary for the gradual dissolution of the strong bond between child and mother. The myelinization of long motor tracts makes possible bipedal locomotion that, in turn, leads to the child's first attempts to explore the world without the mother's immediate aid, the first step in the "psychological" process of the child's discovering the fact of his or her individuality. These biologic determinants of changes in object relatedness could be traced on through the childhood years. Perhaps, however, another example of the biologic basis for changing psychological processes exists in examination of biologic cycles. Adults are fairly well fixed in daily rhythms of such things as sleeping (and dreaming within a sleep period), feeding, maximal alertness, diurnal endocrine output, and the like. Childhood development involves a gradual achievement of this adult cyclicity. The calmer psychological status of older children as compared to infants, therefore, may be dependent to some degree on increasing biologic regularity. Roffwarg and coworkers noted changes not only in the amount of sleep but in the amount and sequencing of rapid eye movement (REM) sleep during early childhood development.[18] They suggested that the large amount of REM sleep (with presumed dreaming) in early infancy is necessary as a source of endogenous stimulation for CNS development. Of course, the diminishing amount of sleep time and REM sleep allows an infant to be more responsive to the caretaker's ministrations, thus furthering the process of attachment.

THE EFFECT OF GENERAL HEALTH STATUS ON DEVELOPMENT

The level of general health and the smooth process of growth and development are important issues to be assessed by a clinician. Any organism undergoing such massive and rapid change is particularly vulnerable to stressors that can impede these changes. Physical illness, trauma, or disability, therefore, can be a major problem.

Reviewing all the preceding biologic aspects of child development makes clear the importance of knowing where a given child should be along a continuum of biologic development, or if deviation has occurred, of designing remedial programs to help the child get back on the normal path. If, for example, either of the two hypothetical children previously described had demonstrated abnormalities in the process of physical development, or had impediments to further development, the clinician would want to assess these problems and plan appropriate remediation. Billy was adopted, and little genetic history is available. The clinician learns, however, that his mother was alcoholic and was drinking during pregnancy. Billy had some delays in developmental milestones that suggest uneven neurological maturation. His daily habits and rhythms had always been irregular. He developed asthma at age three. Amy's history suggests normal progression of biologic development. She also, however, had asthma. Because she was depressed, an extensive genetic history was obtained that did not suggest a family depressive trend.

Psychodynamic Aspects of Childhood Development

Just as the process of biologic maturation may be traced through predictable stages, so can psychological or psychodynamic changes be traced. Again, knowledge of these normal stages is necessary to determine whether or not a deviation from the usual course exists. A comprehensive review of these stages, which is beyond the scope of this section, can be found in several sources.[4–6, 19–38] This section offers an abbreviated outline to be used as a template against which to measure the progression of a given child.

Although certain seminal thinkers (e.g., Darwin, Locke, Rousseau, and St. Augustine) concerned themselves with the question of how the normal child predictably progresses into adulthood, it was Freud who first described stages of childhood development. Erikson also outlined predictable stages, corresponding in approximate age to those of Freud, but he added an emphasis regarding social development to the psychosexual focus of Freud.[19,20] Erikson conceptualized a series of psychosocial crises based on developmental needs of the child and the response of the people in the environment. Anna Freud validated the concept of psychosexual stages through naturalistic observation of children.[21] Freud's, Erikson's, and Anna Freud's work all propose an early supportive attachment between mother and child as necessary to further progression. Bowlby and Ainsworth through naturalistic observation verified the development of this close attachment between mother and child.[22,23,24,25] Mahler described the process of the child's graduated emancipation from the mother (again, in predictable stages), a process leading ultimately to the child's ability to conceive of himself or herself as a separate person.[26] Kohut traced predictable stages in the development of narcissism.[27] Piaget was more interested in the ways that children think than in their psychosexual development or their ways of relating to primary others.[28] It is interesting that he also described stages in the development of the thinking process from the most primitive, concrete, and magical way of interpreting the world, to an ability to conceive of the world in its most complex abstract meanings. Kohlberg has used Piaget's conceptual framework to describe stages in the development of moral sensibility.[36]

The scandalous brevity and selectivity of this review of powerful thinkers belie the prodigious amount of data and theory generated by them and others. Yet studies of child development are not at a stage at which a comprehensive model can be synthesized, a model explaining all observations regarding the developing child. Nevertheless, it is possible to synthesize some tenets, or assumptions, with which most professionals interested in children's development would agree. Extracted from the works of these pioneers and others are some of these important assumptions.

One important assumption is that a mother's experience of her pregnancy, labor, and delivery is critical to how she perceives, accepts, and nurtures her newborn infant. Therefore, a child born to a mother unprepared for pregnancy, unsupported in her pregnancy, or experiencing serious emotional or physical turmoil during pregnancy might be considered at risk. Similarly, a child born to a mother unavailable to the child because of depression or medical complications after delivery also would be one about whom the clinician would be concerned.

A second assumption is that a child who is going to progress through the normal stages of psychological development must first form an extremely close, and mutually satisfying, relationship with the mothering person. The child enters the world in what Mahler dramatically termed a normal autistic stage, i.e., a stage of being unaware of the existence or importance of another person.[26] It is thought that there are certain critical periods occurring early in life in which reciprocal sets of relating behaviors occur between mother and child.[29] An example used previously was a baby's recognition of the face of the caretaker reflexively causing smiling which then elicits nurturing behavior. The clinician is concerned about evidence of a mutually stimulating and satisfying mother-infant fit. One important digression is that infants and children are known to have different types of temperaments.[30] Some infants are cuddly and easily soothed; others are irritable. A given mother may be able to form an optimal attachment to a child of one particular temperament, but not to another.

Freud, of course, described the early period of the child's life, extending until about the first birthday, as a stage of orality.[20] That is to say, one of the child's primary modes of obtaining pleasure, as well as relating to the caretaker, is through sucking, eating, biting, mouthing, and other such oral behaviors. The child also relates through vestibular and tactile stimulation as well as through sight and sound. In any case, the attachment between mother and child usually becomes so close that Mahler, again with dramatic emphasis, described this phase as a normal symbiosis. During this period, according to Erikson, the child establishes a sense of basic trust if the caretakers are reliable and meet the needs reasonably well.[19]

Another important assumption is that further psychological development is dependent upon the child and caretaker being able to separate, in graduated moves, from their extremely close relationship. This period of separation takes place in a fairly predictable pattern, and at the end of this period (approximately three years of age), the child should be able to evoke an internal image of the caretaker as is needed for a feeling of well-being under the stress of new experiences; the child develops a concept of himself or herself as an individual separate and distinct from the caretaker. Freud's stage of anality fits within this period of time. It is true that the child gains great satisfaction and independence from learning to control the bowels. Also, the child gains a sense of mastery of other abilities such as walking, playing, and expressing through languages. Erikson describes the task during this period as the establishment of a sense of autonomy.

Another assumption is that once a sense of autonomy has been achieved, the child needs to come to terms with the triangular nature of the relationship with parents. This triangular relationship, as Freud noted, occurs at a time when the child develops a particular interest in genital sensation. The child often develops a relationship having a romantic quality with the parent of the opposite sex. Some storminess in behavior results when the child realizes that the romantic fantasy of being able to grow up and marry the parent of the opposite sex will not achieve fulfillment. Erikson summarizes the basic conflict of this phase as "initiative versus guilt." If an adequate solution is found so that guilt does not overwhelm initiative, the guilt helps turn the child away from useless sexual strivings, and the child becomes able to use initiative in learning to master the environment. This period of development can involve some significant stress for the child and both parents. Indeed, it is often a period in which parents begin to worry about some behavior in the child that is difficult to manage. Usually this phase of development is resolved by time, maturation, and common sense child management techniques. The child emerges in a calmer state, having decided to identify with the parent of the same sex rather than possess the parent of the opposite sex, and having internalized a code of moral behavior similar to that of the parents.

Lastly, around the school age, the child usually becomes steady in mood and behavior, pliable, and more educable; this state continues until the onset of puberty. With resolution of the competitive struggles within the family, the child gains much increased psychic energy for direction in other areas. It is this conflict-free energy that the child directs toward producing things, completing school work, and trying to understand the world. Freud called this period latency, because conflict about sexuality is usually obscured from parents, although children continue to think and learn about their bodies and sex. The period is certainly not latent with regard to the enormous expansion of the child's knowledge about the complexity of the world. Piaget demonstrated massive cognitive changes during this period of life. Erikson described the primary task of this period as overcoming feelings of inferiority and becoming industrious, mastering the job of enormous learning. School-age children develop more complex social relationships with peers and nonparental adults. The school-age child joins clubs, athletic teams, and church groups. More mature defenses against anxiety (e.g., obsessive compulsive mechanisms, reaction formations, and sublimations) become prominent. The ego of the school-age child undergoes some changes, most prominently characterized by displacement, an increased ability to manipulate symbols and use fantasies in an adaptive fashion, and a better capacity to distinguish fantasy from reality. This period in the child's life is one in which much goes on internally; conflicts with parents are what really become more latent.

This brief review serves to remind readers of the active, progressive development in which a child is immersed. The clinician evaluating Amy and Billy would note that they are of different ages and would want to determine if they are at expected points along this line of development. Billy has always been a temperamentally difficult child, being excessively irritable. His early relationship with his mother was not satisfying to either of them. He has always had a poor ability to modulate his aggression. At age six he has a seductive and manipulative relationship with his mother and a distant and competitive one with his father. His sense of right and wrong has always been variable. He shows no signs of developing the pliability and industriousness of a school-age child.

Amy was a cuddly infant, and she and her mother early formed a mutually dependent relationship that has continued to be very close at her present age of ten. She had previously gained good control of her aggression, had an adequate sense of right and wrong, and had applied herself well in school. She was, however, somewhat of a loner. Her early signs of pubescence began at the same time as the appearance of periodic outbursts of aggressive behavior, suggesting a poor acceptance of growing up and of emerging sexuality.

Familial and Sociocultural Factors

A child is so molded by the social system in which he or she exists that it is important to understand the significance of a social system and to take its forces into account. Although the nuclear family is the system of primary importance, other important systems include the extended family; the peer group; school and formal extracurricular group activities; and in a broader perspective, socioeconomic class, culture, and religion.

THE FAMILY

The family constitutes the primary crucible in which the child's personality formation takes place. The child is so dynamically connected with the family that his or her behavior says as much about family functioning as about the child's. The family's values and ways of relating are slowly internalized as the child progresses. The child's development is the result of the intricate orchestration of drives, defenses, and environmental gratifications and frustrations, all leading to internalization of personality structure; the balance between these forces is mediated mostly by the family. The child is so embedded in the family context that trying to assess his or her status without assessment of the family's functioning is similar to trying to assess the tonal qualities of a single musical instrument being played within a symphony orchestra.

Just as the child grows through successive stages of development, family systems may progress through different levels of maturation. Anthony and Benedek have noted predictable changes in the mother and father as they progress in their parental roles.[39] Research suggests that some parental styles of dealing with children (e.g., an authoritative style) are more optimal than others (e.g., an authoritarian or laissez-faire approach).[40] Research has also demonstrated that families can be placed along a continuum of competence, from extremely pathologic to extremely competent, based on evaluation of such important interactional variables as the way in which power is handled, clarity of communication, the ability to be empathic, and others.[41] Certain patterns of pathologic interactions are likewise delineated in a growing literature on family systems.[42] The point is that professionals are in a position to be much more sophisticated in evaluation of families and understanding the impact of the family on the child.[38]

The extended family may be a source of influence on the child. For example, grandparents may influence the child directly or, through their support of the parents, indirectly. Grandparental support may be particularly important to single parent or other types of nontraditional families. In addition to offering such support, available relatives often help the child to develop a sense of heritage and continuity.

PEER GROUP

The peer group becomes an increasingly important support system as the child grows. After the child has mastered the sibling support system, peer contact is increasingly sought. Healthy relationships with peers require a capacity to hold onto one's identity while at the same time finding gratification in a modified identity as part of a group. The secure child makes this transition easily and finds real support in the new system. The insecure child may respond by withdrawing or becoming a bully. Establishing relationships with peers should help the child with such tasks as beginning separation from parents, solidifying an autonomous identity, and supporting self-esteem.

SCHOOL AND ACTIVITIES

School and organized extracurricular activities constitute the child's first experience outside the family in formal social institutions. School may offer the first extended experience of relatedness to nonparental adults. The child is also confronted with increasing expectations of compliance with rules and social order as well as expectations of competition and achievement. Extracurricular activities offer gratification for the development of skills and talents as well as further chances for social interaction. Because in unstructured situations boys tend to group with boys and girls with girls, these formal activities often allow sustained contact between sexes.

SOCIOECONOMIC CLASS, CULTURE, AND RELIGION

Just as the child is more dependent upon the primary family than is an adult, there is more likely to be significant molding by the values of the broader social system. The child is, therefore, influenced by such things as socioeconomic class values, cultural values, and religious values.[43,44] Socioeconomic class tends to define position, power, and patterns of behavior. It influences educational expectations, career choice, lifestyle, dress code, tolerance for aggression, tolerance for expression of sexuality, types of child discipline, age at the time of beginning work, age at separation from family, age at marriage, and even age of first pregnancy. The definition of what constitutes the nuclear family is also affected, e.g., lower socioeconomic class families are more frequently multigenerational. Working class parents frequently stress conformity to external standards, whereas middle class families stress self-direction and responsibility.[45] Lower class children tend to encounter greater diversity of cultural expectations as they move from home to neighborhood, school, and community. They perceive less coherence in the nature of the world and more often feel failure and devaluation; they less often have a competent role model.[45] As the child grows older, cultural and religious forces become more important. The child is certainly influenced by the dominant American system of values, including such things as independence; hard work; and the high value placed on family, youth, physical strength, attractiveness, competition, and success. Within this dominant culture, the child's particular ethnic heritage modifies the meaning of existence as an American. In addition, religion offers a learned set of rituals, explanations for that which is otherwise inexplicable, and a sense of mankind's connectedness. Religious affiliations may influence self-concept and lifestyle as well as types of pathology and degrees of acceptance of psychiatric treatment.

Clearly, the child's functioning must be assessed as to its meaning with respect to his or her relationship to family, peers, school, and broader cultural forces.[46] The two children, Billy and Amy, are of different family situations, socioeconomic classes, and ethnic groups. Billy is adopted into a middle class Caucasian family in which the parents are in significant conflict. Though Amy's mother is divorced, both parents work together well regarding Amy's needs. In addition, she has a very supportive extended family, and their support helps mitigate the deleterious effects of poverty. It is likely that these differences, and others that will be detailed, may lead to significant differences in their treatment needs.

Data Necessary for Effective Treatment Planning

In gathering data about a child, the clinician needs to know both what is going on within the child and how the child is affected by external forces. One convenient format for cataloging needed data includes learning about individual functioning; family relationships; peer relationships; school and extracurricular activities; socioeconomic, cultural, and religious influences; and the child's physical status.

INDIVIDUAL FUNCTIONING

One might assess the functioning of the individual child as if that functioning were not influenced by the surrounding social system, at the same time being aware that the severe limitation of such a myopic view must be corrected by gathering data at other levels. In evaluating the child, a large number of variables must be assessed with respect to phase specificity and age-related balancing of forces. For example, self-esteem would be more dependent on parental praise for the young child, but should be more internalized for a child of the school years.

There are many schemes for organizing information about the psychodynamic functioning of a child. One time-proven scheme is a traditional psychoanalytic one using five conceptual frames:

1) the dynamic, the question of psychic forces being in conflict
2) the topographic, the degree to which the problem is unconscious or available to consciousness
3) structural, the balancing of forces between the id, ego, and superego
4) economic, how psychic energy is being used, i.e., toward healthy adaptation or to maintain pathologic defenses at the cost of a loss of normal adaptation
5) genetic, a chronologic assessment of the development of the disorder[47]

In addition to this psychodynamic evaluation, an assessment of mental status is needed that attends to the child's cognitive level, ability to maintain attention, verbal skills, thought processes, ability to relate, affect, mood, orientation, presence of observing ego, capacity for empathy, and the extent to which symptoms are dystonic.[48,49]

A thorough history of development is important to determine if problems represent a chronic process or a more reactive one, as well as whether symptoms represent a fixation at a given stage of development or a regression from a previously achieved stage. It is necessary to understand the neonatal experience, the child's temperament as an infant, the nature of the nurturing experience during infancy, and the child's fit with mother. One would want to know the child's pattern of establishing rhythmicity. Developmental milestones are an indication of neurological maturation. One wishes to note sudden shifts and patterns in expression of aggression or sexual drives. Nonspecific ego strengths (e.g., impulse control, frustration tolerance, and the ability to bind anxiety) need to be assessed. Functioning within the conflict-free sphere of the ego (interest and hobbies, extracurricular activities), and the extent to which the child receives gratification in these activities are noted. In evaluating young children, it is particularly useful to consider specific lines of development, e.g., attachment to and separation from parents.[50,21] How has the attachment experience proceeded? How is separation tolerated, e.g., beginning school? Other such specific lines are development of self-skills, development of increasingly accurate reality testing, and development of more mature relationships to peers and authority figures.

With regard to symptoms of psychological distress, the clinician needs to clarify the number, duration, intensity, and form of the symptoms (how bizarre). The clinician also needs to note whether the child perceives the symptoms and is pained by them, and the degree to which family members and other important persons are troubled by the symptoms. If the child and important others are troubled, it is more likely that they will form a partnership with the treating professional to bring about change.

FAMILY RELATIONSHIPS

It is very important to generate data about the family. The family needs to be understood as an interactional system. Change in one part of the system may be compensated by change in another. This fact is important because bringing about temporary change in the child may result only in the development of difficulties in another family member. These homeostatic forces, which are more prevalent in troubled families, tend to maintain a certain degree of difficulty within the system, and this problem dictates that the family must be well understood in a holistic manner. Evaluation of a family system attends a wide number of interactional variables. Just a few examples of such variables are the handling of power, the ability to communicate clearly, the ability to be empathic, intergenerational boundary setting, and prevailing family mood. A detailed description of such variables is presented by Lewis, et al.[41]

Maximum information about a family is obtained by evaluating that system at different levels. Therefore, in addition to understanding what the family is like as a functional, interactional system, the clinician needs to know what family members are like as individuals.

Thus, beyond the evaluation of processes within the whole family system and evaluation of individual family members, it is important to note specific issues of the child's place and function within the family. For example, how autonomous is the child with respect to phase of development? That is, what are the family's expectations about growing up and what support (or infantilization) is offered to the individual child? If the child demonstrates troublesome behavior, how characteristic is this behavior in the family? Is it acting out the family's covert wishes? Is it defensive, such as a child taking part in becoming a scapegoat to preserve the parents' troubled marriage? Who is the family member(s) with whom the child identifies? Because identification is usually never complete, does the identification that is established have healthy or pathologic attributes? Are the child's basic needs for a sense of safety and nurturing being met or neglected? Is the child in danger?

PEER RELATIONSHIPS

Data need to be gathered about the child's relationship with peers. Does the child have a friend? Is there affiliation with a group? If so, is the position within the group one that brings gratification, or does the child fill the position of a scapegoat? Can the child play fair with friends? Can the child channel aggression with friends?

SCHOOL AND ACTIVITIES

In evaluating the child's adaptation to school, the clinician assesses both academic performance and social adaptation. Assessment of the level of academic functioning may involve intellectual assessment, done clinically or by psychometric testing. Poor performance in school may be explained by a variety of factors other than low intellect, such as a specific developmental delay (learning disability), motivational problems related to internal conflicts (e.g., stubbornness and refusal to produce), motivational problems related to internal conflicts that leave inadequate energy for academic pursuits, and low sociocultural expectations about academic achievement. In assessing the child's social adaptation to school, the clinician notes the child's reaction to imposed expectations regarding use of time, producing work, and following rules.

SOCIOECONOMIC, CULTURAL, AND RELIGIOUS DATA

The socioeconomic class of the family can be defined by assessing the parents' level of education, occupation, and income. The clinician needs to know if the family embraces the modal values of the socioeconomic class in which it exists. What are the family's expectations about relating to authority, handling aggression, tolerance for sexual expression, attitudes about money, and attitudes about educational or vocational achievement? Will the family tolerate a deviant value orientation of a youngster? What is the family's religious affiliation? Do all family members embrace the same? Is the religious affiliation used as a social support system, or to instill values, or both? Is religion used in a helpful or destructive way? For example, are religious teachings used to augment the child's sense of worth, or are there conflicts about religion in the child relevant to his or her current problems?

PHYSICAL STATUS

In assessing the child's physical status, data are needed about any genetic loading the child may have for mental illness or intellectual retardation. Data are needed about possible noxious influences during the mother's pregnancy and about the birth experience and postpartum period. A careful history must note growth and changes in physical competence; this is particularly important for severely disturbed children or in the evaluation of very young children. In these cases, a history should contain a careful evaluation of the infant's neurophysiologic organization and its effect on mother-infant reciprocity. With regard to early history, certain physical disorders are especially important (e.g., projectile vomiting, diarrhea, failure to thrive, colic, asthma, orthopedic problems, and disfiguring skin disorders).

A current medical history is important to note if there are any physical handicaps or illnesses that may have particular effect on the developmental process, e.g., an orthopedic problem affecting locomotion, a sensory deficit (blindness or deafness), a specific developmental delay (dyslexia, or an articulation problem). If the child has any physical illness, it is important to note if it is exacerbated by emotional stress and also to note the family's response to a child's illness.[51] If the child is on any medications for a physical disorder, their individual side effects, interactions, as well as meaning to the child and family need to be assessed.

Procedures for Gathering Data

Procedures employed in gathering information vary considerably according to the child's age and the nature of problems. There is no "right" way to conduct a child evaluation, no simple cookbook with a guaranteed recipe. There are, however, commonly used core procedures that provide the clinician with much information. Even these commonly used procedures may be carried out with considerable variation in technique. For example, the individual interview is usually considered one of the central processes of a child evaluation. Yet this interview may be directive or nondirective in nature. It may involve a predominant emphasis on play or an emphasis on vis-à-vis discussion. It simply may involve observation, as with an infant.

This section on gathering information could be organized in two ways: either to list commonly used procedures and those data that are most often elicited by such procedures, or to focus on what data are needed and what procedures are most effective in gathering those data. The former method lends itself more easily to a dogmatic prescription for a child evaluation. The latter organization is thus used.

As noted previously, one organizational scheme used to assess the types of data needed includes:

1) the functioning of the individual child
2) family relationships
3) peer relationships
4) school and extracurricular activities
5) socioeconomic-cultural-religious data
6) physical status

In the course of obtaining these data, a considerable number of procedures may be used. The following are particularly helpful: individual sessions, both playroom and interview; interviews with parents, individually and jointly; family interviews; reports from pediatricians; reports from school; formal psychological testing; educational testing; and the assessment of drawings.

INDIVIDUAL FUNCTIONING

Sources of information about the functioning of the individual child are varied. Some information comes from the child; some from the parent; some from reports from pediatricians or other treating professionals; and some from teachers or coaches.

As in other medical subspecialties, one knows most of what is pertinent to the assessment after taking a careful history. Historical data concern genetic vulnerability, problems of pregnancy or at delivery, neonatal status, temperament, mother-infant reciprocity, rhythmicity, developmental milestones and other indicators of the regularity of developmental progression, responses to stress, family relationships, peer relationships, and school functioning. Some fairly good indicators of strengths (intellect, impulse control, frustration tolerance, and secondary thinking) are available in a carefully taken history. Other issues assessed in the history are moral functioning, likability, object relations, mood, and day-to-day style of life. Special symptoms are often first noted during early history taking, e.g., enuresis, encopresis, cruelty to animals, preoccupation with fires or fire-setting, difficulty with speech, bizarre feeding habits, tics, compulsions, phobias, bizarre thinking patterns, and many others. As noted, some of the history may be obtained from the child, but invariably this history must be augmented by interviews with the child's caretakers and others.

The clinician knows a tremendous amount after taking a good history and is usually able to begin to formulate a dynamic picture of the child's difficulties. Information is available about the child's intelligence and also regarding whether any symptoms are accepted or alien to the child. The clinician should also have a preliminary idea of whether the defensive structure involves withdrawing patterns of behavior or patterns of behavior that involve high levels of objectionable activity. After taking the history, the clinician would have a high degree of suspicion of organicity or psychotic functioning if present. Also, the clinician should have some idea of the child's general motivation for change, ability to explore problems with some insight, and ability to observe his or her own behavior and evaluate the meaning of it. The clinician would have an idea of whether the child might have significant conflicts over learning in school but be able to participate with gratification in clubs or organized sports.

The professional would spend time alone with the child for reasons other than obtaining a history, e.g., assess the child's orientation, memory, goal-directedness of thought, judgment, the ability to abstract, the level of intellect, store of general information, affect, and mood.[49] Goodman and Sours have written about how these basic mental status attributes can be gathered even with very young children.[48] With younger children, a higher preponderance of play would be used in the individual sessions in order to assess their attributes. In the individual sessions, the clinician might gather data on the child's self-concept and body image by asking the child to draw a picture of himself or herself. The Draw-A-Person test is a formal psychological drawing procedure that can be used further to assess self-concept.[52]

Participating in play with the child in order to gather information is one of the child psychiatrist's most coveted skills. Play is used to allow the child to express the most deeply felt impulses, defenses, conflicts, and concerns. Because a child often is not able to talk about these issues, the clinician allows the child to express himself or herself through the displacement and symbolism of play. For example, a child may not be able to discuss fears and distortions about sexuality, but can use parental surrogate dolls in suggestive symbolic themes of play. The clinician experienced with children understands norms of play themes for children of different ages. Paying respect to these norms, the clinician follows themes with a given child to gather evidence of unconscious processes much as one might follow associations of ideas with an adult. The first individual session is frequently frightening for the child, who may not well understand the nature or purpose of the assessment procedure. Therefore, several sessions are necessary before the child feels comfortable enough to behave naturally and discuss, or play out, important themes. Thus, the richest material usually emerges during the second or third interviews.

With certain selected children, the clinician may need to supplement information gathered in individual sessions with information gathered by formal psychological testing.[53] Such testing is required when the basic clinical assessment leaves significant questions unanswered. Testing can answer many questions regarding overall intelligence (Wechsler Intelligence Scale for Children, Revised), special developmental delays (Illinois Test of Psycholinguistic Ability), and neurologic impairment (Bender-Gestalt). Projective techniques often uncover underlying concerns and defenses (Children's Apperception Test, Rorschach). Projective tests attend as well to ego weaknesses, regressive trends in thinking, capacity for human relatedness, extent the symptoms are uncomfortable, motivation, capacity for making an alliance, general character style, and many other variables.

As noted, a wealth of information about the child's individual functioning may come from parents, teachers, pediatricians, or other knowledgeable persons. The procedures for obtaining information from these persons will be noted later.

FAMILY RELATIONSHIPS

Information about the family may be obtained during history taking and by interviewing parents or other family members individually, but the knowledge gained by these procedures is enhanced greatly by meeting with the entire family in a semistructured or nonstructured format. Such family sessions often demonstrate how power is managed and in whom it resides, the presence of coalitions, and intergenerational boundaries. Family mood, capacity for empathy, ability to nurture, styles of imparting discipline, and many other variables may be assessed in this manner. These variables are usually not well assessed by asking the family about them; family members usually tell the truth as they know it, but often have major blind spots. The clinician gains the most information by observing not what they say but how they relate. Understanding may be enhanced by observing the family function fairly typically as they perform a task, e.g., planning something together. Formal scoring techniques have been developed for assessing families in this manner.[41] Some clinicians gather additional information by visiting the patient's home, where they develop a feeling for the family in the natural environment.[54]

PEER RELATIONSHIPS

Because peer relationships tell so much about the child's intrapsychic functioning, this issue must be assessed carefully. The clinician has four sources of information about peer relationships:

1) reports from the child and themes of play related to peer relationships
2) reports from the family
3) reports from teachers
4) psychological testing

In the individual sessions, the clinician notes whether the child mentions a friend, has the ability to describe this peer, and is able to look at conflicts with peers with any understanding. The clinician notes whether the reports from parents, teachers, or testing psychologist are concordant or discordant with the child's perceptions.

SCHOOL AND ACTIVITIES

The child's adaptation to school and extracurricular activities is assessed with regard to both performance and social adjustment. Because a child's school performance is so important to self-esteem, this issue must be evaluated with care. The clinician utilizes reports from the child, the family, and the teachers to answer several questions. Is a child's academic success commensurate with his or her clinically assessed intellectual functioning? Is success diminished by the presence of a specific learning disability found clinically? Is there a motivational problem? In certain circumstances, the clinician may augment the knowledge obtained from interviews and reports by requesting psychological testing to determine the level of intelligence and determine possible unconscious conflicts about learning. In addition, specific educational tests can be employed that differ from the more standard psychological tests in that they focus specifically on the developmental level of learning skills and the child's level of achievement. This testing answers important questions. Is the child on grade level? Is the child learning but unable or unwilling to demonstrate it in school? Is there a specific learning disability?

The child's social adjustment can be assessed by inquiring about this issue with the principal or teachers. Teachers frequently send reports that focus more on achievement than on social adjustment, or the reverse. The clinician may desire to follow up the report with a telephone call to make sure that both issues are well assessed. Teachers can note such things as a child's level of anxiety, self-deprecatory trends, ability to maintain attention, activity level, or any unusual behavior. In some instances in which the child's school adjustment is a pertinent issue, the clinician may learn a great deal through a school visit. Information about the child's involvement in formal extracurricular activities helps with the understanding of the child's conflict-free sphere, sense of belonging and identity, as well as the ability to develop and enjoy skills.

SOCIOECONOMIC, CULTURAL, AND RELIGIOUS DATA

The professional would assess the socioeconomic, cultural, and religious forces directed at the child by first obtaining demographic historical information. He or she would then evaluate how the child is affected by these broad forces in order to answer the important questions outlined in the preceding section. If the clinician believes that there is important material about the value orientation of the family that cannot be tapped by the usual manner of inquiry, there are formal assessment instruments that may be used.[55] Occasionally, the family may suggest securing information from a priest, pastor, or rabbi.

PHYSICAL STATUS

Obtaining the child's history is the first step in learning about the physical status. Reports from teachers or coaches frequently offer important information about the child's coordination and athletic skill. This information can be augmented by the clinician's observations in individual sessions in which the child is asked to perform a task requiring physical dexterity. Certainly reports about the child's health status from the pediatrician or other physicians who have treated the child are needed. A current physical examination may be completed by the psychiatrist or by a pediatrician. In some situations, special examinations may be required by physicians in other specialties or by other health professionals, e.g., a neurologist, an ophthalmologist, an otolaryngologist, a speech pathologist, a physical therapist, an orthopedic surgeon, or others, depending upon the type of problem that needs further special assessment. The physician may obtain routine laboratory tests of blood and urine as well as standard radiologic tests. Special tests (e.g., chromosomal studies) if an abnormality is suspected, or an amino acid screen to rule out amino acid disorders, and so on, may be needed. Full body radiographs may be used to look for old healed fractures if abuse is suspected. An EEG may be obtained to rule out a seizure disorder. Of course, which tests are ordered depends upon the clinician's clinical judgment and the nature of the disorder.

Conclusions and Overview Regarding Treatment Planning

Once the clinician has used the appropriate procedures to collect data in all clinically pertinent areas, the task is to design an effective treatment plan. The first chapter of this volume addresses the importance of careful treatment planning as well as the theoretical underpinnings of this process. Treatment planning is a task of such complexity that its precise definition is difficult. A comprehensive report by the Committee on Child Psychiatry of the Group for the Advancement of Psychiatry (GAP) devoted to the topic of treatment planning for children says: "Differential treatment planning consists of selecting, in order of priority, curative, corrective, ameliorative or palliative approaches to the child patient, his family, and, when needed, his extended environment. Such planning takes the fullest advantage of the available assets in the child, his family and his community."[56]

The authors agree strongly with the essence of the foregoing definition, which is one of the few offered for this complex clinical activity. The authors suggest that there are two basic steps within the task of planning a treatment program. The first step is to formulate the problems and state them in a common sense manner so that they can be understood by the child and those referring the child for treatment. Formulation of the problems should be done so that points of intervention, and a reasonable order of progression of treatment, are clear. The second step is to choose from among the broad spectrum of available treatment modalities those that offer the most effective, rapid assistance in the least restrictive and most cost effective manner.

Having reviewed the good working definition offered by GAP, and having offered the authors' assessment of two basic steps involved, it would be convenient if it were possible to offer a process for this task that would be agreed upon by all child mental health professionals. Several reviews of this process are available in the literature.[34, 56-59] While these approaches are similar in scope, none of them approaches the topic in exactly the same way. These differences again suggest that the process of treatment planning is complex, that it must be based upon clinical experience, and that it can be well carried out in several different but compatible ways. This overview offers yet another format for carrying out the process following the two basic steps noted, i.e.,

1) formulating the problem
2) choosing the best method of treatment

FORMULATING THE PROBLEMS

By this stage in the evaluation process, data have been gathered in six basic areas: the child's individual functioning; the functioning of the family; the child's relationship to peers; the child's performance in school and in formal extracurricular activities; the child's socioeconomic, cultural, and religious experience; and the child's physical status. This format offers a convenient organization for defining problem areas.

Once the clinician has determined the existing problem in each of these six areas, it must be decided if all problems require intervention. Only rarely do all problems encountered warrant formal treatment. It should be noted, however, that there are children and families with such serious and deeply ingrained pathology that an attempt must be made, if there is to be any expectation of beneficial change, to design a high impact program with therapeutic interventions aimed at all major problems. Fortunately, with children it is usually possible to design treatment approaches for selected problems that the clinician determines would, if approached correctly, precipitate improvement in other areas.

Another issue that needs to be addressed, if more than one problem is present, is the order of approach. All problems do not necessarily need to be approached simultaneously. Several factors can be taken into account in determining the order of attack. First, any problem representing an emergency to the child's life or health (e.g., parental abuse), of course, requires immediate intervention. Other problems may not be life-threatening emergencies, yet are also urgent. For example, acute school phobia in a young child needs to be handled in an urgent manner, otherwise it could become a chronic problem and precipitate a multitude of additional problems that interfere with the child's further development. Secondly, the order of attack is often determined by the clinician's assessment of the point of maximum leverage. Even though Problem A may be more serious than Problem B, the clinician may determine that neither the family nor the child is ready to receive assistance with Problem A, but would form a partnership with the clinician to approach Problem B. The clinician would hope that once the child and family experienced some benefit with Problem B, they would be encouraged to seek help for Problem A. Therefore, two factors would affect the clinician's decision about the point of maximum leverage:

1) the alliance (i.e., what problem do the most people want to see solved?)

2) maximum benefit (i.e., what problem, if solved, would offer the most benefit for all to see, and so encourage further efforts?)

Other than ordering a plan of attack based upon an assessment of whether an emergent or urgent situation exists and deciding upon the point(s) of maximum therapeutic leverage, there is no "right way" to determine an order of attack. Any ordering that is dictated by such things as good clinical judgment based on experience, reasonable evaluation of cost effectiveness, reasonable evaluation of time commitments, and evaluation of the patient's and family motivation would be proper.

Let us evaluate the two hypothetical patients presented earlier. The clinician obtains the following information after seeing each child and their mother for one evaluative session:

BILLY

Billy is a six-year-old Caucasian child from a middle class family. He has two sisters, four and ten years of age. Billy was adopted when he was two months old. Although knowledge of his biologic parents is incomplete, it is known that his mother had espisodic alcoholism, and she was thought to have been drinking during her pregnancy. The labor and delivery were normal, and the neonatal status was robust. In spite of his normal early status and his rapid growth, he was twelve months old before he pulled himself into a standing position and eighteen months old before he walked without excessive clumsiness. He was almost two before his speech was clear or he used sentences containing anything other than a subject and a verb.

Billy's family appeared troubled. His mother and father had arranged their lives so that they saw little of each other. On those occasions when they did spend time together, they argued. They had separated for a period of one week this past year. They had very different styles of relating to their children. Billy's mother tended to be very giving and allowed the children to run over her. She then pleaded helplessness to her husband in facing the stress of the children. The father preferred not to be involved with the care of his children, but could not avoid those occasions when his wife called him in as disciplinarian. On those occasions he sometimes lost his temper and spanked his children cruelly.

Prior to entering school, Billy fought with his siblings a lot, and he was more difficult to discipline than his sisters. He also stole their belongings and hid them, and stole coins from his mother's purse. Yet it should be noted that Billy expressed considerable tenderness and caring for his sisters and mother, and he often expressed significant shame and guilt after hurting them or stealing from them.

Recurrent asthma developed when Billy was three; it was worse in the spring. The asthma responded erratically to bronchodilator medication. Recurrent trips to the emergency room were frightening to Billy and his parents.

More serious problems began to develop as soon as Billy entered school. Billy had not been involved in any formal preschool training so that the school entry was a new experience for him. The teachers commented almost from the time of his entry that he was extremely hard to manage. He got into fist fights with his classmates after either provoking them or setting himself up to be picked on by them. He was discriminating in his fighting because he was never involved in altercations with the two boys with whom he had had special friendships for several years. The teachers also noted that Billy seemed distant and sad; none of the activities that gave pleasure to the other children seemed to please him. They thought that perhaps his sadness was related to a learning problem. Toward the end of the first grade, it was very clear that Billy was not handling letters and words with the skill of his classmates. The teachers recommended testing to determine whether Billy had a specific type of learning problem. When tested, Billy volunteered to the educational diagnostician that he had few friends, and he wondered if his parents and siblings really loved him. Shortly thereafter Billy was caught shoplifting, and the parents then sought psychiatric evaluation and care in an attempt to avoid threatened legal retribution.

Amy

Amy is a black girl, aged ten, the only daughter of a woman who eked out a living as a domestic worker. Amy's parents divorced when she was less than two. However, the divorced parents had worked out an amicable agreement with regard to financial issues, visitation, and overall support of Amy.

The pregnancy with Amy was uncomplicated as was the labor and delivery. Her neonatal development was normal and her developmental milestones were all within the average ranges. Amy had no particular behavioral problems as a small child, although the mother did note that she seemed to have a very low level of energy, seemed to have little self-confidence in facing novel situations and new tasks, and she demanded an excessive amount of her mother's support in these new situations. Mother had no problem giving such support because she had no other dependents to whom she was responsible and she avoided social relationships with men. Amy did have problems playing with other children. She seemed not to know how to share and would withdraw to the pleasure of her own company. During these times of withdrawal, she appeared to be quite sad and her attention would seem to be focused on some distant thought. Amy actually had no close friends prior to her entry into school, but after beginning school she befriended one girl with whom she had a close and caring relationship. She continued to be unusually close to her mother. Her relationship with her father was congenial but distant. She had an unusually warm relationship with both of her maternal grandparents who lived close by.

In school, Amy consistently received poor marks for reading. An evaluation by the school educational diagnostician disclosed a specific problem with reading. The diagnostician believed the child's problem did not require any special attention other than the mother's reviewing reading with her each day after school. Another thing noted at school was that Amy tended to be shy and a loner. She did have one close girlfriend in the neighborhood with whom she had maintained a caring relationship for years. During the summer between the third and fourth grade Amy experienced two stressors. She noted an exacerbation of asthma, a problem she had experienced transiently on three or four occasions since the beginning of first grade. Secondly, she experienced a very rapid spurt in growth, development of secondary sexual characteristics, and the beginning of menstrual periods. She was extremely sensitive about her early pubertal development. Upon entry into the fourth grade the teachers commented that they were concerned about Amy because of her increased withdrawal, her lack of pleasure in any activities, and her "spacing out." Of most concern was her severe irritability. She was easily provoked. If she was made fun of by classmates because of her physical changes, Amy struck them, injuring several rather severely. Amy was also discovered in the school bathroom breaking some window panes. When asked why she had done that, she sobbed and then in a rage flew at the school principal with her fists. It was because of these problems and their repetitive nature that the school principal asked Amy's mother to have her evaluated by a psychiatrist. Amy's mother initially deferred that recommendation and preferred instead to try to get some advice and counseling from her pastor. It should be noted that Amy's mother and Amy were very actively involved in the activities of their church. Only after the pastor consulted the school principal did he advise Amy's mother that he agreed with the principal's recommendation for psychiatric help.

The clinician spent but one evaluative session with each child and mother, and yet was able to gather enough descriptive information about symptoms and their duration to arrive at the following working diagnoses:

Axis I	1. 321.23	Conduct Disorder, Socialized, Aggressive (Principal Diagnosis)
	2. 300.40	Dysthymic Disorder
Axis II	1. 315.00	Probable Developmental Reading Disorder
Axis III	1. 493.0 (ICD-9)	Childhood Bronchial Asthma
Axis IV	Degrees of Stress—Moderate—4	
Axis V	Level of Adaptation in Last Year—Poor—5	

Both Billy and Amy received the same diagnoses because their clinical symptomatology fits the criteria for those diagnoses. Yet it is likely that when the clinician gathers additional data it will become clear that the most effective treatment programs for Billy and Amy may be quite different.

The clinician must gather considerable additional data as outlined previously, according to the procedures that lend themselves to the gathering of such data. First, however, an important point must be made: a clinician evaluating a given child and family need not gather all of the data or use all of the evaluative procedures outlined. This would be neither practical nor in the interests of the patient and his or her family. Good judgment is necessary to determine specific areas concerning any child needing in-depth evaluation. For example, the clinician evaluating Billy would probably want to look more carefully for the presence of any constitutional and biologic aberrations. He or she would also want to look for evidence of problems in attachment and problems of the mother-child fit based upon the patient's adoption or a difficult temperament. Problems in these areas may have clinical relevance and lead to ideas for treatment of Billy. The clinician would certainly want to evaluate Billy in some depth with regard to the presence of a neurologic condition. With regard to Billy's family, further evaluation clearly is indicated to determine whether his mother and father are capable, or willing, to bring about any change in their relationship. The clinician would certainly want to know whether Billy's asthma was being treated as optimally as it might be. He or she would want to know more about Billy's peer relationships to determine what is wrong and what might be done to be helpful. Amy's preliminary history, on the other hand, does not suggest the need for an in-depth evaluation into constitutional or neurologic deficits nor an in-depth evaluation into the nature of Amy's early attachment to her mother. Certainly Amy's current relationship with her mother needs evaluation as does Amy's current conflicts about early pubertal development, relationships with peers, and ideas about sexuality.

Let us assume that the evaluating clinician has used the appropriate procedures to elicit the most relevant clinical data. The following is a schematic listing of problems in six defined areas. Obviously, some of these problems are readily observable as behavior. Some of them involve a degree of psychological abstraction and psychodynamic hypothesis-building based upon the additional information derived from proper assessment procedures.

PROBLEMS

	BILLY	AMY
Individual	1. Depressed 2. Breaks rules of society, hurts people 3. Conflict about passivity and dependency, based on helplessness during periods of asthma; made worse by mother's infantilization	1. Depressed 2. Breaks rules of society, hurts people 3. Conflict about bodily changes

	4. Identification with explosive father	4. Identification with mother who has conflicts about men and sex
	5. Hurts people everywhere (home and school), and aggression has become a way of life	5. Hurts people at school
Family	1. Emotionally divorced parents; may be an unalterable problem	1. Mother conflicted about men and sex and conveys covert messages to daughter not to grow up
	2. Excessive coalition between mother and son, excluding father	2. Absence of marital coalition or siblings to help Amy separate from mother
	3. Father is impulsive and frightening	
	4. Conflict with siblings	
Peers	1. Controlling and domineering, fights when he doesn't get his way	1. Keeps peers at a distance
School	1. Reading disability, severe	1. Reading disability, minor
	2. Problems with authority and all rules, long-term problem, provoked by minimal stress	2. Breaks rules episodically when severely stressed, recent onset
Sociocultural, Religious	1. Isolated family	

Physical	1. Asthma, recurrent, moderately severe; significant source of stress to Billy and his family	1. Asthma, not a serious problem
	2. Uncoordinated	2. Early puberty

STRENGTHS

The clinician has elicited data in order to outline areas of major difficulty. Nevertheless, it is hoped that he or she has also become aware of some areas of strength; assessments of strength are equally important for proper treatment planning. For Amy and Billy, such strengths might be listed as follows:

	BILLY	AMY
Individual	1. Intelligent	1. Intelligent
	2. Able to form an attachment	2. Able to form an attachment
	3. High level of energy	3. Wants help to understand and change her situation; she is pained by it
	4. Likability	
	5. Responds to firm limits clearly stated	
Family	1. Invested in seeing that Billy receives help	1. Invested in seeing that Amy receives help
Peers	1. Able to make and keep a friend	1. Able to make and keep a friend
School		1. Adequate academic performance
Sociocultural, Religious		1. Can seek support in church
Physical	1. Good physical health other than noted	1. Good physical health other than noted

The order of problem solving needs to be determined. There exists nothing emergent or life-threatening in either of these situations, but there certainly is some degree of urgency because both children are hurting others and are involved in certain illegal activities.

Billy has ingrained psychological problems. He has severe difficulty with peers. Although evaluation has revealed he is bright and can maintain attention for extended periods of time, he is having difficulty in school. He has physical problems needing attention. Of all these problems, the one requiring the most immediate attention is his violation of the rules of society and hurting others; he has already been in significant difficulty. Both he and his family are in agreement that his problem requires immediate attention. Although he has some significant personal strengths, he needs more external supports and control. He and his family are also in agreement that he needs more help than he is getting with his reading disability, because his inability to read is one of the things that is causing him to be so sad. He and his family are also in agreement that his asthma is a problem that causes significant stress to all. He has shown that he can make and keep a few friends, but he has problems with peers that need attention. He and his family believe that this is a problem with which they would like some help later. It is also clear that the family system is extremely troubled; however, the evaluation has demonstrated that the parents are not particularly concerned about the emotional divorce or the family's social isolation, nor do they want to do anything about it.

Amy has ingrained psychological problems. There are also certain difficulties between her and her mother. She is isolated from peers. She has problems in school. She has asthma. She has had an early pubescence that has caused her significant stress. Of these problem areas, Amy describes most clearly her concern about her early bodily changes and her concerns about sexuality. She is also able to talk about her conflicted and excessively close relationship with her mother. Some personal strengths are evident through her ability to talk about wanting to change these things. She does not seem particularly concerned about her distance from peers and has maintained one close friend. She is not concerned about her minor reading disability, which she corrects with extra homework. Her own assessment would suggest that priority be given to problem solving in the area of her conflict about bodily development and the relationship of that problem to her periodic depression and episodic anger, which precipitates antisocial activities. Her own assessment would suggest that priority also ought to be given to helping her resolve her excessively conflicted relationship with her mother. Mother seems willing to make necessary changes.

CHOOSING THE BEST METHOD OF TREATMENT

Having selected the pertinent data and formulated a list of clinically relevant problems and strengths, the clinician's next step is to choose, from among the multitude of treatment modalities available for children, those thought to be most effective for a given problem in a given child. It is beyond the scope of this chapter to delineate all modifications for children of the five basic therapeutic modalities described previously in this volume. All that is possible is a cursory listing of subtypes of treatment for children within each of these major modalities. We will also list a strategy of environmental modification. A child is profoundly influenced by the milieu, and the clinician must be aware of the power of changing environmental forces. The reader interested in further review is referred to articulate expositions of the indications and contraindications for each of these modalities of treatment.[42,57, 60-67]

Psychodynamic therapies

Psychodynamic therapies can be offered either to the child or to other members of the family. With regard to the child, these therapies can be defined along a number of different dimensions.[68] Those described by the editors in the initial chapter could be modified and related to child therapy as well as to therapy with adults. Such therapy can be described in terms of how directive or nondirective it is, and whether it is designed to shore up ego weaknesses through supportive techniques or, alternately, help the child to gain insight into unconscious processes and modify them. It can be described along the dimension of the relative use of play as compared to direct discussion, the former being more appropriate with younger children. Therapy can be described in terms of the amount of use of specialized techniques, e.g., a mutual story-telling technique, the squiggle technique, and similar methods.[67, 70, 63]

It is often optimal to provide individual psychotherapy for other members of the child's family, and such therapy would be defined along the dimensions described in Chapter II of this volume. An additional descriptive dimension that might be added is the relative amount of guidance offered to parents in managing their child as compared to the amount of self-understanding, or understanding the dynamics of the child, that is sought.

Group therapies

Again, group therapies can be described according to the dimensions outlined in the third chapter of this volume. For children, additional descriptors can be used to indicate the amount of focus on play or activities as compared to focus on discussion and understanding of problems.[64] The composition of the group can also vary in terms of being of the same sex or with both boys and girls. Composition can also vary with age and types of problems of the group members. One commonality of all types of group therapies is the potential to be helpful in terms of improving peer relationships.

Biological therapies

For children, two major thrusts of biologic therapies should be considered. The first is that of any medical care used to treat and improve existing physical problems, chronic illnesses, or congenital defects. The other type of biologic therapy, aimed more specifically at psychological problems, is that of psychotropic medication.[66, 71] Complete description of the use of psychotropic medication in children is a task beyond the scope of this chapter. It should be noted, however, that there are significant differences in the use of psychotropic drugs with children and adults.[72] For one thing, some medications are used in children for purposes for which they are not commonly used in adults. An example of this approach would be the use of methylphenidate or amphetamine stimulants for treatment of an attention deficit disorder. As another example, certain tricyclic antidepressants in small dosages may be helpful in the treatment of bedwetting. Antidepressants also may be used in the treatment of depression in children. Major tranquilizers may be used in the treatment of psychotic symptoms in children. The control of seizures by the use of anticonvulsives is important. The point here is that many different medications may be used; however, the tolerance of children to these medications varies with individual children. The reader is referred to Wiener and others for a more complete description of these therapies.[73, 66, 71]

Behavior therapies

In addition to those descriptions offered in the preceding chapter and others in the vast behavioral literature, it should be noted that one type of behavior therapy often used with children is parental counseling regarding the rewarding of good behavior or the deconditioning of bad behavior.[61, 62] Formal behavior modification programs may be used for objectional behaviors, e.g., enuresis. These programs are particularly useful with mentally retarded or autistic children.

Marital and family therapies

Three primary forms of these therapies would be relevant to the treatment of children and their families. The first is parent counseling with regard to techniques for managing the child's problems. The second is conjoint therapy for improving marital conflicts that may be affecting the child. The third is family therapy involving the parents and child, and perhaps other siblings, to bring about a change in relationships within the family system. Work with parents is crucial in designing appropriate treatment plans and has been well described in other works.[74, 75]

Environmental modification

As noted, it is important for the clinician dealing with children to recognize the powerful effect of changing the child's environment.[76] The following are some types of modification, listed in order of increasing degree of change:

1) Recommendations with regard to changing school programs, e.g., moving a child from a regular classroom to a special classroom
2) Changing schools
3) Involving the child with extended family or extrafamilial adults
4) Involving the child in clubs and groups

5) Involving the child of divorced parents with a Big Brother or Big Sister
6) Leaving the family and living with a relative
7) Leaving the family and going to boarding school
8) Placement in residential treatment
9) Placement in hospital

The clinician, after considering clinically relevant data, formulating a list of problems and strengths, and considering the available treatment modalities, must devise a treatment plan. As noted previously, there is no one correct treatment plan for a given child. There may be several effective treatment modalities for a given problem. Also there is no one correct answer as to what problems should be approached first, or if approached sequentially, in what order. That important statement having been made again, plausible treatment plans for each of our patients are offered:

TREATMENT PLANS

	BILLY	AMY
Individual	1. Individual psychotherapy of an emotive, supportive educative type	1. Individual psychotherapy of a dynamic, insight-oriented type
Family	1. Parental counseling of a supportive, educative, and guiding nature	1. Family psychotherapy of a dynamic, insight-oriented type for Amy and her mother
Peers		1. Church community service group
School	1. Liaison between treating physician and school personnel 2. Special tutor for reading	1. Encourage special relationship with a female teacher

Sociocultural, Religious	1. Encourage family's increased involvement in some kind of community activity	1. Treating clinician would establish liaison with pastor to help Amy be better able to make friends
Physical	1. Re-evaluation of status of asthma by a pediatrician	1. Re-evaluation of asthma and discussion of the physical changes of puberty by a consultant pediatrician
	2. Involvement of Billy in physical activities	

The reader will note that a treatment plan has been devised for Billy that approaches problems in five areas. Clearly, Billy has some significant problems of his own. Individual psychotherapy would probably be helpful if it allowed him to emote feelings, provided support, and served an educative function. Because of Billy's tendency to prefer action to verbalization, it would be expected that a large part of the therapy process would be carried out in the modality of play. The therapy would be aimed at two primary goals: 1) helping Billy to verbalize feelings instead of acting on them, and 2) clarifying options for more adaptive behavior in his environment. The individual therapy would need to be augmented with help to the parents. They would meet with the treating clinician and through support, education, and guidance would be helped to manage Billy's behavior more effectively at home. They could be taught some basic techniques of behavioral modification, such as giving a tangible reward for a day of nonaggressive behavior. Much of this better management would come about as a result of helping the parents to establish a coalition for offering support and discipline. In particular, the clinician might help the father use less aggressive forms of discipline and encourage the mother to be more firm in limit setting. The parents would also be helped to establish a better relationship with school personnel and so create a working partnership for more effective management of Billy's behavior in school. There are significant problems in the family that are not being attended to by this approach, primarily because of the clinician's assessment of lack of motivation. With regard to Billy's relationship with peers, nothing formal is planned at the beginning, although it might be helpful for him to be involved in Cub Scouts or some other type of activity after he has achieved some improvement in his school behavior. Billy's involvement in a formal psychotherapy group certainly might be considered after he has achieved better control of his aggression. The clinician would also establish a working relationship with the school personnel so that he or she might be advised of Billy's status and be able to offer encouragement or advice to the staff with regard to their management of him. Some simple behavioral modification techniques might be applied in the classroom. Billy would need to work with a tutor to improve his reading skills. The family is encouraged to develop support systems in the community. With regard to Billy's physical needs, his asthma needs to be reassessed in order to establish better control. His poor coordination can be improved through his involvement in physical activities (e.g., tumbling or other nonaggressive athletic endeavors). When he has gained better control of his aggression, involvement in competitive team sports might be helpful. Consideration should also be given to the use of psychotropic medication. At some point Billy might benefit from the use of a medication from one of three classes: stimulants, tranquilizers, or antidepressants. The clinician designing the above treatment plan would, however, probably defer the decision to use a drug until the effect of the other interventions could be evaluated. Another clinician might well design a treatment plan with a primary emphasis on a psychopharmacologic approach.

Billy has had his problems for a long time, and his parents have had a very inconsistent style of managing him for an equally long time. The clinician, therefore, might have some concern that Billy's behavior may be beyond the control of the family even if they receive skillful support. It may well be that Billy ultimately needs greater environmental controls that may involve placement of him outside of the home in, e.g., a residential treatment setting. Yet neither Billy nor his family would like to try that option in the beginning, and they certainly deserve a trial of outpatient treatment as has been outlined.

Treatment intervention might be offered for Amy in all six areas.

The primary treatment would be individual therapy along with therapy with Amy and her mother. A dynamic, insight-oriented, individual psychotherapeutic approach primarily involving discussions, with limited use of play for relationship building, fun, and necessary periodic retreats from anxiety-laden discussions, would be indicated. This psychotherapy would be aimed at two primary goals: 1) developing awareness and mastery of feelings about growing up to be a woman, and 2) increasing awareness and mastery of growing up and giving up mother. A psychodynamic, insight-oriented approach to family therapy involving discussions of sexual identity, growing up, and separation would be helpful. These touchy subjects are ones that Amy and her mother have not been able to approach previously. Amy's involvement with peers might be improved by encouraging her to socialize in an environment that is comfortable for her. Therefore, involving her in some type of task-oriented children's activities at church would be attempted. Later, Amy might be encouraged to increase her involvement in age-related extracurricular activities. Group therapy might also be considered at a later time once Amy has gained increased confidence with other children. The clinician might also establish an alliance with Amy's school and with her pastor, who could help with integrating the child with her peers. The clinician might want to collaborate in designing a behavioral approach to increasing Amy's socialization. Arrangements might be made for Amy to discuss issues of concern with a favored woman teacher or with her pastor. A clinician might consider pharmacologic treatment for Amy, with particular consideration to improving her depressed mood; however, a major mood disturbance is not central in her clinical picture. Amy would benefit from discussing the physical changes of puberty with a pediatrician, who could also assess if her asthma is under the best control.

It is hoped that the preceding examples will bring a real clinical feeling to the process of gathering pertinent data and synthesizing those data into a list of problems and strengths on the basis of which a rational treatment plan can be devised.

It should be apparent from the foregoing illustrations that children present certain problems for treatment planning. They are highly affected by the milieu in which they live, thus very careful attention must be given to forces within the family, the peer group, and the school, as well as other aspects of the environment.

Another point to be repeated is that a child's diagnosis offers very little in terms of what treatment should be offered. We can devise more and more sophisticated diagnostic systems and still find that increased diagnostic elegance does not dictate optimal treatment approaches. The changing developmental needs of children means that two children of different ages, but with the same diagnosis, usually require vastly different treatment approaches. The fact that children are so strongly molded by environmental forces, and that the forces affecting two different children may be so divergent, again, indicates that similar diagnoses do not necessarily call for similar treatment plans.

It must be re-emphasized that two skillful clinicians might generate the same data and synthesize the same or a similar list of problems, yet devise different treatment plans for a given child. At this point in our quest for increasingly effective treatment for children, there is no single correct approach.

We have a responsibility to be advocates for the needs of children who do not have the ability to judge how appropriate a treatment plan might be. A child is not as likely as an adult to complain about a poor treatment plan. Even if the child did have the capacity to judge the treatment plan, he or she would not have the social power to change it. This places an especially great burden on the clinician to listen well, evaluate skillfully, and choose a treatment approach based on the individual child's and the family's needs—not upon an ideologic commitment to a favored form of treatment or treatment designed as a result of external pressures from parents, school, other social agencies, the institution with which the professional is affiliated, or those who pay for treatment.

REFERENCES

1. Sameroff, A.: Early Influences on Development, *Merrill-Palmer Quarterly of Behavior and Development*, 21(4):267-294, 1975.
2. Spitz, R.: Hospitalism: An Inquiry into the Genesis of Psychiatric Conditions in Early Childhood, *Psychoanalytic Study of the Child*, I:53-74, 1945.
3. Gesell, A., and Amatruda, C. S.: *Developmental Diagnosis* (2nd ed.), New York: Paul B. Hoeber Medical Division, Harper & Row, Pub., 1947.

4. Gesell, A., and Ilg, E.: *Child Development*, New York: Harper & Row, Pub., 1949.
5. Lewis, M.: *Clinical Aspects of Child Development*, Philadelphia: Lea & Febiger, 1971.
6. Mussen, P. H., Konger, J. J., and Kagan, J. (eds.): *Child Development and Personality*, New York, Evanston & London: Harper & Row, Pub., 1980.
7. Stoller, R. J.: The 'Bedrock' of Masculinity and Femininity: Bisexuality, *Archives of General Psychiatry*, 26:207-212, 1972.
8. Korner, A.: Sex Differences in Newborns with Special Reference to Differences in the Organization of Oral Behavior, *Journal of Child Psychology and Psychiatry*, 15:19-29, 1973.
9. Korner, A.: The Effect of the Infant's Stage, Level of Arousal, Sex, and Ontogenetic State of the Caregiver, in M. Lewis, and L. A. Rosenblum (eds.): *The Effect of the Infant on its Caregiver*, New York: John Wiley & Sons, 1974.
10. Lewis, M.: State as an Infant-Environment Interaction: An Analysis of Mother-Infant Interaction as a Function of Sex, *Merrill-Palmer Quarterly of Behavior and Development*, 18(2):95-121, 1972.
11. Kety, S. S., Rosenthal, D., Wender, P. H., Schulsinger, F., and Jacobson, B.: Mental Illness in the Biologic and Adoptive Families of Adopted Individuals who have become Schizophrenic: A Preliminary Report Based on Psychiatric Interviews, In R. R. Fieve, D. Rosenthal, and H. Brill (eds.): *Genetic Research in Psychiatry*, Baltimore: Johns Hopkins University Press, 1975.
12. Winokur, G., Clayton, P. J., and Reich, T.: *Manic Depressive Illness*, St. Louis: C. V. Mosby, 1969.
13. Bernard J., and Sontag, L. W.: Fetal Reactivity and Sound, *Journal of Genetic Psychology*, 70:205-210, 1947.
14. Stott, D. H., and Latchford, S. A.: Prenatal Antecedents of Child Health, Development and Behavior, *Journal of the American Academy of Child Psychiatry*, 1:161-191, 1976.
15. Pasamanick, B., and Knobloch, H.: Retrospective Studies on the Epidemiology of Reproductive Causality: Old and New, *Merrill-Palmer Quarterly on Behavioral Development*, 12:7, 1966.
16. Drillien, C. M.: Physical and Mental Handicaps in the Prematurely Born, *Journal of Obstetrics and Gynaecology in the British Empire*, 66:272-278, 1959.
17. Metcalf, D. R.: Organizers of the Psyche & EEG Development: Birth through Adolescence, in J. D. Noshpitz (ed.): *Basic Handbook of Child Psychiatry*, Vol. I, "*Development*," New York: Basic Books, Inc., 1979, pp. 63-71.
18. Roffwarg, H. P., Muzio, J., and Dement, W.: Ontogenetic Development of the Human Sleep-Dream Cycle, *Science*, 152:604-619, 1966.
19. Erikson, E.: *Childhood and Society*, New York: Norton, 1969.
20. Freud, S.: *Three Essays on Sexuality* (1905), Standard Edition 7, London: The Hogarth Press, 1953, p. 168.
21. Freud, A.: *Normality & Pathology in Childhood: Assessments of Development*, New York: International Universities Press, 1965.
22. Bowlby, J.: *Attachment and Loss: Attachment*, Vol. I, New York: Basic Books, Inc., 1969.

23. Bowlby, J.: *Attachment and Loss: Separation*, Vol. II, New York: Basic Books, Inc., 1973.
24. Ainsworth, M. D. S.: The Development of Infant-Mother Attachment, in B. Caldwell and H. Riccinti (eds.): *Review of Child Development Research* (Vol. 3), Chicago: University of Chicago Press, 1973.
25. Ainsworth, M., Bell, S., and Staytor, D.: Individual Differences in the Development of Some Attachment Behaviors, *Merrill-Palmer Quarterly of Behavior and Development*, 18:123-143, 1972.
26. Mahler, M., Pine, F., and Bergman, A.: *The Psychological Birth of the Human Infant*, New York: Basic Books, Inc., 1975.
27. Kohut, H.: *Analysis of the Self*, New York: International Universities Press, 1971.
28. Piaget, J.: *The Origins of Intelligence in Children*, New York: International Universities Press, 1952.
29. Lewis, M., and Rosenblum, L. (eds.): *The Effect of the Infant on Its Caregiver*, New York: John Wiley & Sons, 1974.
30. Thomas, A., and Chess, S.: *Temperament & Development*, New York: Brunner/Mazel, 1977.
31. Spitz, R.: *The First Year of Life*, New York: International Universities Press, 1965.
32. Stone, J. L., Smith, H., and Murphy, L. (eds.): *The Competent Infant*, New York: Basic Books Inc., 1973.
33. Duska, R., and Whelan, M.: *Moral Development: A Guide to Piaget and Kohlberg*, New York: Paulist Press, 1975.
34. Rutter, M.: *Helping Troubled Children*, New York: Plenum Press, 1975.
35. Sarnoff, C.: *Latency*, New York: Jason Aronson, Inc., 1976.
36. Noshpitz, J. (ed.): *Basic Handbook of Child Psychiatry*, Vol. I, "*Development*," New York: Basic Books Inc., 1979.
37. Bemporad, J. (ed.): *Child Development in Normality & Psychopathology*, New York: Brunner/Mazel, 1980.
38. Belsky, J.: Early Human Experience: A Family Perspective, *Developmental Psychology*, 17(1):3-23, 1981.
39. Anthony, E. J., and Benedek, T. (eds.): *Parenthood: Its Psychology and Psychopathology*, Boston: Little, Brown and Company, 1970.
40. Baumrind, D.: The Contribution of the Family to the Development of Competence in Children, *Schizophrenia Bulletin*, 14:12-37, 1975.
41. Lewis, J., et al.: *No Single Thread: Psychological Health in Family Systems*, New York: Brunner/Mazel, 1976.
42. French, A.: *Disturbed Children and Their Families*, New York: Human Science Press, 1977.
43. Harrison, S., McDermott, J., Wilson, P., and Schrager, J.: Social Class and Mental Illness in Children: Choice of Treatment, *Archives of General Psychiatry*, 13:411-417, 1965.
44. Clausen, J.: Sociology and Psychiatry: in A. M. Freedman, H. Kaplan, and B. Sadock (eds.): *Comprehensive Textbook of Psychiatry*, Baltimore: Williams and Wilkins, 1975, pp. 373-382.

45. Kohn, M.: *Class and Conformity: A Study in Values*, Homewood, Ill.: The Dorsey Press, 1969.
46. Looney, J., Blotcky, M., and Oldham, D.: Assessing Psychological Symptoms in Adolescents, *Southern Medical Journal*, 71(1):1197-1202, 1978.
47. Nagera, H.: The Developmental Profile: Notes on Some Practical Considerations Regarding its Use, *Psychoanalytic Study of the Child*, 18:511-540, 1963.
48. Goodman, J., and Sours, J.: *The Child Mental Status Examination*, New York: Basic Books, Inc., 1967.
49. Simmons. J.: *Psychiatric Examination of Children*, Philadelphia: Lea and Febiger, 1969.
50. Flapan, D., and Neubauer, P.: *Assessment of Early Child Development*, New York: Jason Aronson, 1975.
51. Anthony, J.: The Impact of Mental and Physical Illness on Family Life, *American Journal of Psychiatry*, 127:136-138, 1970.
52. Koppitz, E.: *Psychological Evaluation of Children's Human Figure Drawings*, New York: Grune and Stratton, 1968.
53. Gittelman, R.: The Role of Psychological Tests for Differential Diagnosis in Child Psychiatry, *Journal of the American Academy of Child Psychiatry*, 19:413-438, 1980.
54. Freeman, D.: The Home Visit in Child Psychiatry, *Journal of the American Academy of Child Psychiatry*, 6:276-293, 1967.
55. Rokeach, M.: *The Nature of Human Values*, New York: The Free Press, 1973.
56. Group for the Advancement of Psychiatry: *From Diagnosis to Treatment: An Approach to Treatment Planning for the Emotionally Disturbed Child*, Vol. VIII, Report No. 87, September, 1973.
57. Adams, P.: *A Primer of Child Psychotherapy*, Boston: Little, Brown and Company, 1974.
58. Harrison, S.: Child Psychiatric Treatment: Status and Prospects, in J. Noshpitz (ed.): *Basic Handbook of Child Psychiatry*, Vol. III, "*Therapeutic Interventions*," New York: Basic Books, Inc., 1979, pp. 3-20.
59. Cohen, R.: The Approach to Assessment, in J. Noshpitz (ed.): *Basic Handbook of Child Psychiatry*, Vol. I, New York: Basic Books, Inc., 1979, pp. 485-504.
60. Axline, V.: *Play Therapy*, New York: Ballantine Books, 1947.
61. Graziano, A. (ed.): *Behavior Therapy with Children*, Vol. I, Chicago: Aldine—Atherton, Inc., 1971.
62. Graziano, A. (ed.): *Behavior Therapy with Children*, Vol. II, Chicago: Aldine—Atherton, Inc., 1975.
63. Gardner, R.: *Psychotherapeutic Approaches to the Resistant Child*, New York: Jason Aronson, 1975.
64. Slavson, S., and Schiffer, M.: *Group Psychotherapies for Children*, New York: International Universities Press, 1975.
65. McDermott, J., and Harrison, S.: (eds.): *Psychiatric Treatment of the Child*, New York: Jason Aronson, Inc., 1977.
66. Noshpitz, J. (ed.): *Basic Handbook of Child Psychiatry*, Vol. III, "*Therapeutic Intervention*," New York: Basic Books, Inc., 1979.

67. Pearson, G. (ed.): *A Handbook of Child Psychoanalysis*, New York: Basic Books, Inc., 1968.
68. Haworth, M. (ed.): *Child Psychotherapy: Practice & Theory*, New York: Basic Books, Inc., 1964.
69. Gardner, R.: *Therapeutic Communication with Children: The Mutual Story-Telling Technique*, New York: Jason Aronson, Inc., 1971.
70. Winnicott, D.: *Therapeutic Consultations in Child Psychiatry*, New York: Basic Books, Inc., 1971.
71. Gittelman-Klein, R.: *Recent Advances in Child Psychopharmacology*, New York: Human Sciences Press, 1975.
72. Minde, K. K., and Weiss, G. C.: The Assessment of Drug Effects in Children as Compared to Adults, *Journal of Child Psychiatry*, 9:124-133, 1970.
73. Wiener, J. (ed.): *Psychopharmacology in Childhood and Adolescence*, New York: Basic Books, Inc., 1977.
74. Arnold, L. (ed.): *Helping Parents Help Their Children*, New York: Brunner/ Mazel, Inc., 1978.
75. Slavson, S.: *Child-Centered Group Guidance of Parents*, New York: International Universities Press, Inc., 1958.
76. Barker, P.: *The Residential Psychiatric Treatment of Children*, New York: John Wiley & Sons, 1974.

Chapter Seven

Special Perspectives on Treatment Planning for Adolescents

John E. Schowalter, M.D.
and
Susan M. Fisher, M.D.

Introduction

Many therapists do not want to treat adolescents. More than other developmental periods, adolescence is a time when vast changes occur not only physically, but socially and emotionally as well. Acts of rebellion, running away, attempted suicide, violence, dramatic sexual expression or repression, the development of life-threatening eating disorders, and great fluctuations in self-esteem are encountered in a more unremitting cadence by those who treat adolescents than by those who treat younger children or older adults. Furthermore, many adolescents do not want to be treated. These points, coupled with the fact that minors are legally under the authority of parents who may wish them to be treated against their will or who countermand the adolescent's desire to be treated, are among the most obvious difficulties facing the therapist involved in treatment planning.

It is helpful to begin with a definition of what will be discussed. The definition of treatment planning as outlined in 1973 by the Group for the Advancement of Psychiatry (GAP) will be used.[1] Treatment planning is defined as "the process which takes place between the diagnostic formulation and the ultimate treatment recommendations." In this chapter, for practical purposes, adolescence will represent the years between the onset of puberty and age eighteen. Operationally, this includes most patients in grades seven or eight through twelve. Although by many definitions adolescence extends for a somewhat longer time, the age of legal majority seems to be a reasonable demarcation point for purposes of treatment planning. It is also important to realize that in most states adolescents below the age of majority can attain majority rights by leaving their family home and care and being declared a "mature" or "emancipated" minor.

Because so many changes take place within a span of seven or eight years, some authors have suggested the designation of subperiods, e.g., early, middle, and late adolescence. Although these categories are helpful in certain types of research, we have decided not to be slavish to this custom. As will be clear, the lines of social, psychological, and physiologic development are so variable, even in normal adolescents, and the pendulum swings of progression and regression so common, that the clinician is best served by conceptualizing adolescence as a multilayered, frequently changing whole, rather than as distinct segments that are or are not attained.

The richness as well as some of the perplexities inherent in the overlap of, and the vacillations between, the physiologic, psychological, and social dimensions of adolescence will be evident in the next three sections of this chapter. It is good for the therapist to keep in mind that adolescence is a time of great variety and change, but that there are also definite developmental scaffoldings available that can help us to understand behavior that might otherwise seem excessively random or chaotic.

Also, it will become clear that this chapter focuses on those developmental aspects of adolescence that a therapist should be familiar with in order to formulate an appropriate treatment plan, but the chapter will not be prescriptive. In addition to developmental issues, a treatment plan is based on the diagnosis plus the objective effectiveness and the therapist's subjective view of the available treatments. A good treatment plan must be flexible and amenable to revision if warranted by new information. Rigidity in treatment planning (e.g., prescriptions) is especially inappropriate when working with adolescents. Preset constraints as to how an adolescent is regarded, the exact treatment to be used, and the length of time the treatment will take assume a greater specificity of approaches and a greater understanding of the human brain and mind than are justified.

Common Biologic Issues

We now know that children are not really latent during the so-called latency period. Especially in the cognitive and social areas, tremendous development and change take place. In biologic growth, however, the years between the beginning of primary school and puberty are characterized by a progression that is relatively orderly and unsurprising. Girls and boys are of similar height and weight, and there is relatively little difference in sex hormone production.

With the onset of puberty, all of this changes. First, however, we must ask what puberty is and what defines its relationship to adolescence. Puberty refers to that period of biologic change as an individual makes the transition from child to adult, the most obvious change being the development of the secondary sex characteristics. Adolescence refers to that period following the onset of puberty when certain psychosocial changes take place leading to one's acceptance by society as an adult. The beginning of puberty, therefore, often coincides with the beginning of adolescence; however, the physiologic changes of puberty are usually completed by the mid to late teens, whereas adolescence is usually thought to meld rather imperceptibly into young adulthood a few years later. Exactness of definition or a specific timetable of events is seldom available for this age period.

Both the fact and the timing of the onset of puberty are important for the clinician to keep in mind. The sequence of change is quite uniform within each of the sexes, but the timing of the initiation of puberty varies greatly within and between sexes. On the average, girls begin puberty two years before boys. Within a sex, puberty is considered to be normal if it occurs within two years before or following the mean. Therefore, a late-developing boy may enter puberty six years after an early-developing girl, and both are still considered to be within the normal range.

The first easily noticeable pubertal change is a growth spurt. Usually, growth speeds up in girls when they are about age 9 1/2 and in boys at about age 11 1/2 years. Because of this age differential, most girls of eleven and twelve years are taller than age-mate boys.[2] Both boys and girls can be anxious about what they perceive as a size misalignment, but between the ages of thirteen and fourteen boys catch up, subsequently becoming taller and heavier than girls. Development of abilities in cognition and logic do not necessarily occur earlier in adolescents with early growth spurts, thus it is important for the therapist not to mistake size alone as an indication of mature understanding.[3]

Breast development begins in most girls during the latter part of their tenth or beginning of their eleventh year and, at about the same time, pubic hair also begins to appear.[2] The formation of breasts is the first anatomic change noticeable, even when dressed, that differentiates girls from boys. Human beings are the only primates whose breasts develop before the first pregnancy. With regard to attracting a male's initial sexual interest, breasts are probably the female's most important sex characteristic.

For most girls, the most striking sign of puberty is the menarche. This occurs two years after the beginning of breast formation and on the average in the United States shortly before the thirteenth birthday; however, it is considered normal for the menarche to begin at any time between ten and fifteen years of age.[2] Largely because of better nutrition, menarche now occurs more than two years earlier than it did in 1900, although the trend toward earlier menarche may now have ceased.[4] Thus, it is important for the clinician to realize that the increase in early teenage sexuality, and sometimes pregnancy, is due to physiological as well as psychosocial factors. Some girls consider the onset of the menarche an achievement or a relief and find monthly menstruation an organizing event; other girls are ashamed of or angry at having their period. In general, how a girl feels about being female is the most important determination as to whether menarche is perceived as a positive or negative occasion.

The adolescent's level of cognition or judgment is independent of sexual maturation. That the relative lack of judgment and intelligence does not slow down sexual development is demonstrated in the classroom writing of a 10 1/2 year-old girl the day *before* she had her first period. At the time she was in a special class and had a full scale, but probably falsely low, IQ of 56. She wrote, "Red makes me think of a beautiful color. I like the color red. I wish I had a boyfriend because he would give me a nice red rose. Red is my favorite color. I have a red dress in my closet. I have a red crayon. I have a beautiful red book in my home. My heart is red. My blood is red. I have red nail polish." Whether or not vaginal spotting had been the stimulus for her "outpouring" (she denied it), this girl demonstrated poignantly the wonder, pleasure, and excitement of menarche.

With the onset of puberty, privacy becomes very important to most young people. Questions about sex and body functioning are much less likely to be answered truthfully, if at all. At this and at probably all ages, sex (or at least love) is much more fragile and, therefore, a more sensitive indicator of adjustment than is work. Love requires greater risk-taking and exposes vulnerability. Early adolescent dating and sex play are often based more on acquiring social prestige or fulfilling curiosity about anatomy than on a true emotional relationship. Indeed, most people in early adolescence would rather be *preoccupied* with sex than occupied with it, and some can love humanity but not a human being. It is also important to keep in mind that adolescent sexuality may stimulate a sexual response in the therapist. Old scars and fixations in the therapist may be reopened giving rise to a wish to act out in the countertransference frustrated fantasies from one's own adolescence. The presumption that an adolescent's sexual understanding and desire are comparable to such feelings in adults, and the stimulation of countertransference reactions, are the most common difficulties therapists have with their adolescent patients' burgeoning sexuality.

The fact of sexual maturation must also be kept in mind when arranging for inpatient treatment. The sexes should not be together in a way that is threatening or over-stimulating. Even within same-sex wards, respect and opportunity for privacy are very important.

Pubertal sexual changes in boys are not as dramatic as in girls. Pubic hair forms as the penis and testicles enlarge. The voice deepens. Axillary and facial hair appear. Nocturnal ejaculations are common, as is masturbation, from the early to the mid-teenage years. Despite the availability to boys and girls of much literature concerning the fact that masturbation is not harmful to body or mind, the classic fear of the development of insanity (as well as acne, poor eyesight, and so on) resulting from masturbation is surprisingly resilient. Therefore, the therapist should be aware that the adolescent might be wondering whether or not masturbation was a factor in his or her illness and whether abstinence is necessary for successful treatment. In addition, for a fairly large subgroup of adolescents, masturbation raises the specter of homosexuality. As the result of recent publicity, homosexuality is being regarded increasingly as normal behavior, but the fear of being homosexual, especially among boys in early adolescence, is still common. Although it should be kept in mind as a possible treatment complication, homosexual panic occurs only rarely in the transference with adolescent patients. In general, early adolescent patients work better with therapists of the same sex. By the time the patient reaches the mid-teens, the choice of a therapist based on sex is usually not crucial, unless deemed so by the adolescent's individual psychodynamics.

Whereas pubertal girls show the more obvious sexual body changes, boys accelerate more in size and strength. A boy's muscle mass doubles between ages eleven and seventeen.[5] This rather suddenly acquired, enhanced ability to run, throw, and hit has practical implications for the clinician. For example, FBI statistics show that almost 50 percent of rapes and murders are committed by adolescents.[6] Longitudinal studies show that the frequency of violent crimes varies directly with the proportion of the population that is in the adolescent group.[7] For many adolescents, especially boys, trial actions with their muscular equipment are as important as trial actions with their sexual apparatus. The outpatient therapist engaged in treatment planning will find it useful to inquire as to the patient's involvement in motoric activities. Helping the angry, hostile, or depressed adolescent to become involved in exercise, athletics, or other active endeavors is often therapeutic. For inpatient treatment planning, it is crucial to have space for these activities as well as the help of an interested and vigorous staff if one is to provide appropriate motoric outlets.

Vast developmental changes occur in the brain as well as the rest of the body during adolescence. One way this is expressed is through cognitive performance. Most intelligence tests use sixteen or seventeen years of age as the cutoff after which all ages are lumped together as "adult." In Piagetian terms, the adolescent increasingly thinks in the mode of formal operations.[8] For example, he or she has a better grasp of time, can form hypotheses, and has an interest in what is potential as well as what is real. Although recent studies suggest that not all adolescents reach the stage of formal operations even by the end of high school, many older adolescent patients have an enhanced capacity for psychological mindedness.[9] Therefore, compared to children, adolescent patients often can better understand interpretations that deal in symbols (e.g., a cigar is not always a cigar) and the concept of defense mechanisms (e.g., projection, displacement, reaction formation, and the like). Unfortunately, many adolescents who can understand interpretations and insights resist doing so, and others so enjoy thinking about thinking that intellectualization becomes a major resistance. A mature comprehension of time begins to develop during adolescence. When this is present, the patient is much better able to plan for the future, including delaying present gratification for future advantage. Many adolescent patients, however, have great difficulty in thinking of themselves in the future. Even the age of thirty seems remote.

For example, a pediatric endocrinologist asked for a consultation on a fifteen-year-old boy who was recently diagnosed as diabetic. A result of the patient's massive use of denial was his inconsistent attention to insulin usage and prescribed diet. In a few months he had experienced both diabetic acidosis and insulin shock. Consultation was requested because warnings linking noncompliance with a greater likelihood of later complications went unheeded. Although during the consultation sessions a good rapport was gained and the patient's denial lifted in part, he seemed genuinely unable to think of himself as ever being age thirty-five. By arranging for him to visit the internal medicine diabetes clinic and to speak with thirty- to thirty-five-year-old patients who had complications ranging from minor to severe, the boy was much better able to project himself into the future. The combination of brief insight therapy and confrontation with his own future was helpful. With a greater understanding of the reasons for doing so, he began to follow his medical regimen much more carefully.

Schizophrenia is a relatively rare illness in childhood, but it begins most frequently during adolescence and early adulthood.[10] While not proven, it seems likely that the type of thinking that becomes available during adolescence is a factor in the age of onset of schizophrenia. The susceptible individual feels overwhelmed when the enormous complexity of the world is comprehended cognitively at a time when the sense of aloneness occurring in the midst of what Blos terms the second separation-individuation period is most pronounced.[11] Often there is a florid use of the new ability to hypothesize as well as a countervailing thrust to think concretely. While the origins of schizophrenia are undoubtedly multidetermined, it is helpful for the therapist to be aware that one important deficit in many schizophrenic adolescents is the inability to control their new-found powers of abstraction.

Maturity of brain tissue is also important in planning the use and dosage of psychopharmacologic agents. When medicating children one must remember that all drugs given orally pass through the liver, and that the liver in children is relatively greater in size than in adults. Children age two to ten years usually metabolize drugs faster than adults.[12] This reduces the drug's half-life and intensifies the distribution of metabolites, which, as in the case of imipramine, can be toxic. By the early teenage years, however, metabolism of most psychoactive drugs is similar to that found in adults. Some drugs (such as amitriptyline) that are not recommended for children may be used in adolescents over the age of twelve.[13]

Brain maturity seems important in attention deficit disorder with hyperactivity, a disorder often treated with stimulants. As the brain matures during puberty, hyperactivity becomes a much less common part of the syndrome, and medication is less frequently prescribed or required. If stimulants continue to be demonstrably helpful in prolonging or focusing a patient's attention, however, they remain indicated even after hyperactivity is no longer a problem.[14]

Some Social Considerations of Adolescence

In the previous section on biologic perspectives, and in the section that follows on psychodynamics, we argue that it is simply impossible to present a "pure culture" discussion of "body" or "mind" without reference to the social factors that shape and channel the expression of these two dimensions of the human being.

We shall look at some of the social forces that shape adolescence and try to put them into a wider historical and cultural context. This perspective can be very liberating to the clinician. It can allow us to see that the problems with which we are presented are not inevitable in that particular form, and the broader perspective can be transmitted to patients with greater tolerance and flexibility.

There is much to be said about family life in Western society. The primary task of adolescence in our culture with respect to family life is to separate and individuate, to establish identifications and idealizations, and then to expand and transcend them. The adolescent must shift the primary allegiance from the family of origin to the world beyond the family and then perhaps to a new family.

The unique culture of any particular family, in relation to the larger American culture of which it is a part, enormously affects how these tasks of adolescence are implemented, regardless of the biologic and psychological structure of the individual adolescent. For example, we must always be aware that in a sexual sense, a date alone with a boy or girl has different meanings to the proper immigrant Greek or Chinese family, the tightly-knit Puerto Rican family, and the middle-class Protestant family. There are, within different ethnic, religious, cultural groups, varying attitudes toward an adolescent's career, ambition, sexuality, and autonomous adventurousness. We must try to understand these differences in order to help the patient whose difficulties are best understood against the background of his or her familial expectations. There are, without question, universals in human development, but we are more useful as clinicians if we understand their expression against the cultural field of the patient's larger community.

Each family's mode of operation, style, and values form the primary setting from which the adolescent enters the world. The family is the model whose expansion constitutes the further social development of the adolescent. Families differ not only in their values, ethics, religions, and expectations, but also in their way of valuing interactions with the outside world. A young schizophrenic man's treatment blossomed when he and his therapist finally understood that in the patient's family his desire for peer friendships and acceptance outside his immediate family was viewed by them as a betrayal. Ideally, the value system that develops in adolescence must bridge in a harmonious way the world of the family and the world outside. When it does not, there can be failures and setbacks in development and performance. A black girl, age fifteen and highly talented in music and literature, attended a predominantly white, upper-middle-class suburban school that included in its district her small, rural black enclave. Her grades fell, and her mood seemed depressed. It was soon learned that she believed that her achievements had created a barrier between her and her family. She felt as if she was leaving them behind and being in some way disloyal. There are hints in this vignette of "success neurosis" and "oedipal rivalry," but without appreciating the reality of her cultural dislocation, intrapsychic understanding alone would not have been sufficiently therapeutic, and the positive outcome perhaps minimized.

It may be useful for therapists to bear in mind that the task of adolescents in contemporary American culture, to separate from the family and become fully autonomous individuals, is not a task required in many other cultures, including the highly sophisticated societies of India, Japan, Israel, and China. During late adolescence and early adulthood, individuals in those countries often remain a part of their families or transfer directly to another family. Actually, for these young people to go out into the world as discrete individuals is, in general, culturally atypical, and through most of human history people have not had to do it. Even in American life before the Industrial Revolution, there was far more communal sharing in extended networks of family and work support groups.[15] Recognition of the great stress of this social demand may increase our patience as we see the many teenagers who experience difficulty in achieving autonomy. There is something here quite comparable to our expectations for the level of maturity required for motherhood. Such maturity is rarely achieved by the teenager, but in other cultures the presence of supportive networks compensates successfully.

This expectation of autonomy, the push for financial independence, and the struggle with early sexual maturity conflict with increasingly prolonged education and training. It is difficult to be full grown and unemployed. We have institutionalized our expectations and we have complex preparations for financial independence and social autonomy in an increasingly technological economy. We have adolescents who are sexually mature at age eleven, yet they are not ready to assume fully adult roles until as much as fifteen years later, an entire lifetime away. If the therapist is sensitive to these contradictions and complexities, he or she can explain them as factors contributing to the patient's confusion and be helpful in a practical way in reaching a solution. Frequently, the most mature solution is living with and sharing the inevitability of these frustrations and confusions.

Blacks have entered the mainstream of American culture and there has been a major shift away from an explicitly racist majority; however, continued discrimination and immense psychological burdens remain for individual blacks. Many of these problems become more noticeable to blacks as they reach their teenage years; they grow more openly conscious of social and economic discrimination and of the comparatively poorer educational and medical services available to them. Despite great gains, black and other minority group teenagers face higher risks of unemployment, and they are less hopeful about what is presented by the media as being accessible to all.[16]

Many of the older, formerly isolated immigrant groups have blended into the melting pot of American society, but newer groups challenge some of our biases. There are increasingly large numbers of Hispanic people, and more vocal presentations of the unique cultural perspectives of American Indians. Many psychiatrists tend to view minority cultures as deficient, rather than different. It is important to recognize that "mental health," as we define it, is a part of many different social patterns. Kellam and her colleagues identified 86 different family structures in the families of 1,391 first-grade children living in a low income, urban, black community at the end of the 1966-67 school year.[17–19] They found that objectively rated successful social adaptation in first grade was strongly predictive of later successful adaptation in adolescence as well as later psychological well-being. Shyness, aggressiveness, and learning problems in first grade were predictive of depression, delinquency, and substance abuse in adolescence. (These early predictors were far stronger for boys than for girls, which raises interesting, as yet unanswered, questions about sex differences.)[17,18] Significantly, the children at the highest risk for later problems in adolescence came from "mother alone" families and the presence of certain second adults seemed to have important ameliorative implications. Mother/grandmother families were nearly as effective as mother/father families in producing low-risk children in first grade. The absence of the father was less important than the aloneness of the mother.[19] This suggests that normative family structure, as it has been usually conceived in terms of presence or absence of the father, is too gross a measure. Child rearing practices, the availability of different role models, and a host of other factors affect development of gender identity, role differentiation, self-esteem, and other issues that are of crucial significance for adjustment in adolescence.

Another social factor that is part of understanding adolescents in America today is the emergence in the late 1960s of the feminist movement. It has struck very deep chords, particularly in middle-class women, and seems to be producing major shifts in women's self-understanding and their attitudes toward work and family. Particular attention has been paid to the vicissitudes of aggression in adolescent girls and to their conflicts about achievement and its relationship to their concept of femininity and the possible price of success.[20] They are aware that "normal healthy assertiveness" in males may be called "aggression" in females, and that feelings of guilt and conflict about sexual identity are often associated with achievement and success and require sorting out in uniquely female ways.[21] For many women, self-assertion and career success seem contrary to their ideas of femininity, whereas, in males, self-assertion and career success enhance the sense of masculinity. This is one cultural dimension that must be considered as a social pattern worthy of scrutiny by the patient and the therapist, with the hope of expanding the adolescent female's sense of identity to encompass without guilt such feelings as assertiveness and anger.

Another important sex difference in child rearing is the earlier acculturation of boys, throughout latency and early adolescence, to set out a life plan with a sense of a timetable and an emphatic expectation of total self-sufficiency. Those aspects of the self defined by what one *does* take precedence, while other aspects of the personality may be held in abeyance until the primary work commitment is clarified. As a result, understanding one's internal affective states is not so encouraged in boys, and this can be constricting for their later development. In many girls, the aspects of self-development that deal with individual achievement and self-expression beyond family and child-rearing, or even along with it, are delayed and seen as contradictory to success in marriage and childbirth. It is important for therapists to be aware of these general patterns of child-rearing in the United States so that they can detect and focus on the underdeveloped aspects of how patients see themselves and the world. Compared to recent generations, there are many more choices open to all adolescents in the areas of work, marriage, and sexuality. Numerous recent shifts in consciousness have occurred, the understanding of which can illuminate our appreciation of present-day adolescent experience. For example, there is a certain sense of insecurity created in a generation growing up with the knowledge of atomic warfare. There is the impact of television and the media that encourages passivity in their audiences while themselves being highly stimulating.

There seems to be a distinct watering down of the sense of old-fashioned American optimism, accompanied by a build-up of great faith in technology. Adolescents are aware of increasing numbers of "facts" in every dimension of modern life. This creates a sense that all problems are solvable by technical manipulation, but obviously they are not. In a pendulum swing from this type of thinking, some adolescents are deeply concerned about ecology and conservation; that the earth could become uninhabitable if technology is not controlled is a meaningful concept to many young people. Disasters such as the pollution of the Love Canal or diethylstilbestrol exposure are frightening to young people and can lead them to wonder about their elders' judgment.

Another change in consciousness that affects adolescents is an across-the-board diminution of authority in public and in private. At every level there is an unwillingness to acknowledge authority. People are less likely to do things because they have been told to, or because it is the expected thing to do. Consequently, governance in the nation and family is more difficult. As authority declines, conformity, molded by public opinion, becomes increasingly powerful. Finally, some adolescents feel a sense of superfluousness because of the increasing delay of economic and social independence caused by the longer training or schooling required today to obtain a well-paid job.

Although these social factors can be mentioned only briefly, and some may appear speculative, they all influence our clinical work with adolescents. Many young patients are affected and confused by various social factors, and our experience is that the therapist's sensitivity to this can only enhance the person-to-person dimension so important in the therapeutic encounter.

Common Psychodynamic Issues

As we come to the third and last perspective from which we shall view adolescent development, it becomes increasingly obvious how much overlap is present among viewpoints. The focus of this section is on psychodynamic issues, but affects, desires, and fears that give power to intrapsychic conflicts are brought to awareness through brain fibers and neurotransmitters. On the other hand, the raw materials we use to judge ourselves and others, to understand the present, and to predict the future all have roots outside ourselves, especially in the family. Even the most twisted or fragmented internal representations have their origins in interactions with the environment.

A central shift taking place during adolescence involves the change from viewing oneself as a child within a family or other group ruled by adults to viewing oneself as a mature sexual person able to function independently from one's parents or guardians. As a child, it is adaptive to believe that adults, especially parents, are all-powerful. The belief that shelter, food, and clothing will be forthcoming enhances a child's ability not to worry, to be able to think of other things, and to sleep well. During adolescence, however, the task of emulating a larger-than-life image may seem not only impossible, but presumptuous as well. But if the mental representations of adults, again especially of parents, are transformed into images of shallow incompetents, the budding adolescent can believe that he or she may also realistically aspire to such a goal. Most adolescents' views of adults improve as their own skills and maturity progress.

There recently has been considerable discussion about the meaning and inevitability of "adolescent turmoil."[22] Unfortunately, the term has come to have both a specific and a general meaning, which sometimes causes confusion. Masterson and others have shown that most adolescents with specifically diagnosed psychopathology (e.g., schizophrenia, personality disorders, character neurosis) also show psychopathology when reassessed as young adults, the lesson being that adolescents should not be expected necessarily to "grow out" of their disorders.[23,24] In fact, the younger the age of onset for psychoses, the poorer the prognosis is likely to be.

The other use of the term "adolescent turmoil" refers to general emotional upset associated with psychological separation from the family and the transition to adult societal tasks. It includes self-limited periods of anxiety, depression, self-doubt, rebellion, and so on. Quotes from Socrates and others attest to the fact that teenagers have irked adults for millenia; however, most recent data come from middle-class white males, psychiatric patients, and autobiographies of the artistically gifted. No large, detailed studies are available. Anna Freud and most of the early psychoanalytic writers were convinced that turmoil and rebellion are necessary elements in the adolescent's attempt to break away from how they were seen and how they thought of themselves as children.[25] More recently, Offer, Rutter, and others have persuasively argued that, although rebellion and turmoil are common during adolescence, they are not essential to becoming an interesting and productive adult.[22,26] It is certainly not therapeutic per se to goad a patient into rebellion so that he or she can "grow up." The reason, however, that there are time requirements to qualify for some DMS-III diagnoses is that self-limited periods of anxiety, depression, self-doubt, or rebellion during adolescence should not be assumed necessarily to be evidence of psychopathology or of need for treatment. Wise therapists are aware that developmental goals can be reached by more than one path, and that disturbing adolescent behavior does not always mean that the adolescent is disturbed.

The more structured the society, the easier it is for the adolescent to form a firm identity. On the other hand, the more structured a society, the more limited are the choices available. Whether providing more structure or more freedom, it should be remembered that external sanctions are only part of the situation. Intrapsychic controls are the other part. External limits can be very helpful to the adolescent with poor inner controls, but external permission alone is usually not sufficient to relieve inhibitions until intrapsychic resistances have been modified.

David, age sixteen, was an almost straight-A student who, despite his excellent academic standing, was constantly worried that his performance was poor and would deteriorate. Unable to relax, he demanded frequent reassurance. This pattern of an overanxious disorder had been present for at least three years. He was referred by his pediatrician because David's concerns were becoming more severe. During the evaluation it was noted that the boy's study habits were poor and that his use of time was disorganized. As part of treatment planning, a rigid schedule for late afternoon and evening activities was developed; each half-hour from the end of school to bedtime was assigned a specific task, including free time. This simple maneuver greatly reduced his acute anxiety. Insight psychotherapy pursued the reasons for David's various fears about success and, as reasons for these fears became conscious, he was able to relax his detailed schedule without return of severe anxiety.

John, age fourteen, was shy; although he wanted to make friends, he was afraid to do so. He was referred for evaluation by his parents who had become very frustrated. In order to give John a structured way to gain friends, they had enrolled him in scouts, Little League baseball, community hockey, dancing classes, and the church youth group. In the evaluation it became clear that all of this parental activity undertaken to help him had actually made John feel unwanted and desirous of avoiding people even more. Family and individual therapies were recommended. As John's view of himself over the next six months became more positive and self-assured, he was able to develop two fairly close friends.

It is common for adolescents to observe everything except themselves. Although typical in all patients, in adolescents especially it seems that defense mechanisms are either too rigid or overwhelmed. This either-or dichotomy in intrapsychic regulation is particularly common at this age because of the upsurge of biologic drives and the contradictory societal messages concerning how much autonomy an adolescent should exercise. Overanxious disorders, pervasive developmental disorders, and schizophrenia represent conditions in which defense mechanisms have been overwhelmed, and the patient often must be aided by environmental, psychotherapeutic, and/or chemical adjuncts.

Psychotherapy is helpful in providing an adolescent with a new or more varied panoply of intrapsychic defenses. Psychodynamic defenses for the most part determine the expression of thoughts and actions, and an important aspect of every treatment plan is to review these mechanisms to determine how to reinforce those that are adaptive and modify those that are not. Although everyone uses almost the full array of intrapsychic maneuvers, a major goal of many types of psychotherapy is to enhance their appropriateness and flexibility. This is true even though the therapist may not practice insight therapy or may use different terminology. Defense mechanisms are neither "good" nor "bad," but rather are useful or detrimental depending on how they are applied, some requiring modification more frequently than others. Repression, projection, denial, and splitting are often overused by patients who exhibit poor reality testing. Adolescents who wish to appear mature frequently identify with an aggressor. Reaction formation, intellectualization, and, by definition, sublimation are defenses that often help to facilitate an adolescent's acceptance into society as an adult. The therapist's task, however, is not so much to stamp out certain defenses and lobby for others than it is to help the patient orchestrate their use in the most adaptive fashion possible. This requires knowledge of the patient's basic strengths and environmental circumstances.

> *Sara, age fifteen, came from an intact family of lower socioeconomic status. She did extremely well in school and emphasized the gap between her academic accomplishments and those of her poorly educated parents. Sara's teachers, aware of her constant verbal and occasional physical battles with her parents, referred the family to a child guidance clinic for evaluation. Although Sara's intellect helped her to move toward interests and abilities that enhanced her self-esteem and her likelihood of success in the adult world, it was also used as a defense against her positive feelings toward her parents. She feared that if she admitted her love and continuing sense of dependency she would have to give up her intellectual aspirations. Psychotherapy focused on the fact that Sara's accomplishments did not have to express and stir up only negative feelings. She became interested in learning about possible financial benefits available to her family, her father being unable to work because of a chronic medical condition. Through her investigations, the family's disability compensation was raised substantially, she felt freer to "be smart," and her parents became less critical of her intellectual pursuits.*

In terms of psychoanalytic structural theory, the biologically increased power of the adolescent's sexual and aggressive drives enhances the influence of the id.[25] The sexual maturity of puberty restrengthens the incest barrier. This decreases the adolescent's use of the parents as auxiliary egos and may cause a rebellion against previously internalized superego sanctions associated with the now forbidden parent. Vacillation between primacy of the id and the superego occurs in adolescents who combine a generally ascetic lifestyle with outbursts of uninhibited behavior. Mild versions of this interaction are common. A more striking example of these psychodynamics is present in certain difficult-to-treat patients with anorexia nervosa who go on eating binges.[27] Toward the end of the teen years, a plateauing of sexual energies, a greater clarity of societal expectations, and an enhanced level of cognitive abilities strengthen the ego relative to the id and superego. It is at this time that identity formation takes place.[28]

How adolescents view themselves is largely a reflection of how they believe their parents view them. This, of course, is not always how in fact the parents do view them, thus it is important for the clinician to determine the congruence of reality and psychic reality. When these views are especially asynchronous, the therapist can also expect to be the recipient of large distortions in the transference.

Just as we know that the likelihood of smoking and drinking and the development of antisocial and other traits in adolescents is much more common statistically when parents exhibit the same behavior, normally functioning parents are extremely important for the normal development of the adolescent. When appropriate and the patient is able to respond, identification with the parents is a psychodynamic mechanism that the therapist does well to exploit. Even when adolescents scoff at the influence their parents possess over them, such influence is usually considerable.

Too much or too little parental concern influences adolescents in many ways. Some parents convey the belief that they do not want their child. In early adolescence this is a powerful stimulus to running away. Runaways are often throwaways. To the older adolescent, the feeling of being unwanted is more an impetus toward suicide than to running away. It is important for the therapist to recognize when negative parental feelings have been internalized and to try to counter this situation. But consciously trying to provide a specific "corrective emotional experience" is a less natural and usually less effective approach than generally showing interest and concern. Trying to set up an environment that is specifically opposite that provided by a "bad" parent tends not only to be artificial but also to be unnecessarily conflict-producing intrapsychically.

Problems requiring and complicating psychotherapy occur not only when parents do not care for their adolescent, but also when children are smothered and not allowed to separate or individuate. These adolescents may believe that they should stay under their parent's close care always. They may also not have had the opportunity to learn the social skills necessary to enter the general social arena. Having been overprotected and regarded as perfect without need for substantiation, these teenagers, now faced with either entering the adult world unprepared or remaining tied to their parents, realize their future lies behind them.[29] Such "prolonged adolescence" often ends only with the death of the parents. When these dynamics are present, referral is usually by someone other than the parents, and the therapist may have great difficulty getting the parents to allow the patient to enter an inpatient setting, take medication, or be in outpatient psychotherapy. In such cases, even when individual therapy is desired, family therapy is usually the first approach possible.

The latter part of adolescence is when most people make their initial choices about career, marital, and social goals. Whether one is making the right choices and pursuing them is a major source of developmental anxiety. One's self-esteem is to a large part based on the congruence of one's internal set of expectations and one's performance in the world. A heightened sense of narcissism is common during adolescence and perhaps necessary if one is to take on the many burdens and unknowns associated with starting out at the bottom of the ladder in so many endeavors. An important task toward the end of adolescence is to give up omnipotentiality.[30] It is comforting to think that one can do everything and do it well, but this is the age when priorities must be determined if the tasks of adulthood are to be faced with success. Any commitment, even the most felicitous, necessarily means that one is not doing something else. The commitment to recover from an emotional illness may be difficult for some adolescents to make, because it forces them to make other life choices that they do not wish or feel able to decide on. A treatment plan must recognize this resistance in certain patients. The need to cling to the belief of omnipotence usually stems from feelings of inadequacy, thus enhanced emotional support from the environment is crucial before choices can be made.

A fear of success is also quite common in late adolescence. The most easily recognized psychodynamic is when the adolescent fears retaliation because of others' envy. A less often recognized but common intrapsychic issue for those uneasy with success is the fear of abandonment. These adolescents believe that if they are successful, no one will recognize that they still have dependency needs. Because getting well may be equated with success, the therapist should be sensitive to the fear of success as a possible source of resistance.

Because parents are such an important part of the treatment planning for adolescents, the therapist should understand some of the common psychodynamics of how this developmental stage affects them. The parental wish not to let go, the feeling that a part of the self will be lost, or that the growing up of children augurs one's deterioration and death are common feelings. Some parents have great difficulty with their adolescents' new ideas and enthusiasm for yet another reason. They remember when they were adolescents with similar dreams of grandeur and success, and their old dreams are awakened along with the sense of frustration that these dreams were never realized. The fear these adults have is that if the young people of this generation succeed, it may mean that their own adolescent renunciations were unnecessary. Because we do not have to worry about what cannot or could not change, our (the adult's) sense of frustration lessens if this generation's dreams also fail. Adult criticism is one of the reasons adolescents turn so frequently to peers for support. In treatment planning, the parents' psychodynamics must be considered in regard to what types of treatment are acceptable to them and what types are necessary.

Being an adolescent and feeling special often go together, and the feeling may be good or bad. Because there are so many changes happening at once, and adolescents are most baffled by the intrapsychic ones, they, even more than adults, tend to think of problems as coming exclusively from the environment.[31] The assumption that external problems are easier to fight than internal ones is a powerful deterrent to cooperation with a treatment plan that includes insight psychotherapy. It is wise for the therapist to assume that the early part of this type of treatment usually requires considerable work at forming a treatment alliance. Especially with adolescents there is no such thing as instant alliance, and the fostering of psychological mindedness takes considerable time and patience.

Before leaving this last section on psychodynamic issues, it seems reasonable to say something about the end of adolescence. Although we have used a definition that describes adolescence as ending at the age of majority, other definitions have less time-bound endings. The best set of criteria is from GAP. While many people will never achieve these six accomplishments, they do present ideal goals toward which a therapist and patient can work:[32]

1) attainment of separation and independence from parents
2) establishment of a sexual identity
3) commitment to work
4) development of a personal moral value system

5) attainment of a capacity for lasting relationships and for both tender and genital sexual love
6) an emotional return to the parents based on relative equality

Types of Information Necessary for Treatment Planning

This section will first focus on issues of treatment planning per se, with comment on general developmental factors that affect the planning for adolescent patients, and will then present information helpful in formulating a treatment plan. The final section will address issues involved in using each of a number of specific treatment modalities.

The obvious first question is whether every patient should have a treatment plan. The answer is "of course." To not have a plan for a patient's treatment is not only foolish but is a form of malpractice. More difficult, however, is to decide how elaborate a plan should be for a particular patient. This will be determined in large part by the diagnosis, which includes the information contained in DSM-III, Axes III, IV, and V. The impact of physical disorders and conditions, the amount and type of stress present, and the usual level of the patient's adaptation are important data in helping to decide what services are necessary. Other crucial information includes the patient's sociocultural background and maturity, the therapist's training and style, the treatment setting, and the demands made by accrediting and reimbursing agencies.

In this age of over-regulation, it is important to try to keep a sense of perspective. Goals and objectives can replace the patient as the focus of our attention, and the admission of ignorance is much less harmful than "knowing" things that are either unknown or untrue. In fact, we do not know how well most treatments work, and there is no such thing as a single "best" treatment plan for a patient. For example, the chosen treatment plan for a patient may differ depending on the particular skills or areas of expertise of the therapist doing the treatment. It is a humbling fact that no therapist can deliver all treatment modalities well.

Wishful thinking is often the greatest enemy of realistic treatment planning. Plans are sometimes made on the basis of what the therapist would like to happen rather than what can be done. If others can provide more appropriate treatment, and referral is possible, the best treatment plan is to arrange for the referral. Assuming, however, no change in responsibility for treatment, it is important not to be trapped with promising oneself, the patient, or the family more than can be delivered.

Treatment goals should be determined before plans are developed to reach them. Goals and plans must be reviewed regularly because both often require revision. Revision, rather than seen as *prima facie* evidence of failure, is more often evidence of clinical acumen and flexibility. The notorious lability of adolescent behavior is just why treatment plans for these patients should not be rigid or preordained by some regulatory agency.

Who should do the treatment planning? Although it is not always possible, those who will do the treatment should also do the planning. In private practice the diagnostician, treatment planner, and therapist are usually the same person. This is the most simple model, and the treatment plan may be in the therapist's head rather than on paper. Although the most powerful impetus recently for individual therapists to write down their treatment plan probably has come from fear of malpractice suits, clinical reasons are also compelling. When one's plans are only in one's head, their change may be so fluid as to often be imperceptible. Plans registered only mentally may be adequate, but the therapist does not then usually have the opportunity to review systematically changes in diagnostic and therapeutic thinking. When one's goals and approach are written down (this may require only a few sentences), the changes and the need for those changes can more easily be studied and learned from. That first thoughts are not always the best thoughts is an obvious truism, but it is also instructive to be forced to face its truth in ourselves. In addition to improved patient care, such review often chronicles patterns of miscalculation that lead the therapist to discover a tendency to repeat certain biases or expressions of countertransference.

When more than one person is involved in the treatment offered, it must be decided who is in charge of planning and of treatment reviews. Many clinics and most inpatient facilities now have multidisciplinary treatment teams that are appropriate bodies to plan the treatment. When the planning has been done prior to the patient's arrival or assignment to the team's responsibility, the team should have the prerogative to modify the plan; however, decisions about therapy are usually not best made by voting. While no therapist can deliver services well that he or she does not believe in, the person responsible administratively for the work done must also agree. When therapist(s) and the person legally responsible are not the same, the plan should be developed by the therapist(s) in collaboration with, or under supervision of, the person responsible administratively.

How much to involve patient, parents, and other family members in treatment planning is based on circumstances, but adolescents should be included whenever possible.[33] Even self-destructive, psychotic, or uncooperative adolescents can profit from being asked their opinion about how they should be treated. The responsibility for the plan is the therapist's, but patients who are consulted about their care (even when they decline or berate the therapist for abdicating accountability) tend to be more motivated to make the treatment work. Also, the process of how the adolescent does or does not cooperate with the initial planning and final plan usually contributes to the therapist's understanding of and future planning for the patient. Depending on the adolescent's age and the laws of the state, there may be a legal requirement to include the patient in the formulation of any treatment plan, at least to the point of obtaining consent.

Parents should be included as much as possible, but this is often a complicated issue when treating adolescents. In individual outpatient therapy, adolescents sometimes do not want their parents involved, although the latter are concerned, curious, and paying the bill. When the therapist believes that the parents should be included, one goal of the treatment plan may be to have this accomplished. In other cases, a goal may be to extricate parents who are too enmeshed in their adolescent's treatment and life in general. Pragmatism dictates that, except when it would be dangerous or obviously futile to act otherwise, the therapist includes and excludes those family members necessary to allow the therapeutic process to begin. Once begun, treatment can move toward the optimal rather than just the expedient cast of players.

The degree to which one involves parents in the inpatient treatment of adolescents can also be a thorny problem.[34] When parents refuse to give their consent, it is very difficult in most states to treat a minor. The finding of extreme dangerousness is usually required to obtain a legal commitment over parents' and the adolescent's objections. More frequently, the conflict arises when parents are in favor of hospitalization and of being involved, while the adolescent is not. Whether or not the patient approves, it is extremely useful, when possible, to obtain a full, three-generation history of the family as well as a complete history of the patient from the parental perspective. More often than not, adolescents who protest parents' involvement early in planning and treatment are by the time of discharge convinced that the decision to include them was practical, if not desirable, and an effective example of the reality principle in action.

Adolescents occasionally seek treatment without or against parental wishes. Because laws vary from state to state, clinicians must be aware of their legal rights and obligations in this regard. It is not unusual for adolescents to benefit from treatment without their parents' approval; however, few therapies succeed when done in the face of family opposition.

A line of questioning too often forgotten and best obtained while involving adolescent and parents in treatment planning is a catalogue of the patient's and family's strengths. Knowing how each has coped well (or poorly) with problems in the past is a great help in planning strategies likely to work in the present. Also important for whether or not a treatment plan is likely to work are the parents' and adolescent's aspirations. Success is not likely if the therapist's goals are not similar to these.

Determining why the patient became symptomatic at this particular time, or why treatment was sought at this time (they are not always the same), is often useful in deciding on the earliest foci of treatment.

> *Ann, age thirteen, was referred by her pediatrician. During the previous three months, Ann had lost almost one-third of her weight, but she still worried that she looked too fat. She had amenorrhea and had developed a need to prepare food constantly for the rest of the family. The history revealed that her eating disorder began when a boy started badgering her for a date. She was both flattered and worried about the possibility of sex. At that time she overheard another boy refer to her as "plump." She initiated a diet and*

developed anorexia nervosa. Although numerous other factors were involved in the formation and elaboration of her disorder, the intrapsychic conflicts she had between both wanting to look better and worse, be sexual and abstentious, be grown-up yet still a child were the areas first addressed in treatment. They proved a good starting place for other conflicts, including those within the family.

Sara was a fifteen-year-old only child also referred by her pediatrician. She had lost slightly more than 25% of her weight and still believed that she looked too fat. She had been amenorrheic for six months and had also been on a diet about the same length of time. She insisted on preparing the family supper each night. Sara's recent personal history showed no major changes in her social or scholastic life, but the family history revealed chronic marital strife. Just before Sara began her diet, the parents for the first time seriously considered divorce. Although Sara supposedly did not know this, obviously she did. Since the onset of her starvation period, the parents' concern about Sara increased and their fighting decreased. Following the diagnosis of anorexia nervosa, a treatment plan was formulated that included marital therapy for the parents as well as family and individual therapy for Sara. This outpatient approach was successful, and hospitalization was avoided.

Before proceeding to formal outlines of specific data needed in planning for treatment, there is the practical question of priority with an adolescent who has multiple problems. The first duty, of course, is to protect the patient and others from harm. By far, most therapy is done through outpatient facilities, but day treatment centers, therapeutic schools, residential treatment centers, psychiatric hospitals, and correctional institutions are sometimes necessary. Since separation is a clear message of family failure and takes responsibility from the parents, it should not be done lightly and should be to the least restrictive but effective environment. When in doubt about the possibility of harm, however, it is usually wise to hospitalize the adolescent until the doubt is resolved. For example, one rule of thumb is that if a team cannot decide whether or not to hospitalize by the time its meeting is three-quarters over, it is usually best to do so. Other areas to keep in mind when planning priorities in treatment of multiple problem patients are 1) resistances that are likely to hamper or halt treatment, 2) the symptoms or issues for which there is the greatest motivation for change, and 3) the strengths that the patient and family have used to advantage in the past.

In completing this section, we shall summarize some of the information in manuals developed by the Certification Committee in Child Psychiatry of the American Board of Psychiatry and Neurology, GAP, and the Joint Commission on the Accreditation of Hospitals. These are schematic and inclusive and, therefore, require repetition of an earlier cautionary note. Although one should always try to think of everything, the written treatment plan need only be as complex as the needs of the therapist or the requirements of regulatory authorities. It is never difficult to think of additional things the therapist or treatment team can write down. The danger, already realized on occasion, is that staff time is spent more with paper than with patients, and it is the treatment plan rather than the patient that is treated.

General Indicators of Competent Treatment Planning[35]

1) Involvement of adolescent, family, or other relevant people
2) Acknowledgment and respect of the sociocultural values of the patient and family
3) Appraisal of the readiness and resistances of the family to initiate therapy
4) Identification of appropriate therapeutic goal(s)
5) Appropriate choice of treatment modalities:
   a. treatment based on diagnostic formulation
   b. therapy adapted to the particular situation, available personnel and community resources
   c. improvisation of a practical approach when the ideal is not feasible
6) Choice of an appropriate therapy setting
7) Referral to other treatment sources when necessary

Knowledge Base for Treatment Planning[35]

1) Knowledge of the usual course and prognosis at different developmental levels of the various emotional disturbances
2) Knowledge of the principles, techniques, indications, contradications, and limitations of the various modalities, including

parent counseling and treatment of parents, behavior modification, psychopharmacology, brief psychotherapies, long-term psychotherapy, family therapy, group therapies, milieu therapy, marital counseling, and collaborative therapy
3) Knowledge of other sources of therapy, of the skills and roles of other disciplines, and of techniques of collaboration in treatment
4) Knowledge of the structure, requirements, flexibilities, rigidities, costs, and so on, of the various institutions, or institutional arrangements through which the adolescent's treatment is carried out
5) Knowledge of the various environments, institutional and otherwise, that impinge upon the child in society (neighborhood, school, courts, welfare, medical and public health services) and the part they play in supporting, or interfering with, successful treatment
6) Knowledge of family dynamics, and the way ethnic, cultural, economic, religious, and moral elements in family life can influence prognosis and treatment

Assessment of the Patient[36]

1) Degree of central nervous system or physical impairment
2) Areas of healthy function
3) Capacity for relating to others
4) Capacity for tolerance of anxiety
5) Capacity for conceptualization and communication
6) Developmental phase
7) Personality structure
8) Frustration tolerance
9) Duration of the problem
10) Severity of the disorder
11) "Psychological mindedness"
12) Proportion of reactive to intrapsychic elements
13) Degree of secondary gain
14) Proneness to regression

Assessment of the Family[36]

1) The nature of the family as a unit (stable, cohesive, divisive, close, distant)

2) Family capacity for cooperation with treatment plans
3) "Psychological mindedness" of members of the family
4) The capacity for communications between family members
5) The degree of mental health or ill health of the family as a unit or in terms of the individual members
6) The role of the patient's disorder in the psychic economy of the family (secondary gain, or family misuse of the child's disorder)
7) The relationship of the family to the community (distant, isolated, involved)
8) The subcultural values dominant in the family

Assessment of the Community[36]

1) The attitude of school personnel and their investment in the child
2) Peer relationships and attitudes
3) The juvenile court and its personnel, where relevant
4) Geographic (urban-suburban-rural) and economic factors
5) Cultural, social, recreational, and religious opportunities and practices
6) The range of helping facilities available

Some Standard Features of a Treatment Plan[37]

1) Short-term objectives
2) Long-term objectives
3) Description of services planned
4) Criteria for discharge or transfer to a less comprehensive or restrictive facility
5) Review or revision of the plan

Advantages and Cautions of Specific Treatment Approaches

Before proceeding to the specific psychodynamic, group, biologic, behavioral, and marital and family therapies, there are some general issues to keep in mind.

First, to do well a therapist must be comfortable working with adolescents. It is important that therapists who do not like to work with or who do not work well with adolescents should admit the fact and not force themselves (and the adolescents) to do so. Some therapists have trouble being objective because they believe young people are not as responsible as they were in their own day or because of feelings they have about their own adolescent offspring. Others have trouble being objective because they are too closely identified with the rebellious aspect of adolescence.[38] Therapists in this latter category tend to "fight" the parents and seek vicarious gratification from patient-parent conflicts.

A second bias is not specific to adolescents, but is common in human nature. Problems may occur when there is an ethnic, racial, or socioeconomic difference between therapist and patient. While it is impossible to match therapist and adolescent perfectly, it is possible to work constantly at avoiding bias and to have therapist and patient as compatible as is feasible. Some therapists work well with a wide variety of patients and others do not. Therapists in the latter category should learn their limitations through experience, introspection, or comments from colleagues. All therapists have some biases, but when these are allowed to interfere with judgment, problems develop.

A final cautionary note has to do with sex. Adolescence is the time for burgeoning sexuality and for seeking an out-of-the-family sex partner. The potential for sexual exploitation by the therapist is, therefore, great. When this occurs, there is no treatment, and degradation, loss of trust, guilt, anger, and depression are the likely result.

As is seen from the foregoing, psychotherapy with adolescents can be difficult. The effort, however, is usually worthwhile. A recent review of psychotherapy outcome research with adolescents showed that the median rate of positive outcomes with therapy was approximately twice that obtained without therapy.[39]

THE PSYCHODYNAMIC PSYCHOTHERAPIES

All therapies are psychodynamic to some extent, because all involve one person, either voluntarily or involuntarily, receiving treatment from another. By their nature such relationships tend to foster strong child-parent transference reactions. The importance of the relationship is sometimes forgotten by those not involved in individual "insight" psychotherapy. For example, a recent study of compliance with lithium prescribed by physicians who were experienced with the drug revealed that only 27% of the physicians, compared to 50% of patients, believed that psychotherapy was "very important" in obtaining compliance.[40]

Although psychodynamics are important in all forms of psychotherapy, we are going to focus in this short section mainly on individual, insight-oriented psychotherapy and counseling.

Many young adolescents cannot or do not want to use psychotherapy that is exclusively interpretive. Anna Freud, for example, has commented on how difficult psychoanalysis is for the young adolescent. There are exceptions, of course, and psychoanalysis can be successful with adolescents of any age who are motivated and psychologically minded. Young adolescents who have not yet mastered symbolic thinking, however, may react to interpretations either with incredulity and disdain or with fear that the therapist can read or control their minds. Indeed, a common error of technique is for therapists to try to avoid the adolescent's disdain by giving flashy or "deep" interpretations during the evaluation or the very early sessions of treatment. Even, perhaps especially, if the interpretations are accurate, they commonly terrify the patient, and the treatment may be stopped precipitously.

Other problems common in treating young adolescents are the patients' tendency to rebel against adults (and the therapist is often perceived as an extension of the parents) and to act in a motoric way rather than to think or remember.

A few years of development make the older teenager a much more felicitous patient. At this age adolescents are more likely to seek therapy themselves rather than be brought by parents. Enhanced cognitive skills now make symbolic representations more accessible, and important early childhood feelings and events are less close and, therefore, sometimes less powerfully repressed. All of these factors make introspection and the psychodynamic psychotherapies far more acceptable.

Confidentiality is a very important issue when treating the adolescent and is best brought up early by the therapist. While state laws, therapists' preferences, and situations all vary, one approach is to tell the adolescent that everything discussed in therapy will be held confidential, with three exceptions: 1) if the therapist believes the patient is self-destructive (a definition of "self-destructive" is necessary here—e.g., whether any types of drug abuse are included), 2) if the therapist believes the patient is a danger to others, and 3) if the patient asks the therapist to share information with others. Of course, there will be situations when the therapist knows that information will be shared with parents or other staff, and this should be made plain to the patient. Therapeutic styles and situations are very different, and our main point is to stress the importance of clarifying the bounds of confidentiality, rather than to suggest the same set of boundaries for every case.

A common mistake made by therapists who are uncomfortable with adolescents is to be too passive. Faced with long periods of silence, the adolescent who is unable to be introspective is often flooded with anxiety, made to feel a failure, and is forced to flee the situation. A common mistake made by therapists who are uncomfortable with being adults is to act too much like the adolescent's peer. Acting as if one is not what one is, not only is a confusing model to present to vulnerable patients attempting to discover the truth about themselves, but is easily spotted as phony by adolescents who are better at this than most older or younger patients. When the therapist's masquerade is not acknowledged, it is usually because one or both parties are more interested in a treat rather than a treatment. Problems also commonly arise when therapists view their role or persona as being super parents who will undo all the "damage" done by the biologic parents.[41]

An individual therapy approach that often works well, even with young adolescents, mixes insight with support. As Aichhorn showed more than a generation ago, even recalcitrant adolescents frequently become susceptible to treatment that points out how their actions get in their own way and how learning more effective patterns of behavior is in their own best interest.[42]

GROUP THERAPIES

There are a number of advantages in treating adolescents in group therapy. Peer acceptance is probably more important at this age than at any other. Group therapy allows the therapist to observe the adolescent's behavior directly in interaction with others. Worry that one is unique in having problems is common during adolescence and finding out that one is not alone can in itself be therapeutic. A group is also helpful for adolescents who are loners but do not want to be; however, group therapy for an adolescent who has no wish to give up being a loner usually works badly. Some adolescents can believe observations and accept interpretations from peers more readily than from an adult therapist and can also more easily tolerate peer support. The presence of the group usually dilutes both the positive and the negative transference toward the therapist(s).

Difficulties can arise when treating adolescents in groups. Young adolescents usually do not have the older adolescent's ability to talk and listen for sixty to ninety minutes and carry forward themes from one session to another. They may giggle or show embarrassment and cannot keep on the subject. The therapist can sometimes adapt to these problems by using shorter sessions or by providing food and activities. While the mixture of adolescents with different problems and of different sexes usually is not a difficulty, mixing less and more mature adolescents usually is not workable.[43] Age, of course, should not be the sole criterion for maturity.

Psychotic, very immature, and unsocialized adolescents are usually not primary candidates for group therapy, although it may be part of a total treatment plan. The mixture of individual and group therapy can be very useful for adolescents who need help socializing, but also need a level of support that can only be provided individually.

Because adolescents can gang up on the therapist, and because learning how to separate from parents is an important developmental task, many people who run groups for adolescents use male and female co-therapists.

BIOLOGIC THERAPIES

In general, biologic therapies are never used in isolation but are part of a comprehensive treatment plan. The most self-sufficient biologic therapies involve medical or surgical treatment of biologic dysfunction (metabolic disorders, neurologic disorders, treatment of space-occupying lesions of the brain) that can cause symptoms of mental disorders. Another type of quickly effective biologic therapy is the discovery and discontinuance of drugs (abused or therapeutic) or environmental toxins that cause symptoms of mental disorders.

Electroconvulsive therapy is only rarely indicated; one example would be its use in a depressed patient who is still determined to commit suicide after thorough inpatient treatment with appropriate types of psychotherapy and medication. While it is not possible to say there is *no* indication for psychosurgery during adolescence, the situation would surely be extremely unusual.[44]

Drug abuse is relatively common during adolescence, yet many teenagers balk at taking prescribed drugs. Others, however, are relieved to abdicate all personal responsibility in favor of being medicated. It is important for the therapist to understand the psychological meaning of the drug to the patient, because this may influence the impact of the drug's physiological action. Weissman and others have noted that psychopharmacologic effects are usually enhanced when combined with psychotherapy.[45]

Further, adolescents may experience the side effects of medications more intensely than younger or older patients. Fears of "being drugged" and losing control are worrisome for many teenagers. These patients are particularly prone to stop their medications when their areas of strength are affected. For example, blurred vision and cognitive blunting will be anathema for the patient interested in academics; and lethargy, orthostatic hypotension, and extrapyramidal signs will be especially bothersome to the adolescent athlete. Also potentially counter-therapeutic is the tendency for ejaculatory problems and weight gain with thioridazine, or the impotence and loss of libido sometimes associated with various antipsychotic and antidepressant drugs.[46] While the clinician may see the positive effects of medication as outweighing these and other side effects, the adolescent should be prepared for the specific nontherapeutic actions that are likely to occur. This preparation allows a more active role for the patient and aids the likelihood of compliance.

BEHAVIOR THERAPIES

A certain amount of behavior modification is, of course, present in all types of psychotherapy. More pure forms of this approach are commonly used in adolescents with anxiety, phobias, habit disorders, anorexia nervosa, and psychological factors affecting physical conditions.

The importance to adolescents of feeling in control makes the presentation and approach to behavior therapies crucial. When the patient believes that treatment is done in tandem with the therapist, therapy is likely to be more successful than when it is perceived as delivered through stealth or coercion. Probably one of the most important ingredients gained by adolescents from the skillful use of behavior therapy is an increased sense of autonomy and self-sufficiency.

The dangers of behavior therapy arise most frequently when the treatment is delivered mechanically and without regard for the adolescent's developmental needs for autonomy and identity formation. These dangers have been noted particularly when behavior modification is used as the sole approach to the treatment of anorexia nervosa.[47]

MARITAL AND FAMILY THERAPIES

Because DSM-III does not attempt to classify disturbed dyadic or family relationships, there has been considerable concern that family therapy will lose its recognition as a useful and justifiable treatment approach. This certainly is not the case when treating adolescents, because family relationships are, at times, crucial to the formation and alleviation of the patient's disorder. It is appropriate to consider family therapy when the adolescent's disorder is caused by, or is causing, significant family disruption. Whether family therapy should be employed is influenced by the therapist's orientation, the family's motivation, and the degree of family disruption.

Family therapy has been hampered in the past by detractors who believed it was necessarily inferior to individual psychotherapy, and by advocates who believed all or most children's disorders stemmed from their parents' marital problems. Fortunately, these extreme stands, never justified, are no longer common.[48] Family problems are frequent in homes in which an adolescent has a mental disorder, and family therapy often can be helpful. However, because adolescence is the age in which a major developmental task is extrication from the family, it requires considerable training and judgment on the therapist's part to decide whether treatment is best accomplished through family therapy, individual therapy, or both. Thus, it is very important that therapists who work with adolescents have training in family therapy, and that all those who do family therapy be well trained in the developmental needs of adolescents.

Family therapy is probably more likely to be helpful for younger than for older adolescents, but there are exceptions. The degree of family pathology is another important variable. Family therapy is less often indicated as the *primary* treatment when there is little or when there is massive family disruption. In the former instances, there is usually little motivation, and in the latter, family members may first require medication or individual psychotherapy.

At times, parental marital problems are the main reason for an adolescent's symptoms. When this is the case, marital therapy, with or without treatment for the adolescent, is preferred.

In summary, treatment planning for adolescent patients requires consideration of a wide range of biologic, social, and psychodynamic variables, the interaction of which must be understood within the context of the specific developmental challenges of this important stage of life. Precisely because there is so much going on at this time, well-planned therapeutic interventions have the potential for facilitating profound and long-lasting changes in the life of the adolescent patient.

References

1. Group for the Advancement of Psychiatry: *From Diagnosis to Treatment: An Approach to Treatment Planning for the Emotionally Disturbed Child*, Vol. VIII, Report No. 87, September, 1973.
2. McCammon, R. W.: *Human Growth and Development*, Springfield, Ill.: Charles C. Thomas, 1970.
3. Offer, R.: Normal Adolescent Development, in H. Kaplan, A. Freedman, and B. Sadock (eds.): *Comprehensive Textbook of Psychiatry/III*, Baltimore: Williams and Wilkins, 1980, p. 2442.
4. Zacharias, L., Rand, W. M., and Wurtman, R. J.: A Prospective Study of Sexual Development and Growth in American Girls: The Statistics of Menarche, *Obstetrical and Gynecological Survey*, 31 (Suppl), 325-337, April, 1976.
5. Cheek, D. B.: Muscle Cell Growth in Normal Children, in D. Cheek (ed.): *Human Growth: Body Composition, Cell Growth, Energy, and Intelligence*, Philadelphia: Lea & Febiger, 1968, p. 337.
6. *New York Times*, December 12, 1975.

7. Robins, L. N.: Sturdy Childhood Predictors of Adult Antisocial Behavior: Replications from Longitudinal Studies, *Psychological Medicine*, 8:611-622, November, 1978.
8. Inhelder, B., and Piaget, J.: *The Growth of Logical Thinking From Childhood to Adolescence*, New York: Basic Books, 1958.
9. Elkind, D.: Quantity Conceptions in Junior and Senior High School Students, *Child Development*, 32:551-560, March to December, 1961.
10. American Psychiatric Association: *Diagnostic and Statistical Manual of Mental Disorders* (3rd Ed.), Washington, D.C.: APA, 1980.
11. Blos, P.: The Second Individuation Process of Adolescence, *The Psychoanalytic Study of the Child*, 22:162-186, 1967.
12. Briant, R. H.: An Introduction to Clinical Pharmacology, in J. Werry (ed.): *Pediatric Psychopharmacology: The Use of Behavior Modifying Drugs in Children*, New York: Brunner/Mazel, 1978, p. 3.
13. *Physicians' Desk Reference*, 35th Ed., Oradell, N. J.: Medical Economics, 1981.
14. Laufer, W. and Shetty, T.: Attention Deficit Disorders, in H. Kaplan, A. Freedman, and B. Sadock, (eds.): *Comprehensive Textbook of Psychiatry/III*, Baltimore: Williams & Wilkins, 1980, p. 2538.
15. Bremner, H., Ed.: *Children and Youth in America*, Vol. I: 1600-1865, Cambridge: Harvard University Press, 1970.
16. Spurlock, J., and Lawrence, L. E.: The Black Child, in J. Call, J. Noshpitz, R. Cohen, and I. Berlin (eds.): *Basic Handbook of Child Psychiatry, Vol. I.*, New York: Basic Books, 1979, p. 248.
17. Kellman, G., Ensminger, E., and Simon, M.: Mental Health in First Grade and Teen-Age Drug, Alcohol, and Cigarette Use, *Drug and Alcohol Dependence*, 5:273-304, May, 1980.
18. Kellam, G., Brown, C. H., and Fleming, J. P.: Longitudinal Community Epidemiological Studies of Drug Use: Early Aggressiveness, Shyness, and Learning Problems, in L. Robins (ed.): *Studying Drug Use and Abuse*, New York: Neale Watson Academic Publisher, Inc. (in press)
19. Kellam, S. G., Ensminger, M. E., and Turner, R. J.: Family Structure and the Mental Health of Children, *Archives of General Psychiatry*, 34:1012-1022, September, 1977.
20. Horner, M.: Toward an Understanding of Achievement Related Conflict in Women, *Journal of Social Issues*, 28:2, 157-175, 1982.
21. Notman, M., Nadelson, C., Miller, J., and Zilbach, J.: Aggression in Women: A Re-examination, In Sheila Klebenow (ed.): *Changing Concepts in Psychoanalysis*, New York: Gardner Press, 1979.
22. Rutter, M., Graham, P., Chadwick, O. F. D., and Yule, W.: Adolescent Turmoil: Fact or Fiction? *Journal of Child Psychology and Psychiatry*, 17:35-56, January 1976.
23. Masterson, J. F., Jr.: *The Psychiatric Dilemma of Adolescence*, Boston: Little, Brown and Co., 1967.
24. Weiner, I. B., and DelGaudio, A. C.: Psychopathology in Adolescence: An Epidemiological Study, *Archives of General Psychiatry*, 33:187-193, February, 1976.

25. Freud, A.: *The Ego and the Mechanisms of Defense*, New York: International Universities Press, 1946.
26. Offer, D.: *The Psychological World of the Teenager: A Study of Normal Adolescent Boys*, New York: Basic Books, 1973.
27. Beaumont, P. J. V., George, G. C. W., and Smart, D. E.: "Dieters" and Vomiters and Purgers in Anorexia Nervosa, *Psychological Medicine*, 6:617-622, November, 1976.
28. Erikson, E. H.: The Problem of Ego Identity, *Journal of the American Psychoanalytic Association*, 4:56-121, 1966.
29. Blos, P: *On Adolescence*, New York: Free Press, 1962.
30. Pumpian-Mindlin, E.: Omnipotentiality, Youth, and Commitment, *Journal of the American Academy of Child Psychiatry*, 4:1-18, January, 1965.
31. Geleerd, E. R.: Some Aspects of Ego Vicissitudes in Adolescence, *Journal of the American Psychoanalytic Association*, 9:394-405, July, 1961.
32. Group for the Advancement of Psychiatry: *Normal Adolescence*, Vol. VI. Report No. 68, February 1968, pp. 829-830.
33. Schowalter, J. E.: The Minor's Role in Consent for Mental Health Treatment, *Journal of the American Academy of Child Psychiatry*, 17:505-513, Summer, 1978.
34. Miller, D., and Burt, R. A.: Children's Rights on Entering Therapeutic Institutions, *American Journal of Psychiatry*, 134:153-156, February, 1977.
35. McDermott, J. F., Jr., McGuire, C., and Berner, E. S.: *Roles & Functions of Child Psychiatrists*, Evanston: Committee on Certification in Child Psychiatry of the American Board of Psychiatry and Neurology, 1976, pp. 30-31.
36. Group for the Advancement of Psychiatry: *From Diagnosis to Treatment: An Approach to Treatment Planning for the Emotionally Disturbed Child*, Vol. VIII, Report No. 87, September, 1973, pp. 555, 556, 558.
37. Accreditation Council for Psychiatric Facilities: *Accreditation Manual for Psychiatric Facilities Serving Children and Adolescents*, Chicago: Joint Commission of Accreditation of Hospitals, 1974.
38. Solnit, S. J., Settlage, C. F., Goodman, S., and Blos, P.: Youth Unrest: A Symposium, *American Journal of Psychiatry*, 125:1145-1159, March, 1969.
39. Tramontana, M. G.,: Critical Review of Research on Psychotherapy Outcome with Adolescents: 1967-1977, *Psychological Bulletin*, 88:429-450, September, 1980.
40. Jamison, K. R., Gerner, R. H., and Goodwin, F. K.: Patient and Physician Attitudes Toward Lithium, *Archives of General Psychiatry*, 36:866-869, July, 1979.
41. Schowalter, J. E., and Pruett, K.: The Supervision Process for Individual Child Psychotherapy, *Journal of the American Academy of Child Psychiatry*, 14:708-718, Autumn, 1975.
42. Aichhorn, A.: *Wayward Youth*, (1925), New York: The Viking Press, 1965.
43. Kraft, I. A.: Group Therapy, in S. Harrison (ed.): *Basic Handbook of Child Psychiatry, Vol. III*, New York: Basic Books, 1979, p. 159.
44. Older, J.: Psychosurgery: Ethical Issues and a Proposal for Control, *American Journal of Orthopsychiatry*, 44:661-674, October, 1974.

45. Weissman, M. M.: The Psychological Treatment of Depression. Evidence for the Efficacy of Psychotherapy Alone in Comparison With, and in Combination With Pharmacotherapy, *Archives of General Psychiatry*, 36:1261-1269, October, 1979.
46. Drugs That Cause Sexual Dysfunction: *The Medical Letter on Drugs and Therapeutics*, 22:108-110, December 12, 1980.
47. Bruch, H.: Perils of Behavior Modification in Treatment of Anorexia Nervosa, *Journal of the American Medical Association*, 230:1419-1422, December 9, 1974.
48. Malone, C. A. Child Psychiatry and Family Therapy: An Overview, *Journal of the American Academy of Child Psychiatry*, 18:4-21, Winter, 1979.

Chapter Eight

Special Perspectives on Treatment Planning for the Elderly

Sanford I. Finkel, M.D., Chairman
Elliott Stein, M.D.
Nancy Miller, Ph.D.
Ian Cameron, M.D.
S. Hontela, M.D.
Carl Eisdorfer, M.D.

Chapter submitted by the American Association for Geriatric Psychiatry

Introduction

Who are the elderly? The concept of old age has been significantly altered with time and cultural change. In 1883, German Chancellor Otto Von Bismarck introduced the concept of mandatory retirement, setting 65 as the age of retirement. At that time, approximately 2% of the American population was over the age of 65. In 1980, almost 100 years later, that figure was about 12% with the average expectable life span over 72 years. Moreover, the number and percentage of individuals in the older age range is expected to continue to grow as the average life span lengthens, increasing to 18-23% by the year 2030. In fact, the over-age-75 group is currently the fastest growing segment of the American population. Many factors have contributed to this trend, e.g., birth control, better living facilities, diet and other preventive approaches, and improved medical treatment and prolongation of life. Clearly, even the definition of old age is in flux.

The elderly are a heterogeneous group with marked variations in social status, living conditions, marital and family relationships, income, language, religion, physical functioning, health, occupational status, and interpersonal relationships. With such a diverse population, generalizations are often difficult and sometimes impossible.

The idea that old age is a time of passivity and helpless dependence is false. Old age can be an emotionally healthy and satisfying time of life that may be accompanied by a minimum of physical and mental impairment. There is no necessary parallel between chronological age and psychological state. Few people in Western culture think of old age as a time of potential health and growth, but the elderly have unique developmental work to do. This includes the process of clarifying, deepening, and finding useful what one has attained in a lifetime of learning and adapting; teaching and enhancing the development of younger generations; and developing a sense of self-integration, satisfaction, and completion.

Most Americans over 65 years of age are well-functioning individuals with little or no evidence of mental disorder. Although 86% of the elderly have one or more chronic health problems, 95% are able to live in the community. Their medical conditions are mild enough to enable 81% of them to get around with no outside assistance. They are, however, a high risk group psychiatrically, and a significant minority are likely to develop psychiatric symptoms or illness, either as a result of conditions of recent onset or as a result of longer standing problems. Compared to the rest of the population, the elderly have a high incidence of poverty, serious physical disease, loss of loved ones, and lowered social status. Moreover, older people are more apt to develop depressions, organic mental disorders (dementias), mental reactions as side effects of medicine, and certain paranoid reactions. Although comprising about 12% of the population, the elderly contribute approximately 20% of the nation's suicides. Psychosis increases after 65 with an additional increase after 75. Severe organic mental disorders afflict over one million elderly and appear in less severe forms in an additional two million older persons. Prevalence of depressive disorders in community-based elderly is at least 10%. It is likely that 15% to 25% of older persons demonstrate significant symptoms of mental illness. Because the fastest growing segment of the American population is the group over age 75, we can expect that the number of elderly with psychiatric illness will increase over the next decades.

Despite an increased risk for mental disorder, the elderly are consistently underserved by both private and public mental health sectors. Nationwide, only 4% of community mental health center patients are elderly. Private practitioners and clinics provide but 2% of their services for the elderly. In fact, less than 1.5% of patient care expenditures for mental illness are provided for older people residing in the community. Furthermore, 60% of those elderly who are admitted to state mental hospitals have received no previous psychiatric care, although appropriate outpatient psychiatric services may have prevented hospitalization for many.

These data are particularly disconcerting because the majority of these disorders (e.g., acute brain disorders, depressions, paranoid reactions) are reversible or treatable. Even patients with irreversible conditions, such as primary degenerative dementia of senile onset, can be helped emotionally and socially with proper intervention. Early diagnosis and treatment of these disorders can reduce their impact and delay or prevent a worsening of the condition. Milder conditions such as anxiety states or situational adjustment reactions are particularly amenable to short-term treatment with psychotherapy and chemotherapy.

Given the complexity and lack of homogeneity in the geriatric population, it is vital for the practitioner faced with a diagnostic question to have a broad perspective and a multiple systems approach. In order to construct an adequate and appropriate diagnostic formulation and to plan and institute treatment, the clinician must consider biological, social, medical, and psychological factors in defining the condition that is the focus of attention.

Biological Issues in Aging

In the biological sphere, physiological changes of advancing age should be differentiated from pathological changes. Aging is characterized by the progressive loss of physiologic capacities and functions. Physical strength and the "five senses" tend to decline in old age. Muscle, cartilage, and bone deteriorate as fibrous tissue replaces elastic and muscular tissue. Lung capacity is reduced. Speed of response and reaction time tend to be slower than those of younger people. The margin for stress and individual organ reserve capacity is reduced, and there is a reciprocal increase in healing time following insult. Other examples of age-related changes are the declines in myocardial, pulmonary, hepatic, renal, and endocrine capacities. Generally, each organ system has a diminished functional reserve; however, the distinction between age-related biological changes and specific diseases prevalent in late life is not always clear. For example, calcification of the arterial system is a linear function of age, beginning in early life and continuing to progress slowly. Nonetheless, it has been found that cerebral flow and oxygen consumption do not decline simply with this function of aging, but rather in proportion to the degree of actual cerebral vascular disease.

Many of the so-called "normal" changes of aging may have significant effects on the physical, psychological, and social functioning of the older individual. Appearance is one of the most obvious examples. The skin thins, generally becoming relatively dehydrated, and loses both strength and elasticity. A simultaneous loss of subcutaneous fat exaggerates the dermal changes to give a folded, lined, wrinkled, and lax appearance. The hair grays and thins out in most cases. Variations in pigment are not confined to the hair; the skin often gets darker in some areas as the melanocytes seem to lose the ability to spread out their melanin granules in an orderly fashion. The skin's sensory functions decline, requiring increasingly vigorous stimulation before touch is perceived, while because of social withdrawal and other reasons the elderly are less likely to be touched by others, compounding deprivation.

Visual changes are of great significance to older individuals. The cornea tends to flatten with age, giving rise to an accentuating astigmatism. Fatty deposits yellow the sclera. With increasing age, the ability to increase the thickness and curvature of the lens, in order to focus upon near objects, is gradually lost. This condition is called presbyopia and accounts for the need for corrective lenses for reading and bifocal additions in older people. Furthermore, lenticular yellowing results in a relative loss of ability to perceive colors of the yellow-blue spectrum and a significant reduction in the amount of light received by the retina. These facts, plus impaired after-dark adaptation and reduced pupiliary response to light and accommodation, have significant effects on the visual perceptions and activities of the elderly.[1] They may wear brighter clothes, have difficulty adjusting to the dark when entering movie theaters, and may stop reading.

Physical health, including nutritional status, as well as social status are affected by the functions of the oral cavity. The swallowing process, for example, is affected by the presence or absence of teeth, as is respiration. When many or all teeth are missing without functional replacements or dentures, speech becomes a difficult task that accentuates withdrawal. Too many older persons are labeled senescent and treated accordingly when their only difficulty is an inability to communicate. The aesthetic appearance of an older person is as important to him or her as it is to a younger individual. In the absence of teeth supporting the oral facial structure and the consequent development of an unflattering countenance, a person might not feel comfortable in the presence of family, friends, and others. Loss of taste buds results initially in a diminution of taste perception and frequently proceeds to appetite loss as well.[2] The loss of sweet taste perception occurs before loss of sour or bitter perception. This may lead to a loss of enjoyment in eating or, conversely, to an increased sugar intake with the possible increased tendency to, or exacerbation of, diabetes mellitus.

With age, the heart becomes a poorer pump as the loss of muscle fibers decreases both efficiency and the strength of myocardial contraction. The conduction system changes and other anatomic and biochemical alterations create a cardiopathy of aging. The peripheral vasculature undergoes change as connective tissue becomes less resilient in accommodating the wide changes in arterial pressure. Systolic blood pressure tends to rise, while diastolic blood pressure tends to remain constant or to fall. Postural dizziness with limitations of motion and increased risk for falling may result. Likewise, the elderly individual is subject to a host of pulmonary problems related not only to the biological process of aging, but also to prolonged exposure to a polluted urban and/or occupational environment.[3]

Of all body systems, the gastrointestinal tract most commonly causes chronic distress in the elderly. It may be difficult to distinguish between changes that are intrinsic and those that represent environmental effects acting over long periods. Over half of the complaints arising from this system, however, are of a functional nature without demonstrable organic basis. Such complaints often appear to be related to poor eating and bowel habits or to a preoccupation with food and elimination. In addition, many gastrointestinal complaints such as heartburn, alterations of appetite or weight, and constipation may result from treatment with psychotropic medications. It cannot be forgotten, though, that symptoms of functional distress often mimic those of organic disease, thus careful study to distinguish between these two is necessary. The ability of the gastrointestinal tract to absorb, and of the hepatic system to metabolize, psychoactive compounds is likewise an area of concern for those treating older individuals.[4]

The kidney is affected by involutionary processes with major changes beginning at about age forty. Tubular function appears to be compromised more than glomerular function. This is characteristically demonstrated by a reduced concentrating ability and may result in loss of the normal diurnal excretory pattern with the development of nocturia; however, one-third of patients 65 and older have glomerular and tubular function no different from that seen in younger people, and more than two-thirds exhibit normal glomerular function. These considerations are particularly important because when acute illness ensues, any pre-existing renal disease or advanced involutionary process will add to the diagnostic problems and worsen the prognosis.[5] Fluid and electrolyte balance is also affected by age. The total body water content diminishes significantly. Extracellular fluid volume, however, tends to remain constant and, therefore, constitutes a larger percentage of total body water. Sodium, potassium, chloride, bicarbonate, blood pH and pCO^2 levels are not significantly altered with age, though it may take the older individual significantly longer to correct any imbalance. Such factors become important when considering the use of lithium in an older patient. Likewise, potassium deficiency may be more readily seen in those older patients having common symptoms such as anorexia, vomiting, constipation, diuretic or laxative abuse, excessive sweating, or alterations of fluid intake.[6]

Conditions affecting the lower genito-urinary tract may be of great concern to the elderly. Some degree of prostatism is present in three-fourths of males 65 and over and symptoms such as urinary urgency, frequency, nocturia, or retention can be uncomfortable and anxiety-provoking.[7] Urinary tract and vaginal infections are common. Despite myths to the contrary, the elderly may be fully functional sexually to a late age, but a longer rebound period between erections for men and decreased vaginal lubrication for women may cause distress.

Laboratory data are commonly obtained when evaluating older individuals, but results should be considered in light of the patient's age. Although an older person's glucose tolerance test may show a diabetic-type curve, the patient may not necessarily present clinical evidence of diabetes. The blood urea nitrogen at age 30 to 40 averages 14 mg %; at age seventy it is typically 21 mg %. Glomerular filtration rate and renal plasma flow at age 80 are approximately 50% below the values found at age 20.[6] The serum alkaline phosphatase level in the elderly is often above the younger adult norm.[8] The laboratory and overall health status of the aged, therefore, should not be evaluated in terms of standards for the young adult. Many laboratory findings change with aging, and norms for the elderly are not established. If the standards for the young are considered the criteria for health, most of the aged would be considered ill. It is important that the practitioner does not assume that all elderly are ill and, conversely, does not assume that age alone accounts for all diagnostic findings in older persons.

Social and Environmental Issues in Aging

Demographic, ethnic, religious, cultural, and financial background are all influential in defining and moderating the older person's behavior. The structure and function of the family, as well as the extended network of friends, are factors in determining a person's adaptation to later life. The loss of important members of these support groups may be crucial. Perhaps more than any other support system, the marital relationship may play a decisive role in determining the capacity of the elderly individual to deal with stress; those who have effective and close marriages are less prone to adaptive failure.

Cultural patterns play a great role in determining variations in human behavior. Positive and negative views of older age have changed with differing cultural orientations. The current view of Western civilizations is markedly different from that of Oriental philosophies in which life, aging, and death are approached as part of the process of human experience. In the United States of 200 years ago, powdering the hair white in simulation of age was the height of fashion.

There are now approximately 25 million people over age 65 in the United States. Of these, approximately 45% are over age 75. There are 143 women for every 100 males over age 65, with the ratio changing from about 120 to 100 for ages 65 to 69 to more than 160 to 100 for age 85 and over.[9] Within these groups most older men are married, while two-thirds of the women are widows. Widows outnumber widowers three to one. The average life expectancy at birth for a woman is 74 years as compared to 67 years for a man. For someone who has survived to age 65, the average life expectancy for a woman is 83 years and for a man 78 years.

Racial and ethnic considerations reveal important differences. Although black Americans comprise 10% of the older age group, they only make up 8% of the older age group. The average life expectancy for black females is 67.5 years and for males 60 years. The trend for a shorter life expectancy reverses after the age of 75 when blacks have a greater life expectancy than whites. Approximately 4% of Hispanic Americans are elderly (except among Cuban-Americans where 8.6% are over 65). Estimated life expectancy for the Hispanic American population as a whole (approximately 57 years) is lower than for the general population. Among Asian Americans (including Chinese, Japanese, and Filipino groups), the elderly form 6-8% of their respective subgroups. Information concerning elderly homosexuals and other cultural or distinct subgroups is almost nonexistent.

Geographically, most elderly live in inner cities or rural locales, although there is a continuing trend towards movement of elderly to the Sun Belt states, and an increasing percentage in suburban areas. Of the 40% who live in rural areas, 35% are in small towns and 5% are on farms. Although this group may benefit from clean air, lack of congestion, and neighbors of long acquaintance, they may also suffer from lack of public transportation, fewer social security benefits, relatively higher taxes, and fewer governmental programs. Among older Americans, 67% live with family members, 26% live alone, 2% are living with nonrelatives in the community, and 5% live in chronic care settings. An estimated 30% live in substandard housing. Although two-thirds own their own homes, some of these have become substandard over time and the older individual may lack the funds to repair them.

Fifteen percent of their income comes from accumulated assets of some type, 29% from continuing employment, 46% from retirement programs, 6% from family contributions or veterans benefits, and 4% from public assistance. There are estimates that 16-25% of older individuals are below poverty levels. Of these, 85% are white, but a greater percentage of black elderly are poor, and elderly black females are the poorest of this group with an estimated 47% having incomes below $1,000 per year in 1970.[10]

There are many family and network concerns that affect the elderly. Losses are a particular stress for the elderly. Common losses include the growth and departure of children from the parental home; retirement; relocation to a retirement community; and illness or death of a still older parent, a spouse, a child, or ultimately one's self. These significant psychosocial stresses are frequent and may be implicated in precipitating psychiatric dysfunction. Ongoing work, continuing education, remarriages, and other continuing or evolving foci of interest may affect positively an older person's functioning and well-being.

Retirement is a common example of a potential stress for older individuals and their families. Some view it as the end of useful life, others as a relief from hard work, and some as a chance to do what they "have always wanted to do." Others begin second and even third careers, while some acquire part-time jobs. There are some indications that workers who take early retirement may be less capable of coping with it than they would at a later age.[11] Retirement may have several phases: an anticipatory or preparatory phase, the actual day of retirement, a period of working-through, and a state of adaptation. Individuals who leave a work place may have more difficulty adapting to this break in continuity than individuals, most frequently women, who have spent much of their time working in the home where constancy of environment is maintained. Furthermore, retirement may bring about a new marital situation in which spouses spend more time together than ever before. Some couples find this wonderful; others cannot tolerate it. Role definitions and role models become confused and altered, with adjustments and new interactional patterns developing.[12]

The elderly are frequently victims of crime, especially robbery. This makes them more fearful and withdrawn. Incidents occur in public housing complexes, public transportation, entry ways and laundry rooms of apartment buildings, and on the streets. Checks are stolen out of mail boxes, purses snatched. Perpetrators of the "battered older person syndrome" and crimes committed by relatives or landlords are rarely prosecuted.[13]

Another example of environmental stress is an elderly person's eventual move to an institution such as a boarding home, nursing home, or mental hospital. Often this is the ultimate outcome of a long series of problems. The aged individuals may deny the failure to function in the former environment. Furthermore, the individual's family may experience frustration regarding the older person's inability to cope with physical or mental problems. Irrational anger or guilt may result. The older individual may feel ambivalent, wishing to be close to and dependent upon adult children, then feeling guilt, or resentment, about this dependency.[14] Frequently, an older individual is sent to a retirement or nursing home without his or her knowledge, cooperation, or adequate preparation, e.g., when he or she is sent directly from an acute care hospital. There may be no chance to return home to collect belongings, to check the mail, or to say good-bye to friends or neighbors; there may be no opportunity to anticipate, work-through, or adapt to the demands or implications of this change. Many respond with panic, anger, depression, somatization, or complete withdrawal. Others, given adequate resources and preparation, can make a good adjustment.[15]

Culture shock in a changing technological society can also have a negative impact, as the individual feels isolated in an unfamiliar environment. There may be many benefits, however, that technology can offer the elderly. Emergency equipment, health monitoring devices, and advanced communications apparatus may be placed in an older individual's home. Micro-electronics are incorporated into hearing aids and pacemakers. The future may bring telephones with vision, the ability to shop or go to school from the home, and other techniques to make the home-bound more comfortable in the community for an extended period.

PSYCHOLOGICAL ISSUES IN AGING

Following Erikson's life cycle model, it is helpful to highlight some of the concerns of normal aging in later life.[16] The last three psychosocial states of this model (intimacy versus isolation, generativity versus self-absorption, and integrity versus despair) focus on the ongoing evolution of the psyche. Close affiliation with another individual and establishing patterns of cooperation and collaboration are stressed. Generativity refers to productivity through offspring, work, teaching, and altruism. It involves sustained responsibility for the growth and well-being of one's self and others. Having achieved occupational or avocational commitment and satisfaction, the older individual may serve as consultant or mentor to others, including a concern for preservation of society and culture in general, which may lead to the last developmental stage, integrity. Integrity is personal acceptance of one's self and the way one has lived life that engenders a sense of wisdom, integration, and completeness.

Achievement of this state presupposes successful passage through previous life phases.

Long-standing personality traits need to be differentiated from those of recent onset. Psychological traits developed in earlier years become altered, merging and blending with later traits. Failures in these three developmental phases of adult late years reflect the negative counterparts of these three phases: isolation, stagnation and self-absorption, and despair. These negative outcomes contribute to psychopathology.[17,18,19]

Butler described the important role that self-reflection and reminiscence plays in this developmental process.[20] The elderly person may achieve a constructive reintegration of past and present with acceptance of one's self through a progressive review of past experiences and previously unresolved conflicts.

Older age can be a time of increased awareness and enjoyment as the individual experiences a sense of immediacy that highlights rather than competes with continuity with the past. The reverse of this is disengagement leading to withdrawal and then despair.

Gerontophobia, the belief that aging is something to be feared, occurs as an outgrowth of some of these notions. While aging has been thought of as decline and deterioration, much of the fear generating this myth developed as a result of the distinctly human foreknowledge of one's own aging and eventual death. Also of importance in regard to this myth is the existence of gerontophobic attitudes on the part of some health professionals. Unresolved fears of aging and death may make it difficult for the professional to approach disorders of the aged with both enlightened detachment and compassion.

A myth that must be dispelled is that the elderly are unresponsive to psychiatric treatments. This has been repeatedly challenged and proven false, yet retains the credibility achieved during early psychoanalytic pronouncements that older individuals were not suitable candidates for psychoanalysis. This unsuitability was thought to be related both to an increased mental inflexibility and the volume of material to be analyzed. Not withstanding this, Freud himself remained vigorous, flexible, and creative until his death at age 83. Karl Abraham proved Freud's assertions to be false by successfully treating older individuals, as did followers of the Meyerian school. It is noted that psychiatrists frequently regard younger patients as having a better prognosis than older patients, and that treatment plans for elders are less likely to include psychotherapeutic treatment.[21] Nonetheless, successful treatment of the elderly may be obtained with various forms of therapy: traditional and nontraditional; supportive and insight oriented; psychodynamic; somatic; behavioral; and individual, family, and group treatments.

A common component of this myth is the idea that the primary psychiatric pathology seen in the elderly is related to the development of brain disease and dementia. While the development of various types of organic mental disorders can be an important event in the lives of some older individuals, it is not the most common type of psychiatric problem encountered in this age range. Depressions are the most common psychopathologic states. Adjustment disorders, interpersonal disorders, and personality disorders are common, as are neurotic and psychotic syndromes.

Affective disorders are by far the most common psychiatric impairments of elderly persons. Depression is often overlooked, with its symptoms being interpreted as manifestations of normal aging, as signs of incipient brain impairment, or as realistic responses to life stress, loss, or physical illness.

Results from incidence studies of depressive disorder in the elderly vary widely, largely because of the variable methodological criteria used to classify depressive phenomena in late life. Figures cited in the literature range from 10% to 65% for presence of affective disorder in older age groups. In studies based on *diagnoses* formulated by psychiatrists, clinical depression is most common between the ages of 25 and 65, while investigations using *self-report* indices find the highest rates of depressive symptomatology to occur in persons over the age of 65. These inconsistencies raise serious questions regarding the relative behavioral significance of symptoms versus syndromes, and of examiner ratings versus self-reports.

This concern is especially salient in view of the variety of depressive equivalents that are common in older persons. These are frequently overlooked by the examining clinician, because they differ from the clinical picture typically observed in young and middle-aged adults. The elderly, for example, may present less dramatically than their younger counterparts, tending to exhibit mood states characterized by apathy, emotional unresponsiveness, and inertia.

These behaviors often are simply attributed to the effects of advancing chronological age, rather than to depressive illness. Older individuals may not admit to the presence of depression itself, but rather to problems with somatic symptoms or to impairments in concentration, memory, and new learning. Accordingly, a more extensive exploration of mood state may be neglected by the clinician in favor of a diagnosis of physical disease or one of progressive organic brain disease. Alternatively, disproportionate responses to recent changes in life status, such as retirement with its attendant shift in economic and social roles, or bereavement, are commonly misconstrued as realistic reactions to normal age-linked developmental tasks. While neither retirement nor widowhood is associated with clinical depression in persons with stable histories of psychological adjustment, too often serious clinical responses to these precipitants go unacknowledged and untreated.

Reality factors often play a prominent part in the symptomatology presented by elderly persons. Although somatic complaints are significantly more common in elderly depressives than in younger depressives, well over 80% of all persons over 65 suffer from at least one or more chronic physical illnesses. At times it is difficult to determine whether the somatic complaint presented by an older patient is primarily physiologic or psychogenic in origin, or an interactive mixture of both. Psychiatric symptomatology and physical illness in older persons do not always follow a similar course. Even in the face of crippling somatic illness, depressive disorders in older persons can remit spontaneously or respond favorably to appropriate treatment. In other cases, even when the physical symptoms are alleviated or eradicated, serious and intractible mood disorder can continue. Whether or not an elderly person's somatic complaints appear to be hypochondriacal or physical, the mood state should be carefully evaluated for the presence of an affective disorder. Antidepressant treatment consistent with the patient's medical regimen and physical status should be vigorously pursued, even in the event of an *equivocal* diagnosis of mood disorder, given that elderly individuals with persistent complaints of physical pain and distress are at serious risk for suicide.

Other difficulties in the diagnosis of affective disorder in late life concern a relatively small proportion of elderly depressives who exhibit measurable memory defects and cognitive impairment and who often are mistakenly diagnosed as having a primary degenerative dementia. Approximately 15% of depressives aged 65 and over have been estimated to present with symptoms that mimic those seen in senile dementia of the Alzheimer's type. The clinical picture in "pseudodementia" may include disorientation for time and place, low scores and poor concentration on various standardized psychometric tests, and vague and/or inappropriate responses to interview questions. These patients are commonly misdiagnosed and, in the past, typically failed to receive appropriate treatment. At the height of the illness, *in the absence of other historical data* and having ruled out all other physical or mental derangement, it may be difficult to determine whether the patient is suffering from a dementing syndrome or an affective illness. In these cases, only the progressive or remitting course of illness will reveal the true nature of the disorder. If a psychiatric history is available, the suggestion of a relatively rapid onset, coupled with previous episodes of affective disorder, should lead to the possible consideration of a pseudodementia (depression). In addition, a family history of unipolar and/or bipolar illness, together with inconsistent cognitive impairment, would also contribute evidence for this diagnosis. Depressions in later life are often reversible with prompt and appropriate treatment. When in doubt, the depression should be aggressively treated.

Finally, mixed symptom pictures, reflecting the presence of both organic and functional syndromes, are commonly seen in the behavioral disorders of the senium. Depression, for example, may develop as an early secondary symptom of organic impairment and may exacerbate the performance decrement associated with altered brain function in later life. Elderly individuals with altered brain function and depression have been reported to be a high risk for suicide. Aggressive treatment of these "organic" depressions is also indicated.

The Examination of the Older Individual

What information is needed to evaluate and plan treatment for an older adult? The usual information needed in a psychiatric examination constitutes an integral part of the evaluation of the geriatric patient; however, in view of the alterations mentioned previously, certain facets of the evaluation must be highlighted, while other aspects must be weighed differently from those in younger people.

Beginning with the biological sphere, a medical history, physical examination, and certain laboratory tests are often essential. Prior general health status, illnesses, traumas, and allergies, as well as current illnesses and physical-medical problems, need to be evaluated. A number of medical conditions are commonly associated with such psychological symptoms as disorientation, depressive affect, lethargy, paranoid ideation, and psychomotor changes. Some of these medical conditions include: anemias, congestive heart failure, thyroid dysfunction, Parkinson's disease, diabetes mellitus, infections, vitamin deficiencies, cerebral vascular disorders, seizure disorders, tumors, and alterations in perceptive or sensory functions. Psychiatric symptoms may be the result of an illness (e.g., lethargy in hypothyroidism), a reaction to an illness (e.g., depression after a stroke), or a result of treatment for an illness (e.g., delirium caused by medication). Table 1 lists physical illnesses that can present with psychiatric symptoms.

EXAMPLE: PSYCHIATRIC SYMPTOMS PRECIPITATED BY MEDICAL ILLNESS:

Mrs. A, an 83-year-old woman, visits the doctor accompanied by her children with whom she is living. The children report a five-day history of increasing confusion and disorientation with paranoid ideation, complaining that her behavior has become difficult to control. They are concerned that she is "becoming senile." Physical evaluation reveals that she had a temperature of 101 degrees, and subsequent laboratory data revealed an increased white count. Chest X-ray demonstrates pneumonia for which she receives antibiotic therapy. Within four to five days her condition is much improved, although several weeks pass before her mental status returns to her premorbid level of functioning.

DX: AXIS I —Organic Mental Disorder—Delirium
AXIS II—Acute Pneumonitis

EXAMPLE: PSYCHIATRIC SYMPTOMS PRECIPITATED BY PRESCRIBED MEDICATION:

Mr. B is 74-years-old and living in a nursing home. He has a

TABLE 1
COMMONLY OCCURRING PRESENTATION OF SOME TREATABLE CONDITIONS[22]

Presentation	
Disturbed mental status	Hypoglycemia, myxedema, hypernatremia, hyponatremia, structural lesions of central nervous system (e.g., meningiomas), subdural hematoma, low pressure hydrocephalus, chemical intoxications, drugs (e.g., hypnotics, tranquilizers), vitamin B_{12} deficiency, uremia, hepatic encephalopathy, infections of central nervous system (e.g., tuberculosis, fungal infections, syphilis), fever from any cause.
Fatigue	Hyponatremia (e.g., adrenal insufficiency), inappropriate ADH syndrome, incipient heart failure, hypothyroidism, hyperthyroidism, chronic infection (e.g., chronic bronchitis, tuberculosis), hypokalemia (e.g., secondary to diuretics, ectopic ACTH syndrome), pulmonary emboli, malabsorption syndromes, bleeding from gastrointestinal tract, anemia from any cause, noncompliance.
Depression	Hypothyroidism, hyperthyroidism, hypercalcemia, drugs (hypnotics, tranquilizers).
Syncope	Structural lesions of central nervous system, seizure disorders, cerebrovascular disease, carotid artery syncope, hypoglycemia, hyponatremia, hypokalemia, paroxysmal rhythm disturbances (e.g., secondary to organic heart disease, drugs), gastrointestinal bleeding (e.g., secondary to peptic ulcer disease, carcinoma of ascending colon), hypovolemia (e.g., secondary to diuretic therapy).
Strikingly few manifestations	Sepsis, subacute bacterial endocarditis, pernicious anemia, heart failure, perforated viscus, pulmonary emboli, chronic renal failure depression.

history of severe cardiac illness, as well as hypertension, and receives multiple medications for each condition. After several months of satisfactory adjustment in the nursing home, he becomes increasingly withdrawn with periods of irritability. He has stopped participating in activities and "feels weak." Physical examination reveals no new symptoms. The laboratory data reveal that he has hypokalemia

(Serum Potassium = 2.4 mEq/1). One of his medications for controlling blood pressure has resulted in a loss of potassium and the subsequent development of both the physical and psychiatric symptoms. Potassium replacement results in significant improvement in less than a week, after which he returns to his prior level of functioning.

DX: AXIS II—Hypertension; Hypokalemia

A medication history should include both current and past medications, with notice taken both of the dosage and the frequency with which they were prescribed and the dosage and frequency with which the patient takes them. Favorable and adverse responses to medication, as well as failure to respond, must be investigated. In addition to prescription substances, use of nonprescription (over-the-counter) substances must be evaluated. The older person sometimes obtains these from friends and relatives or may use folk remedies. The elderly have a high per capita rate of medication consumption whether because of a search for the "Fountain of Youth," or as an attempt to alleviate symptoms and suffering, or to achieve improved functioning. Use or abuse of licit and illicit substances including alcohol also must not be overlooked.

EXAMPLE: PSYCHIATRIC SYMPTOMS PRECIPITATED BY UNPRESCRIBED MEDICATION

Mrs. C, a 57-year-old widow, is brought to the psychiatrist having been referred by her physician because she has been demonstrating "bizarre behavior." She has become very secretive and hears voices that instruct her to accumulate large amounts of newspaper and food. Her daughter is concerned that her apartment is becoming a public health hazard and does not understand what has been occurring with her mother. The daughter describes her mother as without psychiatric history, although she has been an anxious person who has had sleep difficulties on and off through the years. Mrs. C initially provides a history that was unremarkable except for the mental status symptoms described above. While questioning about medication, however, the psychiatrist discovers that she has been taking large amounts of bromide – containing sleeping medication purchased from a drug store. Mrs. C is suffering from bromide intoxication pre-

cipitating schizophrenic-like symptoms. Cessation of the medication during a brief hospitalization results in an improvement in her level of functioning.

DX: AXIS I—292.11 Substance (Bromide) Induced Delusional Disorder

Past treatment with psychotropic medications and responses to them is important information to obtain. Syncopal episodes or ataxia, for example, may occur secondary to benzodiazepine use. Tricyclic antidepressants may cause urinary retention or arrhythmias. Neuroleptics may cause dystonic reactions or tardive dyskinesia. The elderly are particularly susceptible to deleterious side effects.

Older persons are also at higher risk for developing psychoses secondary to anticholinergic medications. The clinician must be aware of which medications have anticholinergic effects, as well as the cumulative effects of several medications.

EXAMPLE: PSYCHIATRIC SYMPTOMS PRECIPITATED BY NONPRESCRIPTION MEDICATION

Miss D, a 75-year-old retired bookkeeper with a long history of recurrent depressive illness, comes to the hospital complaining of visions of rabbits and snakes in her apartment. She also complains of recent problems in waking, feelings of fatigue, and occasional urinary incontinence. These symptoms have occurred within the past few days. The patient's mental status is otherwise unremarkable. The patient takes amitriptyline 100 mg. b.s, Stelazine 5 mg. b.i.d., and Cogentin 1 mg. t.i.d. History reveals that she recently had a cold with a cough that caused insomnia. She had taken cold tablets and sleeping pills containing scopolamine. A diagnosis of anticholinergic psychosis is made, the symptoms of which disappear within two days after cessation of medications.

DX: AXIS I—292.12 Organic Disorder—Hallucinosis

While these patients used drugs excessively, other elderly patients may refuse helpful medications. They may have strong negative feelings about a particular medication based on personal experience or that of friends or relatives. They may be fearful of addiction, concerned about being "drugged," or anxious that medication may cause them physical harm. Refusal to take medication may be particularly problematic for those with depressive disorders. A characteristic sense of hopelessness may lead the depressive patient to believe that antidepressants cannot possibly benefit. This, in turn, leads to noncompliance.

A nutritional history is also very important, because psychiatric syndromes may be caused or exacerbated by dietary abnormalities. Essential questions should include: "How often do you eat?" "What do you eat?" "Do you take vitamins?" "Have you gained or lost weight?" "Can you afford a balanced diet?" "Are your teeth (or dentures) satisfactory for eating?" "Do foods taste differently?" "With whom do you eat?" "Does eating alone affect your food consumption?"

Nutritional requirements change with aging. Depressed mood, social withdrawal, and physical weakness may lead elderly individuals to eat poorly, to shop quickly, or to buy "instant" food, leading to poor nutritional intake. Demented patients may forget whether they have eaten or not. The elderly are also participants in food fads and may use dietary supplements, health food products, and vitamins in ways that may affect their health. Many medications cause gastrointestinal symptoms that can influence appetite. Symptoms such as constipation and diarrhea, which may appear to relate to psychiatric problems or treatment, may actually relate to dietary habits. Vitamin C may decrease the serum concentration of phenothiazines. Vitamin B_{12} deficiency secondary to anorexia may lead to confusion or other symptoms in patients with depression.[23] Insufficient calcium intake in elderly individuals may lead to psychological sequelae including psychosis.

The inclusion of appropriate laboratory data is important in a complete evaluation of an older individual, especially if a major psychiatric disorder is present. The differential diagnosis of many of the psychiatric disorders includes nonpsychiatric physical disorders. The likelihood of such an organic etiology markedly increases with age, and laboratory studies may be the only methods of differentiating these. The organic mental disorders are assumed in DSM-III to have specific etiologies. A diagnosis of primary degenerative dementia should be reached by exclusion only.

A standard work-up for organic mental disorders should include: urinalysis, a syphilis screen, a complete blood count, fasting blood

TABLE 2
ANCILLARY DIAGNOSTIC PROCEDURES FOR EVALUATING DEMENTIA BELIEVED DUE TO DIFFUSE BRAIN DISEASE

Test	Rationale
BLOOD TESTS	
Complete blood count	Anemia (megaloblastic or hypochronic), infection
Serological test for syphilis (STS)	Syphilis
Drug levels (barbiturates, bromides, etc.)	Drug intoxication
Electrolytes (sodium potassium, chloride, carbon dioxide, calcium)	Pulmonary dysfunction, renal dysfunction, endocrine dysfunction
Urea nitrogen	Renal dysfunction
Liver function tests (bilirubin, enzymes, ammonia)	Hepatic dysfunction
Serum thyroxine by column (CT4)	Thyroid dysfunction
Vitamin B_{12} and folate levels	Vitamin B_{12} and folate deficiency
URINALYSIS	Renal disease, hepatic disease
ELECTRO-ENCEPHALOGRAM	Unsuspected focal lesion or diffuse cerebral dysfunction
CHEST X-RAY	Infectious process, primary or metastatic tumor, chronic lung disease
SKULL X-RAY	Unsuspected focal lesion, pineal shift, evidence of increased intracranial pressure, disordered calcium metabolism
COMPUTERIZED AXIAL TOMOGRAPHY	Focal or diffuse cerebral atrophy, intracranial masses, hydrocephalus

BRAIN SCAN	Unsuspected focal lesion
ISOTOPE CISTERNOGRAPHY	Impaired spinal fluid flow and absorption
PSYCHOLOGICAL TESTING	Focal or diffuse cerebral dysfunction

sugar, folate and vitamin B_{12} levels, metabolic blood study batteries (including thyroid, hepatic, renal, and electrolyte studies), chest X-ray, electrocardiogram, and computerized axial tomography (CAT scan).

Although electroencephalography and computerized tomography of the head may be very valuable in diagnosing tumors, normal pressure hydrocephalus, or subdural hematoma, it should be noted that these are, to date, not reliable instruments for definitive diagnosis of primary degenerative dementia. It may be that the development of new instruments and/or the forthcoming positron emission transaxial tomography (P.E.T.T.) scanning may be helpful in this regard in the future. It is often possible to reach a specific diagnosis without performing all of these tests, but in some clinical situations it may be necessary to obtain a more extensive evaluation with appropriate medical and neurological consultation.

Other studies may be indicated prior to initiating certain treatments. For example, prior to administering lithium, assessment of cardiac, renal, and thyroid functions are essential. It should be noted that abnormalities are not necessarily contraindications to lithium use, but do require careful medical supervision.

Prior to electroconvulsive therapy, lumbosacral X-rays, electrocardiogram, and medical clearance are valuable. Similarly, cardiac, renal, genito-urinary, and thyroid functions; intraocular pressure; and blood pressure may be important to evaluate prior to psychopharmacologic treatment. For example, tricyclic antidepressants are often contraindicated in patients with narrow angle glaucoma or significant benign prostatic hypertrophy.

EXAMPLE: Depression Relieved by Medication

Mr. E presents with a classic picture of depression. He is 75 and complains of sleep disturbance with early morning awakening, anorexia, a feeling of hopelessness and pessimism about the future, and occasional tearfulness. He had a similar episode fifteen years ago that lasted for many months. He does not recollect the treatment he received at that time, although he remembers he was on medication that helped. No records were available. Although in need of pharmacologic treatment, Mr. E's history indicates marginal prostatic functioning. He has had urinary hesitancy over the past year and a half and, therefore, was followed carefully after administration of an antidepressant medication. After he developed increasing prostatism, the tricyclic antidepressant he was taking was replaced by another. He had not had such symptoms on that medication and made a subsequent good recovery from the depression without further side effects.

DX: Axis I—296.3x Major Depression, Recurrent, with Melancholia

When evaluating the psychological status of the older individual, a thorough psychiatric history is, of course, vital. Additionally, specific questions should ascertain: the person's prior experience of loss, including his or her reactions to these losses, and the adjustment to the aging of friends or relatives, e.g., how did parents age and what were their attitudes about their aging. Sexual history should be obtained routinely, including current sexual involvements, libido, and sexually-oriented interpersonal activity. The existence of environmental stresses (work, retirement, reaction to retirement, moving to a new residence, etc.) and the status of the individual's support systems (family, friends, religious institutions, community agencies, work, groups, etc.) are also important when evaluating an older patient. Relationships with grandchildren should also be explored.

Psychological testing is often a critical component of the evaluation process. Physicians most frequently call for psychometric evaluations in older patients when there is a serious diagnostic question involving the differentiation of dementia from depression. The problem of distinguishing organic from functional states in the elderly is one of the most complex in psychiatry. Symptoms of major affective disorders in late life often mimic those found in organically based dementias and, moreover, mixed symptom pictures, reflecting admixtures of both states, are commonly seen.

In the hands of a clinician skilled in using psychological tests with the elderly, these instruments can be effective in revealing the presence of serious deficits that are well compensated for on a social level or, alternatively, in highlighting the discrepancy between complaint about memory and actual memory performance. Psychological tests can reveal manifestations of cognitive disorders that are secondary to adaptational and emotional problems. Memory complaint, for example, is often exaggerated in the aged and is particularly related to the stereotyped distortion and pessimistic orientation commonly seen in senescent depressive states. The appropriate psychological tests can assist in demonstrating that, despite self-reports of serious forgetfulness, cognitive function may be within normal limits.

Psychological tests can also be exceptionally helpful in providing a baseline indication of the elderly person's performance at the height of illness, in assisting the physician to monitor systematically the fluctuations in the course of illness at multiple points in time, and in reflecting the effects of treatment.

In evaluating the test scores of elderly patients, it is particularly important to take into account the individual's social class, educational level, and degree of test sophistication. The individual's anxiety level, the presence of any visual or auditory deficits, and the nature of his or her interest and motivation may impair the patient's performance. Older persons are often more conservative and more easily fatigued in testing situations than are their younger counterparts, and they may also manifest far greater response variability.

To date, despite major experimental advances in the understanding of memory, the most frequently used clinical instrument for assessing the existence of diminished cognitive capacity in older persons remains the brief mental status type of examination. Many such measures have been designed for use with older populations, with names such as "The Mental Status Questionnaire (MSQ)," "The Short Portable Mental Status Questionnaire,"and others.[25,26] These instruments are objective, easily administered, and are valuable indicators in the differential diagnosis of organic from affective disorders in the elderly.

Such tests comprise relatively gross measures of cognitive function, however, and do not yield information regarding the precise locus of cognitive dysfunction, whether it be in the memory encoding system, in storage and retrieval, or in pattern recognition and sensory processing. While more innovative information processing approaches to the measurement of cognition have emerged in recent years, such measures have been used predominantly with young, healthy, well-motivated subjects in research settings. Few of these tests have been standardized on older persons with psychopathology. Norms remain largely unavailable so that the current clinical utility of these instruments remains problematic.

Many traditional omnibus test batteries (e.g., the Halstead-Reitan) have not been standardized on older populations, and in some instances, may misclassify normal older persons as demented.[27] False positive scores on psychological tests all too frequently lead to acceptance on the part of the clinician of a spurious organic diagnosis, thereby leading to therapeutic nihilism. Moreover, it has been demonstrated in the elderly that common clinical procedures such as the serial subtraction of 7s from 100, the ability to interpret proverbs, or to repeat digit spans or recall the contents of a paragraph in a newspaper story, are poorly related to brain function but strongly associated with level of education.

Of those individual measures that have proven most effective in differentiating organic from functional disorders in late life, the MSQ and the Face-Hand Test have been shown to be both valid and reliable.[25,29] Block Design tests are also useful and have age-based norms.[28] Tests like Trailmaking, the Benton Visual Retention Test, and Raven's Progressive Matrices have been used to good effect with older persons, as have the Graham-Kendell Memory for Designs and the Stroop Color-Word Interference Test.[30,31,32,33,34] The Modified Word Learning Test and Digit Copying Test have been used successfully in differentiating "pseudodemented" from "true" demented states.[35,36]

In conjunction with measures of cognition, it is also good practice when assessing an older person to evaluate his or her functional capacity for carrying out the necessary activities of self-care in daily living. The Activities of Daily Living Scale is useful for this purpose, as is the Comprehensive Assessment and Referral Evaluation instrument (CARE), a semistructured interview specifically keyed to the elderly that includes psychiatric, medical, nutritional, economic, and social items, and yields reliable psychiatric diagnoses.[37,38] The battery has been standardized on both normal subjects and psychiatric patients. The appropriate psychological tests, when used with knowledge and sensitivity, can provide the examining physician with useful clinical data to assist with treatment decisions.

The Kahn-Goldfarb Questionnaire may easily be administered by nonphysician staff who should, however, be trained to weave it into a conversational framework. Scores of 0 to 3 are generally consistent with a severe degree of dementia, 3 to 6 generally consistent with a moderate degree of dementia, and a score of 7 out of 10 or better, mild to minimal dementia.

Key family members, friends, neighbors, or other supporters may be able to offer valuable details of the patient's history and mental status and offer a perspective of changes over time that can aid in making a diagnosis. When making these collateral contacts, information must be obtained and observations made with the awareness that the illness of the identified patient may have major effects on these supporters and, in turn, the patient's network also has significant impact on the patient. Differing perceptions are likely and distortions may occur.

As mentioned previously, psychosocial factors are an integral part of the evaluation of the geriatric patient. These range from place and circumstances of birth through family background, parent and sibling interactions, schooling, psychosexual and psychosocial development, education, military history, occupational history, avocational history and leisure interests, interpersosnal relationships, marital and family history, ethnic-cultural background, past and present residential locations, and the existence or absence of friends and other interpersonal contacts.

Other Clinical Considerations and Data Needed in Establishing Diagnosis and Treatment Planning

PRIMARY DEGENERATIVE DEMENTIA

In arriving at a diagnosis of Primary Degenerative Dementia, it must again be emphasized that only 55% of patients with dementia will eventually prove to have the irreversible, progressive dementia

TABLE 3
A COMPARISON OF THE MSQ AND SIMILAR SCALES

Mental Status Qustionnaire (MSQ)	Disorientation Factor from a Dementia Rating Scale	Short Portable Mental Status Questionnaire (SPMSQ)	The Orientation TEST	A Simplified MSQ	An Abbreviated Mental Test Score	Clifton Assessment Schedule: Inf/ Orien Sect
			Common Items			
1. What is the name of this place?	Where are you now? Are you in a school, a church, a hospital, or a house?	What is the name of this place?	What is the name of this place? What is the name of the ward you are on?	What is the name of this place?	Name of hospital	Hospital/Address Ward/Place?
2. Where is it located? (address)		What is your street address? OR: What is your telephone number?				
3. What is to-day's date?	What is the day of the week?	What is the date today? What day of the week is it?	What day is it?	What day is it?		Day?
4. What is the month now?	What is the month?		What month is it?	What month is it?		Month?
5. What is the year?	What is the year?		What year is it?	What year is it?	Year?	Year?
6. How old are you now?	Disorientation to age (error of at least 5 years)	How old are you?	How old are you?	What age are you? (error more than 1 year)	Age?	Age?
7. When were you born (month)?		When were you born? Month Day Year		In what month is your birthday?	Date of birth?	Date of birth?
8. When were you born (year)?				In what year were you born?		

9. Who is the President of the United States? 10. Who was the President before him?		Who is the President of the United States now? Who was the President before him?			Name of present monarch?	Prime Minister? U.S. President?
Items not Held in Common						
	What is the time of day (morning, afternoon, or evening)? Inability to find bathroom Wandering Disorientation to people: inability to distinguish patients from staff	What was your mother's maiden name? Subtract 3 from 20 and keep subtracting 3 from each new number all the way down	What time is it? What were you doing before coming to this room? What is my name? (as given at beginning of the interview) What did you have for breakfast/lunch? When did you last have a visitor?	What time is it? (error more than 1 hour) How long have you been here? (error more than 25%)	Time to nearest hour? Address given and recall at end of test Year of 1st World War Count backwards 20-1 Recognition of two persons	Name? Color of British Flag?
Authors						
Kahn, R. *et al.* (1951) Kahn, R. *et al.* (1960)	Lawson, J. S. *et al.* (1977)	Pfeiffer, E. (1975)	Irving, G. *et al.* (1970)	Isaacs, B., & Walkey, F. (1963)	Hodkinson, H. *et al.* (1972)	Patte, A. H., and Gilland, C. J. (1975)

implied in this diagnostic category. Even if the history seems consistent, a standard dementia workup should be pursued. As many as 15% of apparent dementias first presenting to a physician will be depressive pseudodementias. Careful screening for vegetative depressive symptoms is important.

Many patients with Primary Degenerative Dementia have no evidence of other emotional or mental disturbance. They present affably and seem either unaware of or unconcerned about their deficit. Others are concerned that their condition will be obvious to others and, therefore, may withdraw socially, avoiding contact with anyone except immediate family members.

EXAMPLE 1: PRIMARY DEGENERATIVE DEMENTIA

Mrs. E, a 70-year-old woman, is accompanied by her brother and sister. They complain that she has been intermittently forgetful over a period of several years. Over the last few months, the forgetfulness has been accentuated. She has wandered off on several occasions and was brought home by the police. Sometimes she talks about the past, but seems to lose track of time and talks about her children as if they were grandchildren. Recently, she has become agitated at home and on one occasion she actually pushed her sister who was trying to calm her down. Following these episodes she feels ashamed, cries, and refuses to talk about them. Most of the time, however, she sits quietly or sleeps. There is no history of psychiatric illness or previous maladaptive behavior. She was very reluctant to come to see a physician. In the office, she tries to present a pleasant facade. She is a neat-looking woman, appearing her age. She smiles, but seems anxious to leave from the time she arrived. She seems to experience the interviewer as being threatening, saying, "Well, I guess that's all we can do." and started getting up to leave. Frequent reassurance is necessary to keep her sitting for the interview. She is guarded and answers questions evasively. There is no evidence of hallucinations, delusions, or sleep or appetite disorders; however, the tension evident during the interview suggests significant anxiety. On mental status testing, she displays impairment in memory. She is able to recall only one of three objects after five minutes and has difficulty recalling what she had for breakfast that morning. She scores five out of ten on the MSQ and that was obtained with much difficulty. The extent to which anxiety impaired her cognitive functioning during the interview was not possible to determine.

DX: AXIS I —1) 290.00 Primary Degenerative Dementia, Senile Onset, Uncomplicated
2) 309.24 Adjustment Disorder with Anxious Mood
AXIS IV—Code 4—Moderate Severity
AXIS V —Level 4—Fair

Many others with this condition have accompanying mental disorders. Severe anxiety, even panic, may occur, particularly during the early phases. The patient may express the fear of dying. Paranoid reactions are also seen. The most common accompanying disorder is probably depression. One investigator states that 25% of all patients with primary degenerative dementia have concomitant depressive disorders.[24] Suicide ideation and intent can be intense, particularly in the earlier phases.

EXAMPLE 2: PRIMARY DEGENERATIVE DEMENTIA

Mrs. F, a 75-year-old woman, is accompanied by her daughter. She took an overdose of medication a short while back and had been briefly hospitalized. She explicitly stated afterward that she wanted to kill herself, though she experiences much shame at her attempt and much embarrassment about the fact that she did not succeed.

Her history indicates that she has been a well-adjusted person, though "a worrier" most of her life. She had no prior history of psychiatric treatment. Two years prior to her suicide attempt, her husband died suddenly. She had been extremely close to him and had admired him greatly. She went into a long and profound period of mourning that lasted over a year, after which time she came to live with her daughter in another city. At that time, she was both feeling and functioning at a good level. Since the geographic move, however, she has become forgetful, and on one occasion had accidentally set a fire in her apartment by leaving a pot on the stove too long. She has a history of many interests in the arts and, in fact, was an author and had taught school. Recently, however, she complains that she has little interest or motivation to continue her educational pursuits and spends a good deal of her day crying.

Mental status evaluation reveals a woman in much psychological pain who appears her stated age. She cries and yet seems to reach out to the interviewer in a state of desperation. She indicates that she is no longer sleeping well, but she cannot recall just when she rises and goes to sleep. She realizes that she has lost much weight, her clothes are obviously too big for her. She expresses pessimism about the future and indicates that her situation is hopeless. Mental status evaluation reveals that she is person-oriented. She is able to remember the year, but not the day or the date. There is also disorientation to place. She scores a 5 on the Kahn-Goldfarb scale.[25] *There is no evidence of hallucinations or delusions. She indicates that although she probably will not try to kill herself again, she wishes to be dead and has strong impulses to commit another act of self-violence.*

DX: AXIS I —1) 296.2x Major Depression, Single Episode
2) 290.00 Primary Degenerative Dementia, Senile Onset
AXIS II —No Diagnosis, anxious and histrionic personality traits
AXIS IV—Code 5, Severe
AXIS V —Level 6, Very Poor

Although DSM-III does not indicate levels of severity of dementias, this patient's dementia is thought to be of moderate severity; however, full evaluation of this important feature must await treatment of her depression with subsequent assessment of the residual deficits.

The clinician is alerted, nevertheless, to the importance of rating severity. This may have very practical implications. For example, a patient who has mild, irreversible dementia might be capable of carefully structured independent living, whereas a patient with a severe level dementia would not.

SCHIZOPHRENIA

Onset of schizophrenia in late life is virtually nonexistent. Though a few persons with schizophrenia continue to have severe psychosis periodically, most individuals with long histories of schizophrenia show decreased symptoms as they age. Affective withdrawal, however, may increase. The elderly schizophrenic person is most likely socially isolated and/or markedly dependent. Development of new symptoms, though, is rare, and the need for psychiatric hospitalization is markedly reduced.

In late life, the boundaries between schizophrenic subgroups tend to diminish or vanish. Elderly people with schizophrenia are, however, at slightly greater risk for developing senile dementia of the Alzheimer's type.

A special problem of elderly schizophrenics is the high risk of developing tardive dyskinesia as well as a poorer prognosis for eventual remission. The aging brain has an increased likelihood of developing neuroleptic-related tardive dyskinesia. Thus, such medications must be avoided except when absolutely necessary.

EXAMPLE: SCHIZOPHRENIA

Mr. G, a 74-year-old male, spent over 30 years in a state psychiatric facility. He had his first psychotic episode at age 21, and over the next decade had several hospitalizations of from three to fifteen months duration. Subsequently, he had several longer hospitalizations, but was discharged from the state facility over fifteen years ago and has not been rehospitalized since that time. He has been living in the community and goes to senior activities several hours each morning, occasionally playing some cards or watching others play. He has almost no social contacts and eats all meals alone. Afternoons and evenings are spent in his room watching television or listening to the radio. He complains of a tightness in his head with voices telling him that he is no good. Sometimes the voice tells him that he is weak and sexually inadequate. Much of his energy is used fighting the voices, trying to still them. At the local community mental health center he is seen monthly to receive his neuroleptic medication. There is no meaningful family contact, and he has no aspirations or motivation to change his current life situation.

DX: AXIS I —295.62 Schizophrenia Residual Type, Chronic
AXIS IV—Code 2, Minimal
AXIS V —Level 5, Poor

PARANOID DISORDERS

Paranoid disorders occur not uncommonly in later life. Acute paranoid disorders in the elderly are more apt to occur in people who are deaf, have had a sudden loss of vision, or are socially isolated. Such disorders also occur in people with underlying acute and chronic depressions and in people with dementias. The latter conditions may not be apparent during the initial evaluation and, in fact, may not clearly emerge until after the paranoid disorder is successfully treated. Some authorities view the paranoid disorder as a defense against underlying depression, whereas others postulate a biochemical and neurophysiological response to stress as the etiology.

On occasion, the elderly person with an acute paranoid disorder may, in the course of treatment, develop a "benign paranoia" in which everyone or almost everyone in the environment is idealized or considered a friend or benefactor.

A paranoid disorder described in DSM-III as "paraphrenia" (sometimes referred to as "late life schizophrenia") is characterized by delusions of persecution, panic attacks, hallucinations (usually auditory), and feelings of passivity that alternate with feelings of hostility and aggression. Orientation is intact and incoherence or looseness of associations is *not* present.

This type of paranoid disorder, described in DSM-III as Paranoia, occurs more commonly in women. There is usually a one- to two-year period of social isolation during which there is an increase in eccentricity and suspiciousness. As the syndrome develops, there is an increasing hostility accompanied by accusations toward others, particularly neighbors, landlords, and young boys. The person believes these individuals are engaged in hostile or illicit activities—such as stealing, drugging or poisoning, being sexually insulting, ridiculing, or trying to influence or control the person's thoughts. Emotional response is usually anger and severe anxiety. Likely behavioral responses include calling the police, suing the alleged aggressor, and complaining to politicians. Despite the intense and often widespread delusional symptoms, such people often develop trusting relationships with one or more persons.

EXAMPLE: Paranoia

Mr. H, a 92-year-old white male, lives alone in a retirement community. He has been widowed for 23 years. He comes to a mental health center, having been referred for "assistance with his problem." His desire is to have the psychiatrist ask the police to have people stop following him. He reports that for the past eight months, since he moved to his new apartment, he has noted people observing and following him. These people include police, neighbors, boys on the street, and the shopkeepers around the corner from his apartment. He is moderately anxious and insistent that the psychiatrist cooperate with his desire to contact the police. The patient is articulate, verbal, intelligent, and denies any hallucinations. He has excellent physical health and denies depression, sleep disturbance, appetite disturbance, or alterations of his daily habits, except insofar as he avoids the people who are watching and following him. He becomes agitated when it is suggested that these symptoms might be of psychogenic etiology. The patient has lived alone for the past 23 years and moved to a new apartment eight months ago when his rent was raised. His time is occupied attending religious services, reading, and painting. He has mild cataract disease, an arrhythmia that is currently under good control with medication, and reports occasional heartburn.

The mental status reveals that the patient, a tall, thin, man with a full, long white beard, is oriented to person, place, and time. His associations are goal-directed. He is verbal and moderately cooperative, and his speech is articulate. He is anxious, but denies depression, hallucinations, delusions, and suicidal ideation. His memory is very good. His intellectual functions, insight, and judgment are good, except as regards his delusional system.

DX: AXIS I —297.10 Paranoia
AXIS IV—Code 4, Moderate
AXIS V —Level 2, Very Good

DRUG ABUSE

The elderly are believed to abuse opioids, amphetamines, and cannabis rarely. Abuse of barbiturates and other hypnotics, however, occurs more commonly. Barbiturate abuse should be suspected in an older person who experiences periodic dizziness, falls, and has symptoms of delirium and/or periodic apathy and withdrawal, alternating with intervals without apparent psychiatric symptoms.

Older persons are more apt to abuse laxatives, analgesics (particularly aspirin-containing compounds), and over-the-counter medications, including antihistamines, anticholinergic agents, and bromide compounds. Recent reports of benzodiazepine abuse characterized by confusion, dizziness, and ataxia have been reported. This drug may cause delirium or organic delusional syndrome. It is not clear to what extent such abuse is volitional and to what extent it results from failure to understand the physician's instructions.

EXAMPLE: SUBSTANCE USE DISORDER

Mrs. I is a 78-year-old childless widow residing alone in her own home. For the past year she has become progressively more isolated, rarely going out, and spending her time reading and watching television. Several of her friends have found her to be irritable, though on other occasions she has been sociable. She has been hospitalized twice following falls during the past year. On one occasion she called a friend who took her to the emergency room and she was subsequently hospitalized. During that time the patient was agitated, confused, and had difficulties with balance. On another occasion she lay on the floor of her apartment for almost twenty-four hours before she called a friend for help. During each hospitalization, her physical condition was found to be unremarkable except for some long-standing evidence of rheumatoid arthritis. She was seen in a psychiatric consultation during her second hospitalization. The history reveals no other complaints except for her difficulty sleeping in recent years. She admits to taking sleeping medication as well as her antiarthritic medication. Originally, she took 100 mg. of secobarbital and found that effective. Subsequently, she began using several pills during the night with usage extended into the day. She admits taking as many as eight a day, though she vigorously denied that this had anything to do with her falls, agitation, or isolation. Mental status evaluation was within normal limits at the time of the evaluation.

DX: AXIS I —305.41 Substance Use Disorder: Barbiturate Abuse

AXIS II —Rheumatoid Arthritis

AXIS IV—Code 1, None

AXIS V —Level 4, Fair

It needs be pointed out that some elderly persons are fearful of addiction or habituation to medication and, thus, may not take medication in proper dosage.

Alcohol abuse affects close to 10% of the elderly population. Rates are higher among widowers, individuals with medical problems, and those in difficulty with the police. The combination of alcohol abuse, depression, and/or divorce is correlated strongly with suicide. Studies indicate that 12% of all elderly patients admitted to psychiatric hospitals, and 20% of all elderly patients admitted to general hospitals have alcoholic problems.[40] Eighty percent of all arrests of people over age 60 is for drunkenness.

PSYCHOSEXUAL DISORDERS

For many elderly persons sexual interest and activity are satisfactorily sustained. Crucial variables are the availability of a stimulating partner, a history of prior enjoyment of sexual activity, and the absence of a disabling illness. Nevertheless, psychosexual disorders such as inhibited sexual desire, inhibited sexual excitement, inhibited male orgasm, and functional dyspareunia are thought to occur more frequently in later life.

Changes in sexual attitudes with aging can be expected to result in more individual expression and variations from the norm. For some people, this will precipitate conflict, and the frequency of sexual dysfunctions seen in later life may increase.

Inasmuch as certain major and minor tranquilizers, antidepressants, and antihypertension medications have been shown to decrease libido and cause impotence, it is particularly important to review current medications.

Disfiguring surgery, such as mastectomy or colostomy, may precipitate a psychosexual dysfunction. Inhibited sexual excitement following prostatectomy is also believed to be psychogenic in origin.

The concept of disuse as a contributing factor is helpful. For example, widows and widowers without a history of sexual dysfunction may develop such a condition when they encounter a new sexual partner after a period of abstinence. Women who have not engaged in sexual activity for several months may initially have decreased vaginal secretion and, thus, experience dyspareunia.

Some patients with dementias experience decreased sexual inhibitions. For a small percentage of demented elderly males, this may result in socially prohibited sexual activity such as exposure of genitals or making overt sexual advances in public. Such individuals may have higher than normal levels of testosterone.

EXAMPLE: PSYCHOSEXUAL DISORDER

Mr. J is a divorced 66-year-old father of two who presents with a chief complaint of impotence that began approximately four months ago after he was rejected by his latest girlfriend, a 26-year-old actress. He had been the vice president of a small corporation until approximately one year ago at which time the company was bought by a larger company and he was fired. Though he has obtained new employment, he has less responsibility and authority. He spoke in an angry, depreciating way about both his current and past employers, and his rage dominated much of the interview. He continued to talk at some length about the many things he accomplished in work that were never appreciated and felt that he should have been president of his previous corporation. He said that his current position was limited by the "petty politics" of others which, in turn, did not allow him to fully demonstrate his abilities.

He had married a "competent" businesswoman in her mid-twenties and subsequently had two children. He divorced after twenty years "because my wife got wrinkly" and because he felt it was time to have a younger woman. Subsequently, he has had many affairs and a few relationships that lasted two or three years, each terminating when he found fault with each partner. He says that they loved him but were deficient either in sensitivity, intelligence, or common sense. Because of his dynamism and intelligence, he has always been able to attract beautiful women. Six months ago he met an actress with whom he quickly became involved. He thought the relationship was proceeding well until she told him that she was in love with another man and was leaving him. It was after this experience that he began having difficulty in attaining erection with most women. Over the last several months, he has been unable to attain and maintain an erection sufficiently to culminate in intercourse. He has had a physical evaluation because he thought the cause might be cardiovascular, indicating that he had had a "mild" heart attack twelve years ago.

Though he has always enjoyed social drinking, for the past two months he has been drinking more heavily, up to a pint of Scotch a day. He has had several minor accidents and, currently, his driver's license has been suspended. He has also missed some work and has been "taking flak from his boss" for not meeting certain deadlines. He feels that his boss is unreasonable and should appreciate having a man of his competence working for him.

DX: AXIS I —1) 302.72 Psychosexual Disorder—Inhibited Sexual Excitement
2) 305.00 Substance Use Disorder—Alcohol Abuse

AXIS II —301.81 Personality Disorder, Narcissistic Personality Disorder

AXIS III—Status, Post-myocardial Infarction by History

AXIS IV —Code 4, Moderate, New Job, Rejection by Girlfriend

AXIS V —Level 4, Fair

EXAMPLE: SOMATOFORM DISORDER

Mrs. K, a 72-year-old woman, has been widowed for 14 years. She had a son and a daughter, but six months ago her son suddenly died of a heart attack. Since that time she has been sobbing and bitter and has withdrawn from many of her activities and friends. For the past three months she has complained of a variety of somatic symptoms, particularly severe abdominal pain that she feels interferes with her ability to participate in activities or be with people. She also complains of "gas," diarrhea, nausea, feeling faint, headaches, and weakness. Nevertheless, she claims her sleep has been satisfactory and her appetite and weight have remained stable. Though she states much concern about her current symptoms, she denies feeling hopeless and having suicidal ideation. She admits to much pain about the loss of her son, but believes it is not related to her physical complaints. Rather, she is concerned that she may have a serious physical illness; she has been seen by several primary care physicians and has had multiple diagnostic procedures. Though she has been assured that she has no serious physical disorder, she is reluctant to accept this because "the pain is too great—there must be something wrong."

Mrs. K is the eldest of six children and had significant responsibilities for the care of her siblings. She states emphatically that she began working in her early teens to help support the financially stressed family. She has always been hard-working and hard-driving

and realizes that she is a perfectionist. All who know her describe her as the perfect housekeeper and cook. She is active in a number of civic and religious organizations and has been the president of several. Although she maintains contact with her daughter and daughter-in-law, they both have described her through the years as being distant and more interested in her activities than in her children and grandchildren. The daughter-in-law, in particular, has been critical about her relationship with her son and Mrs. K's tendency to be "controlling."

Mental status evaluation reveals a slightly obese, impeccably dressed woman who appears younger than her stated age. She was poised and sociable for the most part, although on several occasions she would double over in pain and complain of her terrible "stomach problems." She would ask, even plead, for help. Though she believed there was no psychological component to her illness, she was willing to see a psychiatrist because, "I'll see anybody who thinks they can help me—I know there's something seriously wrong." Medical history revealed a hysterectomy 30 years ago and the diagnosis of peptic ulcer disease 35 years ago. She indicates that her recent X-rays reveal evidence of a healed ulcer.

DX: AXIS I —300.70 Somatoform Disorder; Hypochondriasis
AXIS II —301.40 Compulsive Personality Disorder
AXIS III—History of peptic ulcer disease
AXIS IV—Code 6, *Extreme*, Death of son
AXIS V —Level 5, 2, Very Good

ADJUSTMENT DISORDERS

Adjustment disorders are common among the elderly. This is easily understood given awareness of two basic facts: the elderly are subjected to a relatively high number of psychosocial stressors and the normal, usual, and accustomed methods by which the elderly have previously handled these stressors are more likely to be impaired.

As mentioned previously, the stressors include deaths, illnesses, retirement, relocation, intra- and extrafamilial relationship problems, and alterations of self and object perceptions and representations. The stressors most common to the aged strike at those aspects of the self and the support systems most crucial for coping. The spouse one depended upon may be either dependent or gone; the job that defined one's status, productivity, and goals, and around which time was structured, may be finished; and the helpful friends, relatives, and organizations may have been left behind in another location. A fixed income can deprive many elderly persons of previously enjoyed compensating pleasures.

EXAMPLE: ADJUSTMENT DISORDER

Mr. L is a retired seventy-year-old lawyer who was successful in his work. Six weeks ago he had a mild myocardial infarction and was recently discharged from the hospital. He had been started on several cardiac medications, but is extremely anxious, pacing the floor, and worrying about the future. He is hesitant about going out for fear that he will have another heart attack and states that he will never have sexual contact again to avoid the possibility of recurrent heart problems. Previously he had adjusted well to retirement and had been active with his family, friends, and hobbies. He had never been sick a day in his life, and was unaccustomed to being slowed down.

DX: AXIS I —309.24 Adjustment Disorder with anxious mood
AXIS II —Cardiovascular Disease, Arteriolsclerosis
AXIS IV—Code 5, Severe Physical Illness
AXIS V —Level 1, Superior

ANXIETY DISORDERS

Anxiety disorders occur in later life under a variety of conditions. For some, the loss of mastery and control over the environment leads to feelings of inadequacy and shame which, in turn, lead to the physical symptoms and/or constriction of functioning characteristic of anxiety. For others, overwhelming environmental stress precipitates an anxiety disorder. Still others experience an important loss of external supplies leaving them feeling abandoned, undernurtured, and depleted.

EXAMPLE: ANXIETY DISORDER

Mrs. K, a 66-year-old mother of two, was widowed approximately one year ago. She is brought in by her daughter who is concerned about her mother's withdrawal and is afraid to leave her alone.

Mrs. K is described as having been passive in relation to her dominant husband. The two daughters were often upset about their father's domination and criticism of mother, but she never protested. When father fell ill of cancer two years ago, mother cared for him selflessly and continued to serve him until his death. She had met him when she was seventeen and married him six months later. She had neither worked nor finished high school and is described as a loving but weak mother who had difficulty clearly defining for her daughters their roles as young women. Though they depend on her love and affection, the daughters do not value her advice. Since her husband's death, she has stayed at home, suffering chest pains, dyspnea, and headaches whenever pressed to leave. Though she is quite willing to see her daughters and grandchildren in her own home, she refuses steadfastly to come to her daughters' homes. In fact, she has her groceries delivered and has refused to see her physicians.

Mrs. K appears anxious, indicating immediately that she was willing to be seen by a physician, but it would be necessary in the future to see her in her own home. Nevertheless, she was able to give a history and seemed quite anxious to please. Other than the anxiety and a significant constriction of interests, the mental status evaluation was unremarkable. She describes no medical disorder, other than periods of hypertension that are controlled with medication. At the time of examination, she was on no medication and her blood pressure was 160 over 95.

DX: AXIS I —300.23 Anxiety Disorder, Social Phobia
AXIS II —301.60 Personality Disorder, Dependent Personality Disorder
AXIS III—Essential Hypertension
AXIS IV—Code 5, *Severe*, Loss of Spouse
AXIS V —Level 5, Poor

DEPRESSION

Depression may underlie other psychiatric disorders such as paranoia, substance abuse, and hypochondria, but may emerge in an identifiable way only when the other conditions are under control. It is important to avoid a diagnosis of depression when depressive symptoms appear immediately following a profound loss. Grief reactions (mourning) are a normal part of later life with losses of people, objects, and social roles. If the intensity or duration of such grief is particularly great, the possibility of a depression must be considered. The differentiation between bipolar and unipolar depression is particularly important, inasmuch as treatment may be different for each syndrome. The following contrasts may be noted: unipolar depression has a median age of onset of 60 years, bipolar at age 24; approximately two-thirds of all unipolar depression occurs in women; bipolar depressions are more evenly distributed, and the bipolar patients are more prone to develop hypomanic and manic episodes in response to somatic therapies.

EXAMPLE: Depressive Illness

A 72-year-old retired hypertensive businessman presented with complaints of loss of interest in the stock market, hobbies, and his wife over a period of six weeks. He acknowledges periods of profound sadness, reduced appetite with significant weight loss, insomnia, fatigue, decreased libido, and recurrent thoughts of death without, however, suicidal ideation. He describes himself as usually serious and conservative, and relatively unable to express affection. He tries to be perfect and to control social situations. In the past he had an excessive commitment to work. Since retirement, he has continued an active involvement in his financial interests and in civic activities.

He indicates that his marriage has been worsening for several years, describing his wife as flighty, over-emotional, and helpless under stress. For the past several years she has been angry, distant, and has declined to be sexually involved with him. This change has occurred since his retirement and his increased time at home. Since the onset of his symptoms, however, she has been solicitous and obviously concerned. The couple has one son who is a successful businessman; the patient's relationship with him is distant.

The patient describes his family of origin as very poor. His father deserted his mother when the patient was 12 years of age when, as the oldest child, he had to take considerable responsibility for younger siblings as well as to work part-time while attending school. The patient's father died at age 72 of a stroke, his maternal grandfather had committed suicide, and two maternal uncles were alcoholics. A paternal uncle died in prison after a long period of antisocial behavior. The patient uses alcohol socially.

Physical, laboratory, and neurological studies were negative. The patient's hypertension is being treated with alethyldopa (Aldomet).

After two evaluation interviews, the attending psychiatrist arrived at the following DSM-III diagnosis:

DX: AXIS I —296.22 Major Depressive Episode
AXIS II —301.40 Personality Disorder, Compulsive
AXIS III—Hypertension
R/O Depression secondary to Aldomet
R/O Sexual dysfunction secondary to Aldomet
AXIS IV—Code 4, Moderate psychosocial stress, marital
AXIS V —Level 4, Fair level of prior adaptive functioning

Treatment Considerations

The geriatric practitioner must be flexible and varied in approach. With the enormity of individual variation seen in later life, the therapist must be prepared to utilize a wide array of treatment approaches.

INDIVIDUAL PSYCHODYNAMIC PSYCHOTHERAPY

Psychotherapy is a vastly underutilized treatment modality for the elderly. This group represents the "survival of the fittest" who have incurred losses, life disappointments, and stresses. Episodes of decompensation have a good prognosis with short-term psychotherapy, although if a person's losses require substantial life readjustment, long-term therapy may be required. Most psychotherapy with elderly patients, however, involves the re-establishment of ego defenses that have worked adaptively throughout the person's lifetime.

A common psychotherapeutic goal is eliminating or ameliorating maladaptive coping patterns and strengthening adaptive coping mechanisms that, in turn, promote a sense of control over one's environment. This often means diminished anxiety and/or depressive symptoms.[41]

How does psychodynamic psychotherapy with the elderly differ from such therapy with younger people? In both groups symptom relief, improved functioning, and enhanced self-acceptance and self-esteem are common aims. In younger people more attention is likely to be focused on self-constructed barriers (maladaptive defenses) that cause psychological discomfort and prevent the realization of work and interpersonal goals. In contrast, psychological work with the elderly often focuses on symbolic replacement of a lost other person who was critical to the patient's psychological well-being and provided a sense of stability. For this reason, it is especially important to discover and understand the history and nature of the lost relationship. Because elderly people are more likely to seek an idealized child than a tyrannical parent in the therapist, a sense of warmth and caring is generally helpful. There are, however, notable exceptions. For some, warmth and friendliness may be felt as depreciating or frightening. They may wonder, "Am I really that bad off?" These differences emphasize the therapist's need to view the elderly as individuals and to be prepared to utilize varied approaches.

The long-term patient is often a survivor of decades of psychological problems and various therapies and may be an encyclopedia of local psychiatrists and local psychiatric history. More to the point, many such patients know exactly what they want and need. They have been in therapy continuously or intermittently for an extended time and will direct the therapist in how best to treat them. The important feature is the therapist's willingness to learn. A frustrating situation may arise if the therapist attempts to convince the patient that a different approach is necessary.[41]

"Defeating" the therapist can be a particularly useful strategy for certain individuals who re-establish a sense of control by defeating others. In some, a feeling of impotence and frustration may be alleviated by reducing the importance of a powerful other. Other elderly patients, however, view the therapist as a powerful parental figure who provides gratification and ameliorates symptoms of psychological distress.[42]

Late life losses may make an older person a "stranger unto himself." This sense of alienation from self and environment leads, in turn, to symptoms of anxiety, rage, depression, and paranoia, often accompanied by feelings of frustration and hopelessness. A careful and detailed history-taking or life review allows a person in such distress to reorganize and reorient with the assistance of the therapist. This process makes possible a "return to roots"; it provides gratification and a rediscovery of one's self. In a post-crisis phase, it also permits the exploration and resolution of both old and recent conflicts.

Psychotherapy with the demented elderly is useful and effective if the patient is able to relate affectively to the therapist. It is *not* important that the patient remember the therapist's name; it *is* important that the patient take with him or her the experience of the session—a sense of enhanced self-esteem and warmth.[44] The therapist must be prepared for much repetition and little "new material," knowing that in its preventive and therapeutic aspects the therapeutic relationship can be sustaining and nourishing in itself.

SOMATIC THERAPIES

As previously mentioned, the elderly are especially sensitive to medication and are, therefore, at high risk for deleterious side effects. Thus, lower doses are indicated initially. Although body habits and age must be considered, a usual starting dose would be 40% to 60% of the dose appropriate for a younger adult.

In general, a test dose for a drug is desirable before beginning regular administration, as the elderly have a very high incidence of adverse drug responses. One can start on a daily basis with the smallest unit of the drug available; thereafter, increments can be offered after several days, with the same step-wise process being continued. The expectation is that the final dose will be kept as low as possible consistent with therapeutic effect. In crisis situations, however, judgment may dictate a more vigorous approach.

When employing tricyclic antidepressants or certain neuroleptics, it is important to have a baseline sitting and standing blood pressure before beginning the drug and to repeat this procedure at intervals. A specific complaint of subjective dizziness may alert the psychiatrist to a hypotensive problem.

The most common indications for using antidepressants in the elderly are "endogenous depression," prophylaxis for cyclical depression, and for treatment of the depressions that accompany senile dementia of the Alzheimer's type.

Contraindications to psychotropic medications are few. They include acute myocardial infarction, narrow-angle glaucoma, benign prostatic hyperplasia, and known allergy or family history of allergy to a specific drug.

Antidepressants are not advised as the primary treatment when there is distinct possibility of suicide. Hospitalization is then usually required, and, in more severe cases, electroconvulsive therapy may be indicated. If hospitalization is not feasible or acceptable, a reliable family member must have the responsibility of monitoring the medication, thus reducing the possibility of overdose. Antidepressants may also precipitate psychosis in those with history of manic episodes or schizophrenia.

In grief reactions or reactive depressions with minimal vegetative symptoms, antidepressants are probably of little use. Their value is also limited with patients in whom paranoid and/or hypochondriacal symptoms predominate. Chronic depressive personalities rarely benefit from antidepressants.

Before administering a medication for depression, a physical examination is of utmost importance. Illnesses such as cancer of the pancreas, silent myocardial infarction, endocrinopathy, or alcohol or drug abuse may all present clinically as endogenous depression. A medication review is necessary to rule out a possible contributing medication such as alethyldopa or reserpine. Special attention needs to be paid to prostatic function and intraocular pressure.

One therapeutic issue is whether or not to use a single dose, usually at bedtime. Although this increases patient compliance, it involves the disadvantage that some patients may have severe anticholinergic effects, particularly in the first three or four days, when receiving a single daily dose of an antidepressant.

Several combinations of tricyclic antidepressants and tranquilizers are currently on the market; however, it is generally more difficult to sort out side effects and the realtive benefit of each medication. In addition, such combinations are limited to certain doses only. As a consequence, if a tranquilizer is needed in addition to the antidepressant, it is best to prescribe it separately. This does, however, increase the possibility of noncompliance.

It is important for the physician to know that alcohol, tobacco, barbiturates, and non-benzodiazepine hypnotics increase the rate of metabolic breakdown of many psychoactive drugs and, therefore, decrease drug plasma levels, thus increasing the possibility of clinical decompensation.

It is particularly important to provide the elderly patient with the following information:

1) Written directions on how to use the medication. Ideally, one should make a chart for the patient, listing all current medications and times when they are to be taken.

2) An explanation to the patient of the most common side effects (e.g., dry mouth, which may cause problems with dentures. Patients may be advised to suck on sugar-free mints or to chew gum). Patients also need to be told that they are likely to experience sleepiness and a drugged feeling during the first two or three days.

3) The frequency of visits needs to be explained in advance to increase the likelihood of compliance.

The development of methods for determining plasma levels of many psychotropic drugs is a particularly exciting development. Evidence now exists, for example, that there is a correlation between antidepressant plasma levels and therapeutic response in the treatment of acute episodes of severe depression. Though this has been studied minimally for the elderly, results with younger depressed patients suggest that these same principles apply. The concept of the therapeutic window is one in which the drug is not effective either below or above a certain range.

Plasma levels are valuable in determining if a positive response to treatment is a result of a placebo effect. Such measurements also allow the evaluation of a lack of response and are helpful in questions of compliance and toxicity. One problem is obtaining quality determinations in many geographic areas. The recent development of national laboratories to determine plasma means an increased access for clinicians across the country.

Side effects must be carefully monitored. Dry mouth has been previously described. Other anticholinergic symptoms include constipation, blurred vision, orthostatic hypotension, and acute organic brain syndromes. Those patients with constipation or hemorrhoids should be placed routinely on a stool softener. Those with blurred vision must be carefully monitored; for some, this can prevent reading or watching television and, thus, may increase depression. It is important to warn patients on medications likely to cause orthostatic hypotension (e.g., imipramine, chlorpromazine, amytriptyline) of this possibility and instruct them to sit for five to ten seconds before they arise from a supine position. Acute organic mental disorders may occur in as many as 10% to 15% of elderly who take psychotropic medications; confusion and visual hallucinations are common symptoms in this group.

The role of the family in monitoring medication can be crucial. Their attitude can either facilitate or interfere with treatment. Periodic contact with them is usually important in the course of treating an older person with psychotropic medication.

Most often, medication is gradually decreased following recovery from psychiatric illness. For antidepressants, the decrease in dosage usually begins one to two months after improvement and is decreased over a period of several weeks. For example, if a patient has a satisfactory response on 75 milligrams of a particular medication, he or she could be maintained on this dose for one month, and then the medication decreased by 25 milligrams every other week until discontinued. Approximately 15% of patients will develop recurrent depressive symptoms and cannot be weaned from the medication. For some of these patients, a maintenance dose of 50% of the maximal dose may be necessary indefinitely.

It is unclear why certain patients who do not have cyclical mood disorders are unable to discontinue medications; whether there is a psychological or physiological base for this has not been determined. For some, however, it allows continuation of the relationship with a parental figure (the doctor) that the patient needs.

Lithium is sometimes indicated in older persons suffering from bipolar and unipolar affective disorders. Due to a presumed nephron loss with aging, the half-life will be prolonged, perhaps from 24 to 36 hours, and, hence, a lower dose will be necessary to maintain a satisfactory serum level. A therapeutic maintenance serum level in the elderly patient is between 0.4 and 0.8 milliequivalents per liter, though toxicity has been noted in elderly patients even within the therapeutic range. Fluid intake should be maintained at 2500 cc a day. In addition to regular monitoring of serum lithium more frequently than in younger patients, electrolytes, blood count, thyroid function, creatinine levels, and cardiac status need to be monitored periodically. Before beginning lithium therapy, it is advisable to have a 24-hour creatinine clearance test as a baseline of renal function. Later, if doubt appears regarding renal function, the test may be repeated. If there is a decrease in renal function, small increases in consecutive serum creatinine levels may also be noted.

Electroconvulsive therapy (ECT), whether used on an inpatient or outpatient basis, is an effective treatment for severe depression. There are three indications for ECT in elderly patients:

1) depression with suicidal risk (requiring hospitalization)
2) agitated depression in which verbal dialogue holds little promise, and the lag time in using antidepressants would extend the period of psychological pain
3) intractable depression in which other modalities of therapy have proved ineffective

The number of treatments varies from a median of three to six in the first two groups to over ten in the third.

GROUP THERAPY

Group therapy can also be a valuable treatment modality for many elderly patients. Groups offer a number of advantages for the older person. They diminish isolation by providing opportunities for interpersonal interactions, facilitate the development of new roles or the re-establishment of familiar roles, provide information on a variety of topics from other group members, and afford group support for effecting change or enhancing self-esteem.

Group therapy for the elderly differs from group therapy for younger groups in the following ways:

1) There is usually a predominance of female members.
2) Common themes are loss (physical, social, economic), intergenerational conflicts, and adaptive struggles.
3) There is a greater emphasis on reminiscence and life review.
4) Therapists share more personal information.

5) There is more physical contact—hugging, touching, kissing.
6) There is more tolerance of silent group members.

Attempts to mix demented patients with those with other diagnoses may prove unsuccessful. In general, nondemented patients become anxious, fearful, and sometimes hostile in such circumstances. Especially early in therapy, these "threatened" patients tend not to return to group sessions—it is as if they fear dementia is an infectious illness.

There are several obstacles to outpatient group therapy: transportation (particularly during the winter), group member absence (due to illness and/or vacation), and economics. Paradoxically, even though group therapy is less costly than individual psychotherapy per unit of treatment, its longer-term nature may mean additional cost. Medicare limitations act as a particular deterrent for those of modest means.

BEHAVIORAL APPROACHES

A number of behavioral therapies have been used for the treatment and rehabilitation of elderly patients in recent years. They have been employed in the alleviation of isolated phobic symptoms, for the treatment of dysfunctional behavior in coping with chronic disease, for adaptational problems related to memory failure, and for reduction of maladaptive and/or disruptive behaviors.

To date, few experimental studies have focused specifically on the use of some of the newer behavioral techniques with the elderly. Cognitive behavioral therapy for the treatment of depression, biofeedback for reduction of anxiety states, and multimodal behavioral therapy are examples. Although research in these areas appears to be increasing, reports of behavioral treatment with the elderly focus most commonly on use of contingency strategies and token economies.

If the published literature is any indication, the preponderance of problems addressed by behavior therapists typically take place in institutional settings, with problems being presented as "undesirable" by staff members rather than by older persons themselves. Problems of hygiene, self-care and self-management (e.g., bedmaking, teeth brushing, face washing, shaving, incontinence, and failure to eat, dress, socialize, etc.) appear more likely to be brought to the attention of the behavioral therapist treating the older person than, for example, problems with sexual dysfunction, maladaptive relationships, and dysphoria, all of which present fewer "management" difficulties.

Some behavioral approaches have been quite effective (e.g., in reducing chronic screaming, and in increasing speech, verbalization, and ambulation). Other approaches, such as bowel and bladder training methods, have been applied with mixed success. Some techniques such as "Reality Orientation" do not appear to have effects that are lasting for the patient or that generalize to other self-care or social behaviors, although they temporarily improve functioning and enhance staff morale.

Behavioral techniques can be useful in ameliorating difficult behavioral situations by focusing on the management and maintenance of function in chronic diseases rather than fostering therapeutic nihilism by aiming at curative treatment.

FAMILY THERAPY

When an older person incurs significant losses, mutual misunderstandings between parent and child(ren) are likely to occur. For the elderly parent, the problems are threefold:

1) Having incurred losses (e.g., retirement, illness, decreased income, etc.) the parent looks for alternative sources of satisfaction. The logical and most available resource are family members. The parent often seeks and needs additional time, attention, and support from family members.
2) Losses stir up feelings of frustration, anger, resentment, and sadness. If not internalized or displaced, these feelings are generally expressed to, or directed at, the adult offspring.
3) The elderly parent's need for more attention and support from the children is often accompanied by a sense of loss of the parental role. Shame and resentment about dependency needs may interfere either with effectively communicating such needs to the children or with allowing the children to meet those needs.[45]

The adult offspring often has many other responsibilities: there may be adolescents at home, or heavy financial burdens for college education may require more time at work. Psychologically, the adult offspring is attempting to deal with his or her own feelings regarding the loss of the parent as a powerful figure. Although the intergenerational equilibrium is based on a fuller understanding of the elderly parent's strengths and weaknesses, there remains a residue of childhood that views the parent as omnipotent and omniscient. Thus, the belief persists that "Mother will take care of me when I'm sick," or "Father will help me if I have financial problems." When a parent is undergoing a physical and/or mental decline, this view of the powerful parent is compromised, and a sense of significant loss may result. The usual reaction is a combination of sadness, anxiety, and anger. This is often complicated by guilt about being angry at the parent who is experiencing such difficult times. Denial is common and may interfere with proper assessment and planning.

Thus the stage is set for misunderstandings and hurt feelings. The parent's increased neediness makes the child feel that "Whatever I do is not enough. He (she) always wants more." The parent's expression of frustration is experienced as "I'm always being criticized. Whatever I do seems to be wrong or inadequate." The anger toward the parent results in the parent's feeling rejection, shame, humiliation, and sadness. This, in turn, leads to the adult child's guilt and sadness. What often follows is a transient feeling of closeness and an attempt to express mutual caring: the importance of the parent-child relationship momentarily pushes the problem into the background. Then the cycle begins again.

Short-term family therapy (one to four sessions) is particularly useful for clarifying the issues and feelings that confront both elderly parent and child. This is particularly important when parent and child live together. The development of insight by either party often helps to reduce tension.

A different problem ensues when a parent is unable to remain in the community. The children's level of anxiety and guilt may rise significantly. Conflicts among adult offspring—many of whom may have minimal contact with each other—arise and reflect real issues (Should the parent be institutionalized? Where? When? How should he or she be told? Are there alternatives?). Old family conflicts may emerge: which child will be the parent's "advocate" and which the "bad guy"? Who should put in the most time? Who should get the most credit or the most blame? Whenever possible, it is important to meet with *all* the children (and their spouses, as well as the parent's spouse) to discuss the relevant issues.

Certain practical principles are important in such meetings: the meeting is best scheduled in the evening as the therapist's final session of the day. This gives all family members an opportunity to be present.

Such sessions may take two to three hours in order for interpersonal conflicts and family roles to emerge. What the therapist often observes is a fascinating recapitulation of early family dynamics, understanding of which allows the therapist to better anticipate and plan for complications. The therapist must personally contact all family members whose presence is needed. An absent member who sees himself or herself as the parent's advocate represents a critical snag in effective planning. Trusting one family member to contact others may suggest that the therapist has a special alliance with that person. This approach presupposes the therapist's knowledge of the parent's condition. If the parent's problems are severe, the therapist must be prepared to share the information with the family and deal with their feelings and reactions. Toward this end, the therapist must be "confronting," if necessary. Denial by family members is common. Some family members will insist that a parent who is moderately demented and depressed will be fine if he or she spends the winter in Florida. Such a vacation, in fact, usually results in an intensification of symptoms from both conditions.

A number of other treatment and/or management approaches have gained some popularity in the past few years. Self-help groups, such as widow-support groups for the recently bereaved and Project Assist-type groups for family members of demented elderly, have proven useful. Biofeedback, Yoga, and Transcendental Meditation, any of which decrease anxiety, enhance self-esteem, and/or diminish somatic complaints, are occasionally helpful. Day center services, which may provide monitoring of medication or a therapeutic milieu after medication, are particularly useful. Such settings also allow for an extended evaluation and the opportunity for family relief, as in the case of the family of a demented patient. Occupational therapy, activities therapy, and recreational therapy are useful for providing pleasure and an enhanced sense of worth.

Conclusion

In this chapter, some common biological, social, and psychological aspects of normal aging have been reviewed, focusing on the clinical data necessary to perform a comprehensive evaluation. Considerations particular to the elderly have been emphasized.

An understanding of the aging process, as well as the emotional and mental problems that may occur, is necessary to arrive at proper diagnosis and to provide sound treatment. Only then can we provide the elderly with the care they need and deserve.

References

1. Kasper, R.: Eye Problems in the Aged, in W. Reichel (ed.), *Clinical Aspects of Aging*, Baltimore: Waverly Press, 1972, pp. 391-402.
2. Hudis, M. M.: Dentistry for the Elderly in Health and Illness, in W. Reichel (ed.), *Clinical Aspects of Aging*, Baltimore: Waverly Press, 1972, p. 415.
3. Harris, R.: Special Problems of Geriatric Patients with Heart Disease, in W. Reichel (ed.), *Clinical Aspects of Aging*, Baltimore: Waverly Press, 1972, pp. 45-64.
4. Sklar,: Gastro-Intestinal Disease in the Aged, in W. Reichel (ed.), *Clinical Aspects of Aging*, Baltimore: Waverly Press, 1972, pp. 173-181.
5. Shapiro, W. B., et al.: Medical Renal Diseases of the Aged, in W. Reichel (ed.), *Clinical Aspects of Aging*, Baltimore: Waverly Press, 1972, pp. 199-212.
6. Lindeman, R.: Application of Fluid and Electrolyte Balance Principles to the Older Patient, in W. Reichel (ed.), *Clinical Aspects of Aging*, Baltimore: Waverly Press, 1972, pp. 213-226.
7. Jaffe, J.: Common Lower Urinary Tract Problems in Older People, in W. Reichel (ed.), *Clinical Aspects of Aging*, Baltimore: Waverly Press, 1972, pp. 227-236.
8. Steel, K.: Evaluation of the Geriatric Patient, in W. Reichel (ed.), *Clinical Aspects of Aging*, Baltimore: Waverly Press, 1972, pp. 3-12
9. Butler, R., and Lewis, M.: *Aging and Mental Health*, 2nd Edition, St. Louis: C. V. Mosley and Company, 1977, p.17.
10. Butler, R., and Lewis, M.: *Aging and Mental Health*, 2nd Edition , St. Louis: C.Y. Mosley and Company, 1977, pp. 8-16.
11. Holtzman, J. M., Berman, H., and Ham, R.: Health and Early Retirement Decisions, *Journal of American Geriatrics*, January, 1980, pp. 23-28.
12. Butler, R., and Lewis, M.: *Aging and Mental Health*, 2nd Edition, St. Louis: C. V. Mosby and Company, 1977, pp. 104-105.

13. Butler, R.: *Why Survive? Being Old In America*, New York: Harper and Row, 1976.
14. Verwoerdt, A.: *Clinical Geropsychiatry*, Baltimore: Williams and Wilkins, 1976, p. 227.
15. Chenitz, C.: Adjusting to Institutional Life: Status Passage for the Aged, presented at the 1980 Annual Meeting of the Gerontological Society of America, San Diego.
16. Erikson, E.: *Childhood and Society*, 2nd Edition, New York: W. W. Norton and Company, 1963.
17. Erikson, E.: *Childhood and Society*, 2nd Edition, New York: W. W. Norton and Company, 1963
18. Verwoerdt: *Clinical Geropsychiatry*, Baltimore: Williams and Wilkins, 1976, p. 227
19. Vaillant, G., and Millfsky, E.: Natural History of Male Psychological Health, IX: Empirical Evidence for Erickson's Model of the Life Cycle, *American Journal of Psychiatry*, 137: 1348-1359, November, 1980.
20. Butler, R.: The Life Review: Interpretation of Reminiscence in the Aged, *Psychiatry*, 26: 65, 73, Spring, 1963.
21. Ford, C., and Sbordone, R.: Attitudes of Psychiatrists Toward Elderly Patients, *American Journal of Psychiatry*, 137(5): 171-175, May, 1980.
22. Steel, K.: Evaluation of the Geriatric Patient, in W. Reichel (ed.), *Clinical Aspects of Aging*, Baltimore: Waverly Press, 1972, p. 4.
23. Dysken, M. W., et al.: Drug Interaction Between Ascorbic Acid and Fluphenazine, Letter to Editor, *Journal of the American Medical Association*, 241(9): 2008, May 11, 1979.
24. Wells, C.: *Dementia*, 2nd Edition, Philadelphia: F. A. Davis Company, 1977, p. 260.
25. Kahn, R. L., Goldfarb, A. I., Pollack, M., and Peck, A.: Brief Objective Measures for the Determination of Mental Status in the Aged, *American Journal of Psychiatry*, 117: 326-328, 1960.
26. Pfeiffer, E.: A Short Portable Mental Status Questionnaire for the Assessment of Organic Brain Deficit in Elderly Patients, *Journal of American Geriatric Services*, 23: 433, 1975.
27. Halstead, W. C.: *Brain and Intelligence*, Chicago: University of Chicago Press, 1947.
28. Savage, R., and Hall, E.: A Performance Learning Measure for the Aged, *The British Journal of Psychiatry*, 122: 721-723, 1973.
29. Fink, M., Green, M., and Bender, M.: The Forehand Test as a Diagnostic Sign of Organic Mental Syndrome, *Neurology*, 2: 46-48, 1952.
30. Reitan, R. M.: Validity of the Trail Making Test as an Indicator of Organic Brain Damage, *Perceptual Motor Skills*, 8: 271-276, 1958.
31. Benton, A. L.: *The Visual Retention Test: Clinical and Experimental Applications*, New York: Psychological Corporation, 1963.
32. Raven, J. C.: *Progressive Matrices*, London: H. K. Lewis, 1938.
33. Graham, F. K., and Kendall, B. S.: Memory for Designs Test: Revised General Manual, *Perceptual Motor Skills*, 30: 319-326, 1960.

34. Fuzard, J. L., Wolf, E., Bell, B., McFarland, R., and Podolsky, S.: Visual Perception and Communication, in J. E. Birren, and K. W. Schale (eds): *Handbook of the Psychology of Aging*, New York: Van Nostrand Reinhold, 1977, pp. 497-534.
35. Walton, D., and Black, D. A.: The Validity of Psychological Tests of Brain Damage, *British Journal of Psychiatry*, 30: 270-279, 1959.
36. Kendrick, D. C.: Speed and Learning in the Diagnosis of Diffuse Brain Damage in Elderly Subjects: A Bayesian Statistical Approach, *British Journal of Social Clinical Psychology*, 4: 141-148, 1967.
37. Folstein, M. F., Folstein, S. E., and McHugh, P. R.: Mini-mental state, A Practical Method for Grading the Cognitive State of Patients for the Clinician, *Journal of Psychiatric Research*, 12: 189-198, 1975.
38. The Comprehensive Assessment and Referral Evaluation (CARE) Rationale Development, Vol. 8(1): 9-42, 1977.
39. Gurland, B.: The Assessment of the Mental Health Status of Older Adults, in James Birren, and Bruce Sloan (eds.): *Handbook of Mental Health and Aging*, Englewood Cliffs, New Jersey: Prentice-Hall, 1980, p. 679.
40. Schuckit, M., and Miller, P.: Alcoholism in Elderly Men: A Survey of General Medicine Ward, *Annals of the New York Academy of Science*, 273: 558-571, 1976.
41. Finkel, S.: Experiences of a Private Practice Psychiatrist Working with the Elderly in the Community, *International Journal of Mental Health*, 8: 164, Fall-Winter, 1979-1980.
42. Finkel, S.: Experiences of a Private Practice Psychiatrist Working with the Elderly in the Community, *International Journal of Mental Health*, 8: 164, Fall-Winter, 1979-1980.
43. Goldfarb, A.: Psychotherapy of Aged Persons, *Psychoanalysis Review*, 42: 180, 1955.
44. Finkel, S.: Experiences of a Private Practice Psychiatrist Working with the Elderly in the Community, *International Journal of Mental Health:* 8: 165, Fall-Winter, 1979-1980.
45. Finkel, S.: Experiences of a Private Practice Psychiatrist Working with the Elderly in the Community, *International Journal of Mental Health:* 8: 168-169, Fall-Winter, 1979-1980.

DEC 5 1990	DATE DUE		
MR 31 '93			
AP 10 '96			
MY 07 '96			